THE NATIONAL ACADEMIES PRESS   500 Fifth Street, N.W.   Washington, DC 20001

NOTICE: The project that is the subject of this report was approved by the Governing Board of the National Research Council, whose members are drawn from the councils of the National Academy of Sciences, the National Academy of Engineering, and the Institute of Medicine. The members of the committee responsible for the report were chosen for their special competences and with regard for appropriate balance.

Support for this project was provided by the Agency for Healthcare Research and Quality (AHRQ). The views presented in this report are those of the Institute of Medicine Committee on Data Standards for Patient Safety and are not necessarily those of the funding agencies.

Library of Congress Cataloging-in-Publication Data

Patient safety : achieving a new standard for care / Committee on Data Standards for Patient Safety, Board on Health Care Services ; Philip Aspden ... [et al.], editors.
   p. ; cm.
 Includes bibliographical references and index.
 ISBN 0-309-09077-6 (hardcover)
   1. Medical records—Standards—United States. 2. Medical informatics. 3. Medical errors—Data processing—Standards—United States.
   [DNLM: 1. Medical Errors—prevention & control—United States. 2. Health Policy—United States. 3. Information Services—standards—United States. 4. Patient Care—standards—United States. 5. Policy Making—United States. 6. Risk Management—United States. 7. Safety Management—United States. WB 100 P2975 2004] I. Aspden, Philip. II. Institute of Medicine (U.S.). Committee on Data Standards for Patient Safety.
   R864.P38 2004
   651.5′04261—dc22
                    2004001869

Additional copies of this report are available from the National Academies Press, 500 Fifth Street, N.W., Lockbox 285, Washington, DC 20055; (800) 624-6242 or (202) 334-3313 (in the Washington metropolitan area); Internet, http://www.nap.edu.

For more information about the Institute of Medicine, visit the IOM home page at: **www.iom.edu.**

"Knowing is not enough; we must apply.
Willing is not enough; we must do."
—Goethe

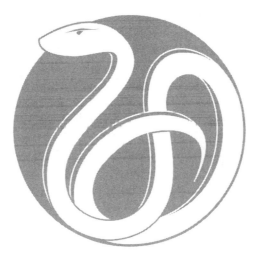

INSTITUTE OF MEDICINE
OF THE NATIONAL ACADEMIES

Adviser to the Nation to Improve Health

THE NATIONAL ACADEMIES
Advisers to the Nation on Science, Engineering, and Medicine

The **National Academy of Sciences** is a private, nonprofit, self-perpetuating society of distinguished scholars engaged in scientific and engineering research, dedicated to the furtherance of science and technology and to their use for the general welfare. Upon the authority of the charter granted to it by the Congress in 1863, the Academy has a mandate that requires it to advise the federal government on scientific and technical matters. Dr. Bruce M. Alberts is president of the National Academy of Sciences.

The **National Academy of Engineering** was established in 1964, under the charter of the National Academy of Sciences, as a parallel organization of outstanding engineers. It is autonomous in its administration and in the selection of its members, sharing with the National Academy of Sciences the responsibility for advising the federal government. The National Academy of Engineering also sponsors engineering programs aimed at meeting national needs, encourages education and research, and recognizes the superior achievements of engineers. Dr. Wm. A. Wulf is president of the National Academy of Engineering.

The **Institute of Medicine** was established in 1970 by the National Academy of Sciences to secure the services of eminent members of appropriate professions in the examination of policy matters pertaining to the health of the public. The Institute acts under the responsibility given to the National Academy of Sciences by its congressional charter to be an adviser to the federal government and, upon its own initiative, to identify issues of medical care, research, and education. Dr. Harvey V. Fineberg is president of the Institute of Medicine.

The **National Research Council** was organized by the National Academy of Sciences in 1916 to associate the broad community of science and technology with the Academy's purposes of furthering knowledge and advising the federal government. Functioning in accordance with general policies determined by the Academy, the Council has become the principal operating agency of both the National Academy of Sciences and the National Academy of Engineering in providing services to the government, the public, and the scientific and engineering communities. The Council is administered jointly by both Academies and the Institute of Medicine. Dr. Bruce M. Alberts and Dr. Wm. A. Wulf are chair and vice chair, respectively, of the National Research Council.

ww.national-academies.org

COMMITTEE ON DATA STANDARDS FOR PATIENT SAFETY

Study Staff

PHILIP ASPDEN, Study Director
JULIE WOLCOTT, Program Officer
SHARI ERICKSON, Research Associate
DANITZA VALDIVIA, Senior Project Assistant
REBECCA BENSON, Senior Project Assistant

Health Care Services Board

JANET M. CORRIGAN, Director
ANTHONY BURTON, Administrative Assistant

Editorial Consultants

RONA BRIERE, Briere Associates, Inc.
ALISA DECATUR, Briere Associates, Inc.

Reviewers

This report has been reviewed in draft form by individuals chosen for their diverse perspectives and technical expertise, in accordance with procedures approved by the National Research Council's Report Review Committee. The purpose of this independent review is to provide candid and critical comments that will assist the institution in making its published report as sound as possible and to ensure that the report meets institutional standards for objectivity, evidence, and responsiveness to the study charge. The review comments and draft manuscript remain confidential to protect the integrity of the deliberative process. We wish to thank the following individuals for their review of this report:

ENRIQUETA C. BOND, Burroughs Wellcome Fund
WILLIAM A. BORNSTEIN, Emory Healthcare
RICHARD BOTNEY, Oregon Health & Science University
CAROL C. DIAMOND, Markle Foundation
HAROLD S. KAPLAN, Columbia University
CLEMENT J. MCDONALD, Regenstrief Institute for Health Care, Indiana University
ROBERT L. PHILLIPS, American Academy of Family Physicians
NANCY RIDLEY, Massachusetts Department of Public Health
WILLIAM B. RUNCIMAN, Australian Patient Safety Foundation, Royal Adelaide Hospital, Australia
PAUL M. SCHYVE, Joint Commission on Accreditation of Healthcare Organizations

Although the reviewers listed above have provided many constructive comments and suggestions, they were not asked to endorse the conclusions or recommendations, nor did they see the final draft of the report before its release. The review of this report was overseen by **Don E. Detmer**, University of Cambridge and University of Virginia, and **John Bailar**, University of Chicago, Professor Emeritus. Appointed by the National Research Council and the Institute of Medicine, they were responsible for making certain that an independent examination of this report was carried out in accordance with institutional procedures and that all review comments were carefully considered. Responsibility for the final content of this report rests entirely with the authoring committee and the institution.

Preface

Just as the health care system has started to come to grips with the threat of patient safety concerns, new data are expanding the scope of the threat. Unintended harm arising from medical management is not limited to the hospital setting; nor is it limited to acts of commission. The Committee on Data Standards for Patient Safety believes that patient safety should be a new standard for quality care—care that is free of unintended injury from acts of commission or omission, in any setting in which it is delivered. Consequently, data standards needed to support patient safety go well beyond the needs of adverse event and near-miss reporting. In this report, we describe a vision of patient safety systems integrated with clinical information systems and recommend strategies to create data standards that support that vision.

The past 2 years have seen three very positive developments with regard to clinical data standards. In October 2001, the Department of Health and Human Services (DHHS) established the Consolidated Health Informatics (CHI) initiative to articulate and execute a strategy for the adoption of health care interoperability standards by federally operated and funded health care providers. Given the purchasing power of the federal government, representing more than 40 percent of health care expenditures in the United States, the incorporation of the standards into government programs will be a powerful and effective means of establishing these standards on a national basis. On March 20, 2003, HHS Secretary Thompson announced that the federal government, including DHHS, the Department of Defense, and the

Veterans Administration, would adopt the first set of standards for the electronic exchange of clinical health information. In June 2003, the Markle Foundation Connecting for Health Initiative published the results of a 9-month collaborative of private- and public-sector leaders that outlined a series of important steps toward the completion and adoption of health care information data standards to enable the sharing of clinical information. A follow-up Markle initiative is likely. Finally, on July 1, 2003, HHS Secretary Thompson announced that DHHS had signed an agreement with the College of American Pathologists to license the college's standardized medical vocabulary system (SNOMED) and make it available without charge throughout the United States. This means that an important clinical data standards building block will be accessible to all in the health care industry.

The recommendations given in this report build on these three major initiatives to provide a road map for the development and adoption of a comprehensive set of national health care information standards that support patient safety.

A number of previous Institute of Medicine studies have called for increased investment in information systems as an essential technology for delivering care in the 21st century. This report, along with the committee's letter report on the Electronic Health Record that was released in July 2003, begins to lay the foundation and framework for a national health information infrastructure. The data standards described in this report refer not only to the actual data elements that populate medical records and patient safety reports but also to a new cultural standard that uses data to continuously improve patient safety. Our report calls upon national leadership to transform the uncomfortable status quo, whereby clinicians practice in a delivery system riddled with latent system failures, into an environment where patient safety is not only state of the art but also a new standard of care.

This report represents the culmination of dedicated effort by several groups of people. I would like to thank my fellow committee members, who have worked long and diligently on this challenging study; the members of the study liaison panel, who helped with our deliberations at three committee meetings; the many experts who provided formal testimony to the committee and informal advice throughout the study; and the staff of the Health Care Services Board who managed the study and coordinated the writing of the final report.

Paul C. Tang, M.D., M.S.
Chair
November 2003

Foreword

This report is at the intersection of two important and complementary streams of Institute of Medicine (IOM) work. One stream is focused on improving the quality of care in America and the other on fostering the use of information technology within the health care system.

The IOM's quality initiative began with the National Roundtable on Health Care Quality, which raised awareness of the overuse, misuse, and underuse of health care services. This was followed by the release of two reports, *To Err Is Human: Building a Safer Health System* and *Crossing the Quality Chasm: A New Health System for the 21st Century*, which put forward ideas for redesigning the health care delivery system to raise the standards of care to the levels of the best clinical practice.

In 1991, the IOM issued the report *The Computer-Based Patient Record*, which called for the elimination of paper-based records within 10 years. A key recommendation of that report was to develop uniform national standards for health care data. A revised edition of the report, published in 1997, reaffirmed the messages of the initial version. Earlier this year, at the request of the Department of Health and Human Services, the IOM carried out a fast-track study that built on ideas from *The Computer-Based Patient Record* to identify the core delivery-related functionalities of an electronic health record system.

Crossing the Quality Chasm calls for a concerted national commitment to building an information infrastructure to support health care delivery. Fundamental to such an information infrastructure are health care data standards. This report puts forward a road map for the development of these standards in the context of delivering high-quality, safe care. I believe that the conditions for implementing this road map are now extremely favorable.

Harvey V. Fineberg, M.D., Ph.D.
President, Institute of Medicine
November 2003

Acknowledgments

The Committee on Data Standards for Patient Safety wishes to acknowledge the many people whose contributions and support made this report possible.

The committee especially recognizes the members of the liaison panel: Jim Bagian, Michael Cohen, Linda J. Connell, Suzanne Delbanco, Marie Dotseth, Frederick J. Heigel, Betsy L. Humphreys, Stephen F. Jencks, Kenneth W. Kizer, Dr. Linda McKibben, Paul M. Schyve, and Janet Woodcock.

The committee benefited from presentations made by a number of experts over the past 2 years. The following individuals shared their research, experience, and perspectives with the committee: Jared Adair, Centers for Medicare and Medicaid Services; Diane Aschman, SNOMED International; James Battles, Agency for Healthcare Research and Quality; Claire Broome, Centers for Disease Control and Prevention; Lynn Chevalier, New York State Department of Health; Gary Christopherson, Veterans Health Administration; John Combes, The Hospital & Healthsystem Association of Pennsylvania; Paul Conlon, Michigan Health and Safety Coalition; Diane Cousins, U.S. Pharmacopeia; John Declaris, The Kevric Company, Inc.; Henry Desmarais, Health Insurance Association of America; Charles Fahey, Milbank Memorial Fund; Loretta Fauerbach, Association for Professionals in Infection Control & Epidemiology; Clive Flashman, National Patient Safety Agency, U.K.; Ellen Flink, New York State Department of Health; Nancy Foster, American Hospital Association; Kathe Fox, The MEDSTAT Group; Margaret Glavin, Resources for the Future; David Hopkins, Pacific

Business Group on Health; Helen Hughes, National Patient Safety Agency, U.K.; Betsy Humphreys, National Library of Medicine; Harold Kaplan, Columbia University; David Lansky, Foundation for Accountability; Kathryn Lesh, The Kevric Company, Inc.; Randy Levin, Food and Drug Administration; Janet Marchibroda, eHealth Initiative; Clement McDonald, Indiana University School of Medicine; Scott McKnight, Veterans Health Administration, Michigan; Gregg Meyer, MGPO Massachusetts General Hospital; Blackford Middleton, Partners Healthcare System, Inc.; Jean Narcisi, American Medical Association; John Oldham, Medical University of South Carolina; Marc Overhage, Regenstrief Institute for Health Care; Wilson Pace, University of Colorado; Donna Payne, Child Health Corporation of America; Susan Penfield, Booz Allen Hamilton; Robert Phillips, American Academy of Family Physicians; Nancy Ridley, Massachusetts Department of Public Health; Karlene Roberts, University of California, Berkeley; John Rother, American Association of Retired Persons; Bill Runciman, Australian Patient Safety Foundation; Julie Sanderson-Austin, American Medical Group Association; Joyce Sensmeier, Healthcare Information and Management Systems Society; Robert Slack, Alcoa; Stanton Smullens, Thomas Jefferson University; Cheri Throop, Child Health Corporation of America; C. Peter Waegemann, Medical Records Institute; and Scott Williams, Utah Department of Health.

The following individuals were important sources of information, generously giving their time and knowledge to further the committee's aims: Andrew Chang, Joint Commission on Accreditation of Healthcare Organizations; Rosanna M. Coffey, The MEDSTAT Group; Carol C. Diamond, the Markle Foundation; Gary Dickinson, Misys Healthcare; Susan Dovey, The Robert Graham Center; Noel Eldridge, Department of Veterans Affairs; Linda Fischetti, Department of Veterans Affairs; Michael Fitzmaurice, Agency for Healthcare Research and Quality; Ellen M. Flink, New York State Department of Health; Douglas Godesky, Department of Health and Human Services; John Gosbee, Veterans Affairs National Center for Patient Safety; Marjorie S. Greenberg, National Center for Statistics; Shirley Kellie, Centers for Medicare and Medicaid Services; Scott A. Laidlaw, DoctorQuality; Ned McCulloch, IBM; Sue Osborn, National Patient Safety Agency, U.K.; Anna Polk, Agency for Health Care Administration, Florida; Wes Rishel, Gartner Research; Frances Stewart, U.S. Navy; Margaret VanAmringe, Joint Commission on Accreditation of Healthcare Organizations; Karen VanHentenryck, Health Level Seven, Inc.; Susan Williams, National Patient Safety Agency, U.K.; William A. Yasnoff, Department of Health and Human Services; and Scott Young, Agency for Healthcare Research and Quality.

The committee commissioned seven papers that provided important background information and insights for the report. Paul Barach, University of Chicago, authored a helpful paper providing an overview of reporting systems. David Brailer, CareScience, wrote an overview of the use and adoption of computer-based patient records in the United States. Richard Cook, University of Chicago, provided a paper on patient safety metrics and analysis strategies. Carol Friedman, Columbia University, authored a paper on natural language processing, while W. Ed Hammond, Duke University, provided a paper on data standards and patient safety. John McDonough, Brandeis University, wrote a paper on organizational systems and hazard analysis. Additionally, Luke Sato, Risk Management Foundation of the Harvard Medical Institutions, supplied a piece on data protection.

The committee also benefited from the work of other committees and staff of the Institute of Medicine that conducted studies relevant to this report. The committee particularly benefited from the efforts of the Committee on the Quality of Health Care in America and the Committee on Identifying Priority Areas for Quality Improvement. The Committee on the Quality of Health Care in America produced the 2000 report *To Err Is Human: Building a Safer Health System* and the 2001 report *Crossing the Quality Chasm: A New Health System for the 21st Century*. The Committee on Identifying Priority Areas for Quality Improvement produced the 2003 report *Priority Areas for National Action: Transforming Health Care Quality*.

The committee would like to acknowledge the particular contributions of Suzanne Bakken, Jonathan Einbinder, and Larry Grandia in developing a standards-based mechanism for an integrated national health information infrastructure (Chapter 2), Brent James in drafting an innovative approach to patient safety systems (Chapter 5) and specific patient safety applications (Chapter 8), and Tjerk van der Schaaf in crafting a model for the collection and analysis of near-miss data (Chapter 7).

Finally, funding for the project came from the Agency for Healthcare Research and Quality (AHRQ). The committee extends special thanks to AHRQ for providing such support, and within AHRQ, to Jim Battles and Rob Borotkanics for their assistance throughout the project.

Contents

PATIENT SAFETY

ACHIEVING A NEW STANDARD FOR CARE

Executive Summary

ABSTRACT

In response to a request from the Department of Health and Human Services, the Institute of Medicine convened a committee to produce a detailed plan to facilitate the development of data standards applicable to the collection, coding, and classification of patient safety information.

Americans should be able to count on receiving health care that is safe. To achieve this, a new health care delivery system is needed—a system that both prevents errors and learns from them when they occur. The development of such a system requires, first, a commitment by all stakeholders to a culture of safety and, second, improved information systems.

A national health information infrastructure is needed (1) to provide immediate access to complete patient information and decision support tools for clinicians and their patients and (2) to capture patient safety information as a by-product of care and use this information to design even safer delivery systems. Health data standards are both a critical and time-sensitive building block of the national health information infrastructure. The Department of Health and Human Services should be given the lead role in establishing and maintaining a public–private partnership for the promulgation of standards for data that support patient safety. The committee considered the status of

1

current standards-setting activities in three key areas—health data interchange, terminologies, and medical knowledge representation. For each of these areas, the committee reviewed the future work needed and recommended a work plan.

To achieve an acceptable standard of patient safety, the committee recommends that all health care settings establish comprehensive patient safety programs operated by trained personnel within a culture of safety and involving adverse event and near-miss detection and analysis. In addition, the federal government should pursue a robust applied research agenda on patient safety, focused on enhancing knowledge, developing tools, and disseminating results to maximize the impact of patient safety systems. Finally, the committee recommends that a standardized format and terminology be developed for the capture and reporting of data related to medical errors.

Since the release of the Institute of Medicine (IOM) report *To Err Is Human: Building a Safer Health System* (Institute of Medicine, 2000), national attention has been focused on the need to reduce medical errors. The health care community and the public at large have come to realize that the nation's health care system is not as safe as it should be.

Every day, tens if not hundreds of thousands of errors occur in the U.S. health care system. Fortunately, most of these errors result not in serious harm but in near misses. A *near miss* is defined as an act of commission or omission that could have harmed the patient but did not do so as a result of chance (e.g., the patient received a contraindicated drug but did not experience an adverse drug reaction), prevention (e.g., a potentially lethal overdose was prescribed, but a nurse identified the error before administering the medication), or mitigation (e.g., a lethal drug overdose was administered but discovered early and countered with an antidote). Sadly, however, a small proportion of errors do result in *adverse events*—that is, they cause harm to patients—exacting a sizable toll in terms of injury, disability, and death.

To Err Is Human focuses primarily on errors that occur in hospitals and is based on the evidence available at the time that report was written. Newly released research indicates the existence of serious safety issues in other settings as well, including ambulatory settings and nursing homes (Gurwitz et al., 2000, 2003). In fact, because the number of outpatient encounters far exceeds the number of inpatient admissions, the consequences of medical errors in the former settings—and the opportunities to improve—may dwarf those in hospitals.

Earlier research on patient safety also focused on errors of *commission* (e.g., prescribing a medication that has a potentially fatal interaction with another drug the patient is taking). However, errors of *omission* (e.g., failing to prescribe a medication from which the patient would likely have benefited) may pose an even greater threat to health. On average, patients receive only about 55 percent of those services from which they would likely have benefited (McGlynn et al., 2003).

It is not possible to quantify the full magnitude of the safety challenge with certainty. The health care sector does not routinely identify and collect information on errors. Experts have challenged the estimates of patient harm attributable to errors, as well as the methodologies used to derive them (Brennan, 2000; Hayward and Hofer, 2001; McDonald et al., 2000; Sox and Woloshin, 2000). As substantial evidence about adverse events continues to accumulate in the United States and other countries (Vincent et al., 2001; Wilson et al., 1995), however, there is no doubt that their occurrence is a serious matter warranting attention. The risks to public safety—and the opportunities for large-scale improvements—are sizable.

As concerns about patient safety have grown, the health care sector has looked to other industries that have confronted similar challenges, in particular the airline industry. This industry learned long ago that information and clear communication are critical to the safe navigation of an airplane. To perform their jobs well and guide their planes safely to their destinations, pilots must communicate with the air traffic controller concerning their destinations and current circumstances (e.g., mechanical or other problems), their flight plans, and environmental factors (e.g., weather conditions) that could necessitate a change in course. Information must also pass seamlessly from one controller to another to ensure a safe and smooth journey for planes flying long distances; provide notification of airport delays or closures due to weather conditions; and enable rapid alert and response to an extenuating circumstance, such as a terrorist attack.

Information is as critical to the provision of safe health care—care that is free of errors of both commission and omission—as it is to the safe operation of aircraft. To develop a treatment plan, a doctor must have access to complete patient information (e.g., diagnoses, medications, current test results, and available social supports) and to the most current science base. The doctor and the patient must also be aware of other environmental factors that affect the ability to implement a treatment plan, such as the availability of hospital beds, current waiting times to obtain specific services, and insurance requirements for prior authorization or use of specific providers. Doctors and nurses armed with information on infectious diseases (e.g., influenza, West Nile virus) can also better counsel their patients about preventive steps that may be beneficial. For patients with chronic conditions, it is critical that information flow freely among all authorized members of the care team (e.g., primary care providers, specialists, pharmacists, home health aides, patients, and lay caregivers).

On the other hand, a salient difference between the work environment of airline pilots and that of clinicians and patients is the level and sophistication of the information technology infrastructure that supports their work. Pilots have immediate access to the information they need to make informed decisions. In health care today, no such information technology infrastructure exists. Only a fraction of hospitals have implemented a comprehensive electronic health record (EHR) system,[1] although many have made progress in certain areas, such as computerized reporting of laboratory results (Brailer, 2003). Rates of adoption of EHR systems are higher in ambulatory settings— probably about 5–10 percent of physician offices—but there is much variability in their content and functionality. Also, only a handful of communities have established a community-wide, secure Internet-based platform to facilitate access to clinical information by multiple providers, not just those within a given institution, such as a hospital or group practice (Institute of Medicine, 2002a).

---

*Better management of health information is a prerequisite
to achieving patient safety as a standard of care.*

The airline industry also learned that for every tragic accident there are many near misses and that much can be learned from analysis of these events. Aviation reporting systems are in place to capture detailed information on near misses (e.g., time, place, individuals involved, nature of event, and circumstances that allowed harm to be averted). Accidents are meticulously documented and investigated by the National Transportation Safety Board.

In recent years, patient safety reporting systems have emerged in the health care arena. Many hospitals now routinely capture information on errors, both near misses and adverse events, as a part of their internal safety

---

[1] An EHR system encompasses (1) longitudinal collection of electronic health information for and about persons, (2) electronic access to person- and population-level information by authorized users, (3) provision of knowledge and decision support systems, and (4) support for efficient processes for health care delivery.

improvement programs. The Joint Commission on Accreditation of Healthcare Organizations (JCAHO) requires hospitals to conduct root-cause analyses of adverse events as part of its accreditation program and encourages reporting of these events to JCAHO. Moreover, about one-half of states have reporting systems that focus on adverse events (Rosenthal and Booth, 2003). Various federal agencies maintain reporting systems as well, including those pertaining to drugs and medical devices, hospital-acquired infections, and blood products. There are also many examples of voluntary reporting systems in the private sector, including those for medication errors and adverse events occurring in hospitals.

The usefulness of these patient safety reporting systems, however, has been limited. As a result of the paucity of EHR systems, most patient safety reports cannot be generated automatically as a by-product of the patient care process. Nor can the lessons learned through analysis of patient safety reports easily be transferred back to the point of care. Without EHRs, reporting systems typically rely on special data collection mechanisms (both human- and computer-based), making reporting a cumbersome, costly, and sporadic exercise. The data collected in these systems are neither complete nor standardized, making it difficult to aggregate the data or identify trends or patterns. Liability concerns also impede participation in many reporting systems.

Patient safety is the prevention of harm to patients.

The development of an information technology infrastructure is essential to improve the safety of health care (Institute of Medicine, 2001). Computer-based reminder systems for patients and clinicians can improve compliance with preventive service protocols (Balas et al., 2000). The availability of complete patient health information at the point of care delivery, along with clinical decision support systems (e.g., for medication order entry), can prevent many errors from occurring (Bates et al., 1998, 1999; Evans et al., 1998). Computer-assisted diagnosis and chronic care management programs can improve clinical decision making and adherence to clinical guidelines (Durieux et al., 2000; Evans et al., 1998).

The committee strongly believes that patient safety is indistinguishable from the delivery of quality care. A new delivery system must be built to achieve substantial improvements in patient safety—a system that is capable of preventing errors from occurring in the first place, while at the same time incorporating lessons learned from any errors that do occur. To achieve such a system capable of providing care that is safe will require a culture of safety and the active participation of all health care professionals, organizations, and patients themselves. A critical component of this new health care delivery system will be the development of an information technology infrastructure.

> **Recommendation 1. Americans expect and deserve safe care. Improved information and data systems are needed to support efforts to make patient safety a standard of care in hospitals, in doctors' offices, in nursing homes, and in every other health care setting. All health care organizations should establish comprehensive patient safety systems that:**
>
> • **Provide immediate access to complete patient information and decision support tools (e.g., alerts, reminders) for clinicians and their patients.**
> • **Capture information on patient safety—including both adverse events and near misses—as a by-product of care, and use this information to design even safer care delivery systems.**

To support the objectives of care delivery that is free of errors and the implementation of robust safety reporting systems, a broad range of patient data will be needed, including demographic information, signs and symptoms, medications, test results, diagnoses, therapies, and outcomes. In addition, to learn from near misses and adverse events, the system must capture such data as the individuals involved, where and when the event occurred, what happened, the likely severity of avoided or actual outcomes, contributing factors, and recovery procedures, as well as reporters' narratives that will reveal the underlying system failure.

ELEMENTS OF A HEALTH INFORMATION INFRASTRUCTURE

As shortcomings in the current health care system have become increasingly apparent, the National Committee on Vital and Health Statistics and numerous expert panels have called for the establishment of a national health information infrastructure to meet many of the nation's needs for safe and efficient care delivery, public health, homeland security, and health research (Institute of Medicine, 2001; National Committee on Vital and Health Statistics, 2001; President's Information Technology Advisory Committee, 2001). It will not be enough for individual providers making independent decisions to invest in information technology because patients often receive services from many different providers and in a variety of settings within and across communities. Components of a national health information infrastructure include EHR systems with decision support, a secure platform for the exchange of patient information across health care settings, and data standards to make that information understandable to all users. A partnership between the public and private sectors will be needed to build this infrastructure (Department of Health and Human Services, 2003a; Institute of Medicine, 2002a; Markle Foundation, 2003).

A previous IOM committee has spoken to the need for strong federal leadership and financial support for a national health information infrastructure (Institute of Medicine, 2002b). Private-sector investments will account for a good deal of the capital required to build this infrastructure, but the federal government also has an important role to play in providing financial support. To achieve the greatest gains, federal financial support should be targeted to three areas. First, federal financial investment should support the development of critical building blocks of the national health information infrastructure that are unlikely to receive adequate support through investment by private-sector stakeholders, including the establishment of a secure platform for the exchange of data across all providers and, as discussed below, maintenance of a process for the ongoing promulgation of national data standards. Second, the federal government should provide financial incentives to stimulate private-sector investments in EHR systems; this might be done through revolving loans, differential payments to providers with certain information technology capabilities, or other means. Third, federal government funding of safety net providers will be necessary to support their transition to a safer health care delivery system.

The Department of Health and Human Services (DHHS) recently commissioned the IOM to identify the key capabilities that an EHR system should possess to support patient safety and quality of care. This committee responded to that request in a letter report entitled *Key Capabilities of an Electronic Health Record System* (Institute of Medicine, 2003a) (see Appendix E). In structuring financial incentives, both public and private purchasers should consider linking provider incentives to the acquisition of EHRs that possess these important capabilities. The letter report also provides a framework that should prove useful to accreditation organizations in establishing standards for EHR systems, as well as to providers in selecting and venders in designing such systems.

National leadership will also be needed to establish and maintain standards for the collection, exchange, and reporting of data to support patient safety. Data standards are both a critical and time-sensitive building block of the proposed national health information infrastructure. In the absence of national data standards, health care organizations will likely be slower to invest in information technology, and the systems that are built will be inadequate to make patient safety a standard of care.

> **Recommendation 2. A national health information infrastructure—a foundation of systems, technology, applications, standards, and policies—is required to make patient safety a standard of care.**
>
> • **The federal government should facilitate deployment of the national health information infrastructure through the provision of targeted financial support and the ongoing promulgation and maintenance of standards for data that support patient safety.**
> • **Health care providers should invest in electronic health record systems that possess the key capabilities necessary to provide safe and effective care and to enable the continuous redesign of care processes to improve patient safety.**

Although the focus of this report is on patient safety, it is important to note that the proposed national health information infrastructure will yield many other benefits in terms of new opportunities for access to care, care delivery, public health, homeland security, and clinical and health services research. Through the use of telemedicine, critically ill patients in small rural hospitals will be able to benefit from round-the-clock remote monitoring by physicians with advanced training in intensive care. Like air traffic controllers, public health officials and clinicians with appropriate information and communication supports will be able to detect earlier and respond more rapidly to infectious disease outbreaks. Enhanced communication and information technologies will allow the health system to make a significant leap forward toward safer care.

A PUBLIC–PRIVATE PARTNERSHIP FOR SETTING STANDARDS

Efforts of both the public and private sectors to invest in information technology are hampered by the lack of national data standards for the collection, coding, classification, and exchange of clinical and administrative data. The establishment of such national data standards must be an ongoing process, including updates to reflect both advances in clinical knowledge and changes in safety and quality reporting requirements.

Establishing and maintaining data standards is integrally linked to the advancement and diffusion of clinical knowledge. The discovery of new knowledge leads to the redefinition of what constitutes best practices in a specific clinical area. Overlooking or failing to adhere to best practices is an important source of errors of omission that lead to morbidity and mortality among patients. In the early 1980s, for example, new scientific evidence became available indicating that medications known as beta-blockers administered to patients at the time of a heart attack greatly reduce the likelihood of a subsequent heart attack (Beta-Blocker Heart Attack Trial, 1982). To be applied speedily and consistently in practice, such new evidence must be translated into a care guideline (e.g., absent contraindications, patients experiencing a heart attack should be prescribed beta-blockers). Hospitals, physicians, and other providers must modify their care processes to be consistent with the new best practice (e.g., the patient's attending physician is responsible for prescribing a beta-blocker to the patient at the time of the heart attack). Information systems must be modified to capture information on the new practice (e.g., the pharmacy system must add this new drug to the formulary), and computerized decision support systems must be modified to issue an alert to the clinician and patient if the patient's record does not include entries substantiating that beta-blockers were prescribed at the time of the heart attack, if appropriate.

Unfortunately, the current health care delivery system lacks well-defined processes for translating new knowledge into practice. Not surprisingly, then, a 1997 study showed that only 21 percent of eligible elderly patients suffering a heart attack had received beta-blockers, and there was a 75 percent higher mortality rate among those who did not receive the treatment than among those who did (Soumerai et al., 1997). Similar examples can be found in virtually every area of clinical practice (Institute of Medicine, 2001; McGlynn et al., 2003). Overall, the toll in terms of lost lives, pain and suffering, and wasted resources is staggering.

As a complement to the present study, DHHS asked the IOM to identify a limited number of clinical areas that might serve as a starting point for public- and private-sector efforts to improve care delivery. In fall 2002, the IOM released the report *Priority Areas for National Action: Transforming Health Care Quality* (Institute of Medicine, 2003b) identifying 20 areas—consisting primarily of leading chronic conditions—that account for a sizable proportion of health care services.

Through the efforts of the Agency for Healthcare Research and Quality (AHRQ) progress is being made on translating knowledge into practice in selected clinical areas, including the 20 priority areas identified by the IOM. As of October 2002, AHRQ had provided support to 13 evidence-based practice centers to develop evidence reports and technology assessments and to work in partnership with other groups to develop practice guidelines and implementation tools (Agency for Healthcare Research and Quality, 2003). In September 2000, AHRQ also initiated the Integrated Delivery System Research Network, which encompasses nine partnership arrangements, each linking health care organizations, research institutions, and managed care organizations for the conduct of applied health services research and the dissemination of findings (Agency for Healthcare Research and Quality, 2002). Nearly all of the 20 priority areas identified by the IOM are being addressed in this ongoing work.

The health care sector also lacks standardized measurement and reporting mechanisms that can be used for routine monitoring of the extent to which health care is safe and effective. In designing and building information technology systems, it is helpful to know in advance the reporting specifications that must be satisfied. As noted earlier, there are many safety and quality measurement and improvement efforts sponsored by health care providers, public and private purchasers, federal and state agencies, and accreditors. Some focus on near misses or adverse events, while others assess compliance with best practices through medical care process and outcome measures. Some noteworthy efforts have been made to encourage standardization of reporting requirements. In late 2003, DHHS is expected to release the first National Healthcare Quality Report, in which an attempt has been made to address the IOM's 20 priority areas. In the future, this report will likely extend to the state and community levels. Likewise, the Quality Interagency Coodinating Task Force, an interagency government committee, has made some progress toward establishing standardized safety and quality measures and tools, some of which have been incorporated into multiple government health care programs. And the National Quality Forum, a public–private partnership organization, has established standardized reporting requirements for various health care settings (e.g., nursing homes, hospitals) and for certain safety-related events, called *serious reportable events* (National Quality Forum, 2002). Much work remains to be done, however. The data requirements for clinical guidelines and for safety and quality reporting must feed into the process used to develop data standards for EHR systems if those systems are to serve as the primary source of information and decision support for providers seeking to follow best-practice guidelines and respond to patient safety reporting requirements.

The National Committee on Vital and Health Statistics (NCVHS), a public–private advisory committee established to provide advice to DHHS and Congress on national health information policy, has for many years recommended that the federal government assume a more active role in establishing national data standards (National Committee on Vital and Health Statistics, 2000). In 1996, Congress passed the Health Insurance Portability and Accountability Act (HIPAA, Public Law 104-191), which mandated standardization of administrative and financial transactions. In 2001, the Consolidated Health Informatics (CHI) initiative, an interagency effort, was established as part of the Office of Management and Budget's eGOV initiative to streamline and consolidate government programs among like sectors (Office of Management and Budget, 2003). DHHS was designated the managing partner for the CHI initiative, with the Centers for Medicare and Medicaid Services taking the lead. The CHI initiative played a pivotal role in the recent decision by the federal government that programs of DHHS, the Veterans Administration, and the Department of Defense would incorporate certain data standards and terminologies (Department of Health and Human Services, 2003b).

The CHI initiative, although off to a very promising start, lacks a clear mandate to establish standards. In addition, the future of the initiative once initial standards and gaps have been identified is unclear. The initiative would also benefit from closer collaboration with NCVHS to ensure the active participation of private-sector stakeholders.

> **Recommendation 3. Congress should provide clear direction, enabling authority, and financial support for the establishment of national standards for data that support patient safety. Various government agencies will need to assume major new responsibilities, and additional support will be required. Specifically:**
>
> • **The Department of Health and Human Services (DHHS) should be given the lead role in establishing and maintaining a public–private partnership for the promulgation of standards for data that support patient safety.**
> • **The Consolidated Health Informatics (CHI) initiative, in collaboration with the National Committee on Vital and Health Statistics (NCVHS), should identify data standards appropriate for national adoption and gaps in existing standards that need to be addressed. The membership of NCVHS should continue to be broad and diverse, with adequate representation of all stakeholders, including consumers, state governments, professional groups, and standards-setting bodies.**
> • **The Agency for Healthcare Research and Quality (AHRQ) in collaboration with the National Library of Medicine and others should**

(1) provide administrative and technical support for the CHI and NCVHS efforts; (2) ensure the development of implementation guides, certification procedures, and conformance testing for all data standards; (3) provide financial support and oversight for developmental activities to fill gaps in data standards; and (4) coordinate activities and maintain a clearinghouse of information in support of national data standards and their implementation to improve patient safety.

• **The National Library of Medicine should be designated as the responsible entity for distributing all national clinical terminologies that relate to patient safety and for ensuring the quality of terminology mappings.**

Without federal leadership in the establishment of standards for data that support patient safety, information technology systems built over the coming decades will be inadequate to support the delivery of safe and effective care. The time to act is now.

Given the sizable purchasing power (over 40 percent of health care expenditures) and regulatory authority of the federal government, the incorporation of data standards into government programs is one approach to establishing national standards. After providing a reasonable time period for health care organizations to comply with national standards identified by CHI, the major government health care programs, including those operated or sponsored by DHHS, the Veterans Administration, and the Department of Defense, should immediately incorporate these data standards into their contractual and regulatory requirements (e.g., Medicare conditions for participation).

AN ACTION PLAN FOR SETTING DATA STANDARDS[2]

The standards-setting process, like any other major undertaking, needs a focus and specific objectives. This committee considered the need for standards and the status of current standards-setting activities in three key areas:

• *Data interchange formats*—standard formats for electronically encoding the data elements (including sequencing and error handling). Interchange standards can also include document architectures for structuring

---

[2]This section covers material that is highly technical. Readers who are not familiar with the various types of data standards may find it useful to consult the list of acronyms and terms at the end of this Executive Summary.

data elements as they are exchanged and information models that define the relationships among data elements in a message.

- *Terminologies*—the medical terms and concepts used to describe, classify, and code the data elements, and data expression languages and syntax that describe the relationships among the terms/concepts.
- *Knowledge representation*—standard methods for electronically representing medical literature, clinical guidelines, and the like for decision support (Hammond, 2002).

Following is a discussion of future work needed in each of these areas and a recommended work plan.

Data Interchange Standards

Because health care data are distributed across several locations (databases), standards for data interchange (i.e., rules for transmitting data from one database to another) are necessary. For messaging standards, a number of mature standards cover the required domains:

- Administrative data (the X12 standard of the Accrediting Standards Committee, Subcommittee on Insurance, Working Group 12)
- Clinical data (Health Level 7 [HL7])
- Medical images (Digital Imaging and Communications in Medicine [DICOM])
- Prescription data (National Council for Prescription Drug Programs [NCPDP] Script)
- Medical device data (Institute for Electrical and Electronics Engineers [IEEE] standard 1073).

These standards[3] were recently endorsed by the Secretary of Health and Human Services. However, there is an urgent need to accelerate the development of the next version of HL7 (version 3.0) to support increased interoperability of systems and comparability of clinical data, as well as patient safety initiatives. In addition to standards, implementation guides, conformance testing, and certification procedures must be developed to ensure consistent application of the standards in commercial systems.

---

[3]Along with the data interchange standards, the Department of Health and Human Services endorsed a terminology for use with laboratory results, the Logical Observation Identifiers, Names, and Codes (LOINC).

Clinical information will continue to appear in textual clinical notes for many years to come. A document architecture standard is needed to enable the interchange of clinical notes and to facilitate the extraction of information using natural language processing techniques. DHHS and AHRQ should support the development of the HL7 Clinical Document Architecture for this purpose. An intuitive and efficient user interface is also an important part of clinical information systems (Shortliffe et al., 2001). User interface tools to facilitate data acquisition are still in the early stages of development, and a number of research projects are under way to resolve technological constraints on the widespread implementation of clinical information systems. Much is being learned from the ubiquity of Web interfaces, and continued research is necessary to design user interfaces that incorporate human factors into the engineering of applications.

When exchanging patient-specific data for clinical and patient-safety reasons, it is imperative that the data be linked to the correct patient accurately and reliably through a unique health identifier (UHI). Without a national UHI, fragmentation of patient data can lead to medical errors and adverse events. Although a UHI was mandated by HIPAA, Congress placed a hold on further action until privacy protection was enacted. Now that privacy and security rules to protect health data have been established under the provisions of HIPAA,[4] Congress should authorize DHHS to take immediate steps to identify options for implementing a UHI system. Consideration should be given to implementing a voluntary UHI system in which patients can elect to participate.

Terminologies

If health professionals are to be able to send and receive data in an understandable and usable manner, both the sender and the receiver must have common clinical terminologies for describing, classifying, and coding medical terms and concepts. Use of standardized clinical terminologies facilitates electronic data collection at the point of care; retrieval of relevant

---

[4]The administrative simplification provisions of HIPAA set forth standards and regulatory requirements for the electronic transmission of data for administrative and financial transactions. The provisions also include standards for privacy and security to protect individually identifiable health information and standards to uniquely identify providers, employers, health plans, and patients. Because the privacy and security provisions were not in place at the time the legislation was enacted, only the employer and health plan identifiers have been implemented.

data, information, and knowledge; and reuse of data for multiple purposes (e.g., disease surveillance, clinical decision support, patient safety reporting).

No single terminology has the depth and breadth to represent the broad spectrum of medical knowledge; thus a core group of well-integrated, nonredundant clinical terminologies will be needed to serve as the backbone of clinical information and patient safety systems. Efforts are now under way within the National Library of Medicine and other key government organizations to evaluate existing terminologies and identify those that should be included in the core set. Patient safety is an important area in which significant gaps in terminology for concept representation exist and for which a new terminology and classification system needs to be developed. The new terminology should be fully integrated with the core set and made publicly available for widespread dissemination and use. The National Library of Medicine should be responsible for dissemination, mapping, and updating of the core terminology standards.

Knowledge Representation

As noted above, to support patient safety, ongoing syntheses of the clinical literature should be conducted to determine best practices for clinical management in the 20 priority areas identified by the IOM. The National Institutes of Health and many private-sector academic and research centers play critical roles in the ongoing generation of clinical knowledge. Various professional associations and AHRQ, working through evidence-based practice centers, contribute to the development of practice guidelines and the identification of best practices. This information is critical to the development of decision support tools that can assist clinicians and patients in making evidence-based decisions. Standards are needed for the representation of clinical guidelines and the implementation of automated triggers.

A Work Plan

Accelerating the development and adoption of standards for data to support patient safety will require a concerted and sustained effort in both the public and private sectors. Leadership and support from the federal government will be necessary.

Recommendation 4. The lack of comprehensive standards for data to support patient safety impedes private-sector investment in informa-

tion technology and other efforts to improve patient safety. The federal government should accelerate the adoption of standards for such data by pursuing the following efforts:

- *Clinical data interchange standards.* The federal government should set an aggressive agenda for the establishment of standards for the interchange of clinical data to support patient safety. Federal financial support should be provided to accomplish this agenda.
  - After ample time for provider compliance, federal government health care programs should incorporate into their contractual and regulatory requirements standards already approved by the secretaries of DHHS, the Veterans Administration, and the Department of Defense (i.e., the HL7 version 2.x series for clinical data messaging, DICOM for medical imaging, IEEE 1073 for medical devices, LOINC for laboratory test results, and NCPDP Script for prescription data).
  - AHRQ should provide support for (1) accelerated completion (within 2 years) of HL7 version 3.0; (2) specifications for the HL7 Clinical Document Architecture and implementation guides; and (3) analysis of alternative methods for addressing the need to support patient safety by instituting a unique health identifier for individuals, such as implementation of a voluntary unique health identifier program.
- *Clinical terminologies.* The federal government should move expeditiously to identify a core set of well-integrated, nonredundant clinical terminologies for clinical care, quality improvement, and patient safety reporting. Revisions, extensions, and additions to the codes should be compatible with, yet go beyond, the federal government's initiative to integrate all federal reporting systems.
  - AHRQ should undertake a study of the core terminologies, supplemental terminologies, and standards mandated by the Health Insurance Portability and Accountability Act to identify areas of overlap and gaps in the terminologies to address patient safety requirements. The study should begin by convening domain experts to develop a process for ensuring comprehensive coverage of the terminologies for the 20 IOM priority areas.
  - The National Library of Medicine should provide support for the accelerated completion of RxNORM[5] for clinical drugs. The National Library of Medicine also should develop high-quality

---

[5]RxNORM is a normalized (standard) form for representing clinical drugs and their components.

mappings among the core terminologies and supplemental terminologies identified by the CHI and NCVHS.

- *Knowledge representation.* The federal government should provide support for the accelerated development of knowledge representation standards to facilitate effective use of decision support in clinical information systems.
  - The National Library of Medicine should provide support for the development of standards for evidence-based knowledge representation.
  - AHRQ, in collaboration with the National Institutes of Health, the Food and Drug Administration, and other agencies, should provide support for the development of a generic guideline representation model for use in representing clinical guidelines in a computer-executable format that can be employed in decision support tools.

PATIENT SAFETY SYSTEMS IN HEALTH CARE SETTINGS

Since patient safety is an integral part of the delivery of quality care, achieving an acceptable standard of patient safety requires that all health care settings develop comprehensive patient safety systems, including both a *culture of safety* and *organizational supports* for safety processes. A key aspect of a patient safety system is a culture that encourages clinicians, patients, and others to be vigilant in (1) identifying potential or actual errors, (2) taking appropriate steps to prevent and mitigate harm, and (3) disclosing appropriate information on errors that do occur to facilitate learning and the redesign of care processes. As noted above, safe care settings are ones that have an adequate information infrastructure to provide clinicians and patients with immediate access to health information. But other organizational supports are needed as well, including trained professionals with expertise in safety and well-designed reporting systems for near misses and adverse events.

The establishment of patient safety systems is in a relatively early stage of development in most health care settings. Some aspects of a patient safety system can be found in all, or nearly all, institutional settings, but this is not the case for ambulatory settings, where the majority of health care is provided.

In general, patient safety systems have been evolving along three dimensions: (1) an expansion of the types of events that are analyzed to include both adverse events and near misses; (2) increased use of automated surveillance, as opposed to relying on clinicians or patients, to identify and report cases; and (3) increased attention to the application of knowledge gleaned from reporting systems to the design of systems that can prevent errors. Traditionally, patient safety systems have detected events through individual reports (e.g., a clinician reports an adverse event to a hospital risk manager), document review (e.g., retrospective review of patient records and death certificates), or monitoring of patient progress. In the future, most events will likely be identified through automated surveillance of clinical data (e.g., identifying patients with unusual laboratory results) as more and more of the important components of the patient record become computer based. Automated surveillance, sometimes called data-driven triggers, offers many advantages, including (1) more immediate identification of events when there may still be an opportunity to mitigate patient harm, (2) identification of larger numbers of adverse events than is possible with methods that rely on individual reports or sampling techniques, and (3) a less labor-intensive approach than individual case finding.

To date, most patient safety efforts have focused on the detection and analysis of events, especially adverse events. Adverse events are certainly important, but as noted earlier, they occur infrequently and, by definition, after patients have been injured. Less attention has been focused on the detection and analysis of near misses, and this relative neglect represents a missed opportunity. Experts believe that for each serious adverse event there are probably dozens of near misses, which might best be described as warning signs. Because near misses occur more frequently, monitoring and analysis of these events provide quantitative insight into the distribution of factors that contribute to the occurrence of and recovery from errors (Billings, 1999). The monitoring of near misses may also contribute to a higher level of risk awareness in the working environment. This increased awareness can lead to proactive efforts and system changes that can increase the probability of preventing errors from occurring. Finally, multiple failures often contribute to a single adverse event, and early detection of the first such failure provides an opportunity to intervene and stop what could become a chain of failures leading up to a serious adverse event. However, none of these patient safety reporting systems for detecting and analyzing adverse events and near misses can function effectively in the absence of universally adopted standards for data to support patient safety.

Perhaps the most important dimension of the evolution of patient safety programs among the three cited at the beginning of this section is an increased emphasis on prevention. Progress along this dimension is closely related to progress along the other two. As reporting and analysis move upstream from adverse events to near misses, more knowledge is discovered about high-risk conditions and patients, thus opening the door to preventive interventions. The committee believes that continued evolution along these three dimensions is critical and that steps should be taken to accelerate the pace of this evolution. All health care settings, not just hospitals, nursing homes, and large group practices, should have mature patient safety systems and cultures.

> **Recommendation 5. All health care settings should establish comprehensive patient safety programs operated by trained personnel within a culture of safety. These programs should encompass (1) case finding—identifying system failures, (2) analysis—understanding the factors that contribute to system failures, and (3) system redesign—making improvements in care processes to prevent errors in the future. Patient safety programs should invite the participation of patients and their families and be responsive to their inquiries.**

Efforts should also be made to develop a rich portfolio of knowledge and tools that will be useful to all health care settings seeking to establish comprehensive patient safety systems. Research in this area should focus on the development of the full range of data-driven trigger systems for the detection and prevention of adverse events. Additional research is also needed to assist health care settings in establishing effective reporting systems for near misses. As noted above, the health care sector has far less experience with such systems than with those focusing on adverse events. The high volume and diversity of reports submitted to near-miss systems pose certain challenges.

> **Recommendation 6. The federal government should pursue a robust applied research agenda on patient safety, focused on enhancing knowledge, developing tools, and disseminating results to maximize the impact of patient safety systems. AHRQ should play a lead role in coordinating this research agenda among federal agencies (e.g., the National Library of Medicine) and the private sector. The research agenda should include the following:**
>
> - **Knowledge generation**
> - **High-risk patients—Identify patients at risk for medication errors, nosocomial infections, falls, and other high-risk events.**
> - **Near-miss incidents—Test the causal continuum assumption (that near misses and adverse events are causally related), develop and test a recovery taxonomy, and extend the current**

individual human error/recovery models to team-based errors and recoveries.
- Hazard analysis—Assess the validity and efficiency of integrating retrospective techniques (e.g., incident analysis) with prospective techniques.
- High-yield activities—Study the cost/benefit of various approaches to patient safety, including analysis of reporting systems for near misses and adverse events.
- Patient roles—Study the role of patients in the prevention, early detection, and mitigation of harm due to errors.
- Tool development
- Early detection capabilities—Develop and evaluate various methods for employing data-driven triggers to detect adverse drug events, nosocomial infections, and other high-risk events (e.g., patient falls, decubitus ulcers, complications of blood product transfusions).
- Prevention capabilities—Develop and evaluate point-of-care decision support to prevent errors of omission or commission.
- Data mining techniques—Identify and develop data mining techniques to enhance learning from regional and national patient safety databases. Apply natural language processing techniques to facilitate the extraction of patient safety–related concepts from text documents and incident reports.
- Dissemination—Deploy knowledge and tools to clinicians and patients.

PATIENT SAFETY REPORTING

As concerns about safety and quality have grown, so, too, have reporting requirements. Performance information can serve a range of purposes. At one end of the spectrum are applications used by public-sector legal and regulatory bodies, such as professional and institutional licensure and legal liability, that are intended to hold health care professionals and organizations accountable. At the other end of the spectrum are applications that focus on learning—both organizational and professional. The feedback of performance data to clinicians for continuing education purposes falls into this category, as does the redesign of care processes by health care organizations based on analysis of data collected by reporting systems for near misses and adverse events. Somewhere between these two ends of the spectrum are applications intended to encourage health care providers to strive for excellence by rewarding those who achieve the highest levels of performance with larger payments and greater demand for their services.

EHR systems should be capable of supporting the full range of applications outlined above. Ideally, performance reports, whether for external accountability or internal quality improvement purposes, should be generated automatically as a by-product of the EHR system. Achieving this objective will require a great deal of standardization of both the information reported and the patient and other data captured as part of the patient care process.

Some progress has been made in the standardization of certain types of performance reporting requirements. For example, there are standardized care process measures (e.g., immunization rates, proportion of diabetics who received an annual eye exam) for health plans, hospitals, and nursing homes (Department of Health and Human Services, 2002a, b; National Committee for Quality Assurance, 2003), and efforts are under way to encourage national adoption of various standardized measurement sets (Kizer, 2001). Far less attention has been focused on the standardization of reporting requirements applicable to reporting systems for near misses and adverse events. These types of reporting systems capture detailed information on specific events. Although sometimes used to produce error rates (e.g., adverse drug events per 1,000 admissions), such reporting systems focus more on the conduct of root-cause analyses to determine the factors that contributed to the event and identify ways of redesigning the care process to reduce the likelihood that similar events will occur in the future.

Most health care organizations must comply with a multitude of reporting requirements for errors. Many public and private purchasers, state governments, and private accrediting and certifying organizations require or encourage the reporting of errors. In addition, many health care organizations have their own internal reporting systems that play an integral role in the organization's quality improvement programs. For the most part, each reporting system determines what types of events are reported, and many also have their own terminology to represent information. As a result, there is little if any ability to share and compare data, and the reporting burden on health care organizations is sizable.

The development of a standardized format and terminology for the capture and reporting of data related to patient safety events (i.e., adverse events and near misses) would improve the usefulness of the data and ease the reporting burden considerably. The standardized format should use the HL7 Clinical Document Architecture and include the reporter's narrative; who was involved; what happened, where, and when; risk assessment of severity and probability of recurrence; preventability; causal analysis; recovery factors; and corrective actions if an adverse event. Standard taxonomies for the domain areas of the report format should be developed. Taxonomies for the sets of contextual variables (who, what, where, outcome, etc.) should be tailored to each domain. The widely used Eindhoven Classification Model— Medical Version should be used as a standard taxonomy to classify root causes identified through analysis of near misses and adverse events. All new terms should be incorporated into the key reference terminology (System- ized Nomenclature of Human and Veterinary Medicine Clinical Terms [SNOMED CT]) of the NCVHS core terminology group, with mappings to higher-level classifications in supplemental terminologies, such as the Inter- national Classification of Diseases (ICD) 9/10 CM E-codes. The National Library of Medicine should be funded to maintain and distribute the patient safety taxonomies. Also, in light of the recently established patient safety initiative of the World Health Organization, additional work on the ICD 9/ 10 CM E-codes should be undertaken to enhance their capacity for repre- senting adverse events and to facilitate international comparisons (World Health Organization, 2002).

An earlier IOM committee recommended that AHRQ establish a na- tional patient safety reporting database containing standardized, deidentified patient data drawn from various public- and private-sector reporting sys- tems (Institute of Medicine, 2001). Before acting on that recommendation, AHRQ will need to develop an event taxonomy and common report format for submission of data to the national patient safety database.

Recommendation 7. AHRQ should develop an event taxonomy and common report format for submission of data to the national patient safety database. Specifically:

- **The event taxonomy should address near misses and adverse events, cover errors of both omission and commission, allow for the designation of primary and secondary event types for cases in which more than one factor precipitated the adverse event, and be incorpo- rated into SNOMED CT.**
- **The standardized report format should include the following:**
- **A standardized minimum set of data elements.**
- **Data necessary to calculate a risk assessment index for deter- mining prospectively the probability of an event and its severity.**
- **A free-text narrative of the event.**
- **Data necessary to support use of the Eindhoven Classification Model—Medical Version for classifying root causes, including expansions for (1) recovery factors associated with near-miss events, (2) corrective actions taken to recover from adverse events, and (3) patient outcome/functional status as a result of those corrective actions.**

- A free-text section for lessons learned as a result of the event.
- Clinical documentation of the patient context.
- The taxonomy and report format should be used by the federal reporting system integration project in the areas for basic domain, event type, risk assessment, and causal analysis but should provide for more extensive support for patient safety research and analysis (Department of Health and Human Services, 2002c).

The event taxonomy and standardized report format are intended to serve as a framework for federal, state, and private-sector reporting systems. AHRQ should also develop tools and guidelines to assist public- and private-sector reporting programs in implementing the common report format and data standards. Furthermore, the development of external data auditing criteria would provide assurance to all stakeholders that data used for reporting are valid and reliable.

THE JOURNEY AHEAD

The committee has laid out an ambitious agenda that has the potential to produce dramatic improvements in patient safety. This agenda is likely to yield considerable benefits in many other areas as well, including public health, homeland security, clinical and health services research, and health professions education.

At the heart of the agenda is the development of a national health information infrastructure, including EHR systems that adhere to national standards for data supporting patient safety in all health care settings. Although the committee recognizes that carrying out this agenda will require a sizable up-front capital investment, we believe its creation is essential not only to patient safety but also to the health of the American people more generally. The committee believes that establishing this information technology infrastructure should be the highest priority for all health care stakeholders.

This is a journey that will take a decade to accomplish and in which the federal government, working in partnership with the private sector, has a critical role to play. The federal government should act immediately to establish the national data standards called for in this report. Although modest financial resources will be required, the committee believes the return on this investment will be very high. Many if not most providers are investing in EHRs. National data standards are needed now to ensure that these systems possess the necessary capabilities to improve patient safety and are capable of exchanging information reliably.

There is little doubt that sizable financial investments will be needed to build the national health information infrastructure. It was beyond the scope of this study to develop estimates of the resources required to accomplish the agenda proposed herein or to evaluate alternatives for providing these resources. The conduct of such an analysis represents an important next step that should be pursued immediately.

Once the basic health information infrastructure has been built, the health care sector should be able to function at a far higher level of safety and efficiency. Many of the factors that lead to errors (e.g., illegible handwriting in clinical records, mistakes in calculating drug dosages, lack of access to information on a patient's known drug allergies) will have been eliminated. Although human analysis of errors that do occur will still be necessary, the information technology infrastructure should greatly reduce the human effort currently required to identify and analyze most errors. Over time, the infrastructure, including health care data standards, will need to evolve to accommodate developments in medical knowledge, technological innovations, and social changes in the way patients and their families interact with the health care delivery system.

Although building the information technology infrastructure is critical to both error prevention and error reporting, the elegance of implementing an EHR system is that it is a single solution to both objectives. Investment in EHR systems is critical to applying much of the knowledge that already exists about error prevention. Robust internal and external reporting systems for near misses and adverse events provide new knowledge that makes it possible to design even safer delivery systems. In building their EHR systems, health care organizations may want to target initial investments to the establishment of key capabilities for which a sizable knowledge base already exists with regard to the prevention of errors (e.g., medication order entry systems significantly reduce medication errors) and in areas in which computerized data will be useful in detecting and analyzing errors. All health care providers should also derive benefits in the near future from AHRQ's efforts to establish standardized error reporting requirements and to conduct applied research that will lead to enhanced knowledge and tools that can be used to improve patient safety.

ACRONYMS

The committee apologizes for the heavy use of acronyms in the Executive Summary and the report itself. Both spoken and written discussion on health care data standards are replete with acronyms. To help the reader, a list of acronyms used in the Executive Summary is provided below; a fuller list is provided in Appendix B.

AHRQ—Agency for Healthcare Research and Quality
CHI—Consolidated Health Informatics (initiative)
DHHS—Department of Health and Human Services
DICOM—Digital Imaging and Communications in Medicine
EHR—electronic health record
HIPAA—Health Insurance Portability and Accountability Act
HL7—Health Level Seven
ICD—International Classification of Diseases
IEEE—Institute of Electrical and Electronics Engineers
JCAHO—Joint Commission on Accreditation of Healthcare
    Organizations
NCPDP—National Council on Prescription Drug Programs
NCVHS—National Committee on Vital and Health Statistics
SNOMED CT—Systemized Nomenclature of Human and Veterinary
    Medicine Clinical Terms
UHI—unique health identifier

REFERENCES

Agency for Healthcare Research and Quality. 2002. *Integrated Delivery System Research Network: Fact Sheet.* Online. Available: http://www.ahrq.gov/research/idsrn.htm [accessed August 14, 2003].

———. 2003. *AHRQ: Evidence-Based Practice.* Online. Available: http://www.ahrq.gov/clinic/epcix.htm [accessed April 25, 2003].

Balas, E. A., S. Weingarten, C. T. Garb, D. Blumenthal, S. A. Boren, and G. D. Brown. 2000. Improving preventive care by prompting physicians. *Arch Intern Med* 160 (3):301–308.

Bates, D. W., L. L. Leape, D. J. Cullen, N. Laird, L. A. Petersen, J. M. Teich, E. Burdick, M. Hickey, S. Kleefield, B. Shea, M. Vander Vliet, and D. L. Seger. 1998. Effect of computerized physician order entry and a team intervention on prevention of serious medication errors. *JAMA* 280 (15):1311–1316.

Bates, D. W., J. M. Teich, J. Lee, D. Seger, G. J. Kuperman, N. Ma'Luf, D. Boyle, and L. Leape. 1999. The impact of computerized physician order entry on medication error prevention. *J Am Med Inform Assoc* 6 (4):313–321.

Beta-Blocker Heart Attack Trial. 1982. A randomized trial of propranolol in patients with acute myocardial infarction. I. Mortality results. *JAMA* 247 (12):1707–1714.

Billings, C. E. 1999. The NASA aviation safety reporting system: Lessons learned from voluntary incident reporting. In: *Enhancing Patient Safety and Reducing Errors.* Chicago, IL: National Patient Safety Foundation.

Brailer, D. J. 2003. *Use and Adoption of Computer-Based Patient Records in the United States: A Review and Update.* PowerPoint Presentation to IOM Committee on Data Standards for Patient Safety on January 23, 2003. Online. Available: http://www.iom.edu/file.asp?id=10988 [accessed December 16, 2003].

Brennan, T. A. 2000. The Institute of Medicine report on medical errors: Could it do harm? *N Eng J Med* 342 (15):1123–1125.

Department of Health and Human Services. 2002a. *HHS Launches National Nursing Home Quality Initiative: Broad Effort to Improve Quality in Nursing Homes Across the Country.* Online. Available: http://www.dhhs.gov/news/press/2002pres/20021112.html [accessed August 19, 2003].

———. 2002b. *Secretary Thompson Welcomes New Effort to Provide Hospital Quality of Care Information.* Online. Available: http://www.dhhs.gov/news/press/2002pres/20021212.html [accessed August 19, 2002].

———. 2002c. *HHS Moves Forward to Establish New System for Collecting Patient Safety Data.* Online. Available: http://www.hhs.gov/news/press/2002pres/20021125.html [accessed August 18, 2003].

———. 2003a. *National Health Information Infrastructure 2003: Developing a National Action Agenda for NHII.* Online. Available: http://www.nhii-03.s-3.net/welcome.htm [accessed May 30, 2003].

———. 2003b. *Federal Government Announces First Federal EGov Health Information Exchange Standards.* Online. Available: http://www.dhhs.gov/news/press/2003pres/20030321a.html [accessed May 29, 2003].

Durieux, P., R. Nizard, P. Ravaud, N. Mounier, and E. Lepage. 2000. A clinical decision support system for prevention of venous thromboembolism: Effect on physician behavior. *JAMA* 283 (21):2816–2821.

Evans, R. S., S. L. Pestotnik, D. C. Classen, T. P. Clemmer, L. K. Weaver, J. F. Orme Jr., J. F. Lloyd, and J. P. Burke. 1998. A computer-assisted management program for antibiotics and other antiinfective agents. *N Engl J Med* 338 (4):232–238.

Gurwitz, J. H., T. S. Field, J. Avorn, D. McCormick, S. Jain, M. Eckler, M. Benser, A. C. Edmondson, and D. W. Bates. 2000. Incidence and preventability of adverse drug events in nursing homes. *Am J Med* 109 (2):87–94.

Gurwitz, J. H., T. S. Field, L. R. Harrold, J. Rothschild, K. Debellis, A. C. Seger, C. Cadoret, L. S. Fish, L. Garber, M. Kelleher, and D. W. Bates. 2003. Incidence and preventability of adverse drug events among older persons in the ambulatory setting. *JAMA* 289 (9):1107–1116.

Hammond, W. E. 2002. *Patient Safety Data Standards: View from a Standards Perspective.* PowerPoint Presentation to IOM Committee on Data Standards for Patient Safety on May 6, 2002. Online. Available: http://www.iom.edu/file.asp?id=9915 [accessed December 16, 2003].

Hayward, R. A., and T. P. Hofer. 2001. Estimating hospital deaths due to medical errors: Preventability is in the eye of the reviewer. *JAMA* 286 (4):415–420.

Institute of Medicine. 2000. *To Err Is Human: Building a Safer Health System.* Washington, DC: National Academy Press.

———. 2001. *Crossing the Quality Chasm: A New Health System for the 21st Century.* Washington, DC: National Academy Press.

———. 2002a. *Fostering Rapid Advances in Health Care: Learning from System Demonstrations.* Washington, DC: The National Academies Press.

————. 2002b. *Leadership by Example: Coordinating Government Roles in Improving Health Care Quality.* Washington, DC: The National Academies Press.

————. 2003a. Key Capabilities of an Electronic Health Record System: Letter Report. Washington, DC: The National Academies Press.

————. 2003b. *Priority Areas for National Action: Transforming Health Care Quality.* Washington, DC: The National Academies Press.

Kizer, K. W. 2001. Establishing health care performance standards in an era of consumerism. *JAMA* 286 (10):1213–1217.

Markle Foundation. 2003. *Connecting for Health. A Public-Private Collaborative: Key Themes and Guiding Principles.* New York, NY: Markle Foundation.

McDonald, C. J., M. Weiner, and S. L. Hui. 2000. Deaths due to medical errors are exaggerated in Institute of Medicine report. *JAMA* 284 (1):93–95.

McGlynn, E. A., S. M. Asch, J. Adams, J. Keesey, J. Hicks, A. DeCristofaro, and E. A. Kerr. 2003. The quality of health care delivered to adults in the United States. *N Engl J Med* 348 (26):2635–2645.

National Committee for Quality Assurance. 2003. *HEDIS®—Health Plan Employer Data and Information Set.* Online. Available: http://www.ncqa.org/communications/publications/hedispub.htm [accessed November 11, 2003].

National Committee on Vital and Health Statistics. 2000. *Uniform Data Standards for Patient Medical Record Information.* Online. Available: http://ncvhs.hhs.gov/hipaa000706.pdf [accessed April 15, 2002].

————. 2001. *Information for Health: A Strategy for Building the National Health Information Infrastructure.* Online. Available: http://ncvhs.hhs.gov/nhiilayo.pdf [accessed April 18, 2002].

National Quality Forum. 2002. *Serious Reportable Events in Patient Safety: A National Quality Forum Consensus Report.* Washington, DC: National Quality Forum.

Office of Management and Budget. 2003. *Consolidated Health Informatics.* Online. Available: http://www.whitehouse.gov/omb/egov/gtob/health_informatics.htm [accessed April 21, 2003].

President's Information Technology Advisory Committee. 2001. *Transforming Health Care Through Information Technology.* Online. Available: http://www.hpcc.gov/pubs/pitac/pitac-hc-9feb01.pdf [accessed May 7, 2003].

Rosenthal, J., and M. Booth. 2003. *Defining Reportable Events: A Guide for States Tracking Medical Errors.* Portland, ME: National Academy for State Health Policy (NASHP).

Shortliffe, E. H., L. E. Perreault, G. Wiederhold, and L. M. Fagan. 2001. *Medical Informatics: Computer Applications in Healthcare and Biomedicine.* New York, NY: Springer-Verlag.

Soumerai, S. B., T. J. McLaughlin, D. Spiegelman, E. Hertzmark, G. Thibault, and L. Goldman. 1997. Adverse outcomes of underuse of beta-blockers in elderly survivors of acute myocardial infarction. *JAMA* 277 (2):115–121.

Sox, H. C., and S. Woloshin. 2000. How many deaths are due to medical error? Getting the number right. *Eff Clin Pract* 6:277–283.

Vincent, C., G. Neale, and M. Woloshynowych. 2001. Adverse events in British hospitals: Preliminary retrospective record review. *BMJ* 322 (7285):517–519.

Wilson, R. M., W. B. Runciman, R. W. Gibberd, B. T. Harrison, L. Newby, and J. D. Hamilton. 1995. The quality in Australian health care study. *Med J Aust* 163 (9):458–471.

World Health Organization. 2002. *Quality of Care: Patient Safety.* Online. Available: http://www.who.int/gb/EB_WHA/PDF/WHA55/ewha5518.pdf [accessed December 16, 2003].

1

Introduction

In 2000, the Institute of Medicine (IOM) released the report *To Err Is Human: Building a Safer Health System*, focusing national attention on the issue of patient safety (Institute of Medicine, 2000). Since that time, the evidence base substantiating the magnitude of the safety concerns addressed in that report has continued to grow, but so, too, has our knowledge of ways to make the health system safer. It has also become clear that the use of information technology must be a core component of any comprehensive strategy to improve patient safety (Institute of Medicine, 2001).

This report is one of a series of reports following from the IOM's *Crossing the Quality Chasm: A New Health System for the 21st Century* (Institute of Medicine, 2001). Its focus is on the role of information technology in improving patient safety, in particular the need for national standards for safety-related data. This introductory chapter provides a brief description of the magnitude of the safety problem, with emphasis on recently released literature; an overview of the response to *To Err Is Human*; a discussion of the vital role of information technology in designing a safer health care system; an overview of the IOM *Quality Chasm Series*, intended to place this report within a broader context of health system change initiatives; a brief review of the charge to this IOM committee; and an overview of the report, including a discussion of essential concepts. The chapter also introduces definitions for key terms used throughout the report, which are summarized in Appendix B.

MAGNITUDE OF THE PROBLEM

It has long been recognized that medical care has the potential to cause harm. However, general acknowledgment that much iatrogenic injury may be due to human error or system failures has been slower to emerge.

Every day, tens if not hundreds of thousands of errors occur in the U.S. health care system. Fortunately, most of these errors result not in serious harm but in near misses. A *near miss* is defined as an act of commission or omission that could have harmed the patient but did not do so as a result of chance (e.g., the patient received a contraindicated drug but did not experience an adverse drug reaction), prevention (e.g., a potentially lethal overdose was prescribed, but a nurse identified the error before administering the medication), or mitigation (e.g., a lethal drug overdose was administered but discovered early and countered with an antidote). Sadly, however, a small proportion of errors do result in *adverse events*—that is, they cause harm to patients—exacting a sizable toll in terms of injury, disability, and death.

To Err Is Human estimates that 44,000 to 98,000 hospitalized patients die annually in the United States and that more than 1 million patients are injured as a result of error. These estimates were based on the findings of studies conducted in Colorado and Utah (Thomas et al., 1999, 2000) and on the Harvard Medical Practice Study conducted in New York State (Leape et al., 1991), extrapolated to hospital admissions throughout the nation. These epidemiological studies helped jump-start a process to define the overall scope of the safety problem. Elsewhere, the Quality in Australian Health Care Study (Wilson et al., 1995) generated similar findings for hospital-based care, as did a preliminary study in the United Kingdom (Vincent et al., 2001).

---

*An error is the failure of a planned action to be completed
as intended (i.e., error of execution) or the use of a wrong plan
to achieve an aim (i.e., error of planning).
An error may be act of commission or an act of omission.*

It is not possible to quantify the full magnitude of the safety challenge with certainty. The health care sector does not routinely identify and collect information on errors. Experts have challenged the estimates of patient harm attributable to errors as well as the methodologies used to derive them (Brennan, 2000; Hayward and Hofer, 2001; Sox and Woloshin, 2000; McDonald et al., 2000). As substantial evidence about adverse events continues to accumulate in the United States and other countries, however, there is no doubt that their occurrence is a serious matter warranting attention. The risks to public safety—and the opportunities for large-scale improvements—are sizable.

To Err Is Human focuses primarily on inpatient injuries arising as a direct consequence of treatment (errors of *commission*, such as prescribing a medication that has a potentially fatal interaction with another drug the patient is taking). Since the release of that report, major studies have been published substantiating serious shortcomings in other care settings and involving errors of *omission* (such as failing to prescribe a medication from which the patient would likely have benefited; see Table 1-1). For example, many adverse drug events occur in ambulatory care settings and in nursing homes, as well as in hospitals. A large cohort study of all Medicare enrollees cared for by a major multispecialty group practice during a 12-month period (1999–2000) identified 1,523 adverse drug events during 30,397 person-years of observation (i.e., 50.1 adverse drug events per 1,000 person-years) (Gurwitz et al., 2003). And a study of 18 Massachusetts nursing homes identified 546 adverse drug events during 2,403 nursing home resident-years of observation (i.e., 227 adverse drug events per 1,000 resident-years) (Gurwitz et al., 2000).

Similarly, a major recent study found high levels of errors of omission in U.S. health care (McGlynn et al., 2003). More than 6,700 adults in 12 metropolitan areas were interviewed during the period 1998–2000 about selected health care experiences. In addition, those interviewed gave written consent for researchers to review their medical records and use the information to evaluate performance on 439 detailed clinical indicators of care for 30 acute and chronic conditions, as well as preventive care. The study focused on identifying instances in which proven, noncontroversial, poten-

TABLE 1-1 Health Care Errors in the United States

Type of Error	Inpatient Care	Other Care Settings
Commission	An estimated 44,000 to 98,000 hospitalized patients die annually in the United States (Institute of Medicine, 2000).	In outpatient care, 50 adverse drug events per 1,000 person-years were found (Gurwitz et al., 2003). In nursing home care, 227 adverse drug events per 1,000 resident-years were found (Gurwitz et al., 2000).
Omission	Patients receive 55 percent of recommended care (McGlynn et al., 2003).	

tially life-saving treatment was not used when it should have been. Overall, participants in the study had received only 55 percent of recommended care. There was little difference in the proportion of recommended preventive care provided (55 percent), the proportion of recommended acute care provided (54 percent), and the proportion of recommended care for chronic conditions provided (56 percent).

An adverse event results in unintended harm to the patient by an act of commission or omission rather than by the underlying disease or condition of the patient.[1]

A cause for additional concern is that errors resulting in adverse events are likely underreported, perhaps by as much as a factor of 20 (Cullen et al., 1995); that is, for every event reported, 20 are not. Such underreporting likely reflects care providers' fear of blame and retribution through litigation and of losing professional respect, their failure to appreciate the extent of iatrogenic injury, and the burden of reporting.

RESPONSE TO *TO ERR IS HUMAN*

In response to *To Err Is Human* and to the ensuing report of the U.S. Department of Health and Human Services' (DHHS) Quality Interagency Coordination Task Force (Quality Interagency Coordination Task Force, 2000), a major federal initiative was launched to reduce medical errors and improve patient safety. Congress appropriated $50 million in fiscal year 2001 to carry out this initiative and directed the Agency for Healthcare Research and Quality (AHRQ) to establish a Center for Quality Improvement and Patient Safety.

To date, AHRQ has funded more than 90 new grants, contracts, and other activities. These efforts are organized into several areas, including clinical informatics, centers of excellence, developmental centers, dissemination and education, reporting demonstrations, working conditions, and integrated delivery systems research networks. Nearly half of the AHRQ funding, $22.9 million, supports 16 patient safety reporting demonstration projects. These projects were initiated in September 2001 and are all sched-

---

[1]This definition makes it clear that the potentially avoidable results of an underlying disease or condition, for example, a recurrent myocardial infarction in a patient who was not given a beta-blocker (an error of omission), should be considered an adverse event.

uled to be completed in August or September 2004. Most are hospital based, but a small number are being carried out in ambulatory and other settings. Additionally, several are focusing on specific clinical areas or conditions, such as end of life, medication usage, diabetes, asthma, chronic obstructive pulmonary disease, congestive heart failure, lipid management, intensive care, and nosocomial infections. In general, the purposes of these demonstrations fall into two categories: (1) evaluation of a new or existing patient safety reporting system and (2) examination of surveillance methods and other patient safety or quality improvement systems to detect injuries or errors and determine the frequency and patterns of errors.

To Err Is Human, along with federal support for patient safety reporting and surveillance activities, boosted existing reporting systems and stimulated new ones. Today in the United States, there are many types of patient safety reporting systems in operation or under development in the public and private sectors (Appendix C provides an overview of selected examples of these reporting systems). Overseas, Australia (Australian Council for Safety and Quality in Health Care, 2001; Runciman and Moller, 2001) and the United Kingdom (National Patient Safety Agency, 2001) are implementing nationwide patient safety reporting systems.

In the United States, the federal government operates many reporting systems in carrying out its public health responsibilities (e.g., the National Nosocomial Infections Surveillance System operated by the Centers for Disease Control and Prevention), its regulatory responsibilities (e.g., the Adverse Event Reporting System of the Food and Drug Administration), and its caregiver role (e.g., the Patient Safety Reporting System of the Veterans Administration). Twenty-one states also have mandatory reporting requirements as part of their oversight processes for hospitals and other institutional settings (Rosenthal, 2003a). One example, the New York Patient Occurrence Reporting and Tracking System, is described in Appendix C. In addition, many health care institutions operate patient safety reporting systems for internal quality improvement purposes, and a few private-sector organizations operate such systems on a national basis.

Of the patient safety reporting systems currently operational in the United States, most focus on adverse events; only a small proportion collect and analyze information on near misses (see Appendix C). None of the federal regulatory oversight reporting systems includes near misses as reportable events. Of the 21 states mandating patient safety reporting systems, only Pennsylvania and Kansas collect information on near misses (Rosenthal, 2003b). Private-sector reporting systems are more likely to collect such information.

A near miss is an act of commission or omission that
could have harmed the patient but did not cause harm
as a result of chance, prevention, or mitigation.

As the number of patient safety reporting systems has grown, it has become apparent that a more consistent, standardized approach is needed to reduce the burden of multiple reporting requirements; to make the systems easier to use; and to allow for the pooling of data, which is especially useful for the early identification of the types of errors that occur infrequently. DHHS has responded to this need in two ways. First, AHRQ contracted for the development of technical specifications to integrate the many reporting systems that are operated by federal agencies (as discussed in Chapter 9). Second, AHRQ asked this IOM committee to provide guidance on whether certain aspects of reporting (e.g., types of events, information provided on those events, reporting formats, and definitions of data elements) should be standardized (as discussed below).

THE IMPORTANCE OF INFORMATION TECHNOLOGY IN DESIGNING A SAFER HEALTH CARE SYSTEM

The overarching objective of all patient safety reporting systems is to obtain information that can be used to design a safer health care delivery system. As more and more has been learned about the factors that contribute to the occurrence of errors, the focus of the patient safety movement has moved upstream from detecting and analyzing errors to redesigning the care delivery environment to prevent errors. Indeed, patient safety *is* the prevention of errors.

In recent years, it has become increasingly apparent that major improvements in safety will be achieved only if a stronger information infrastructure is built. For example, the reporting and analysis of adverse drug events in hospitals have led to the identification of the following common factors associated with errors: a decline in renal or hepatic function requiring alteration of drug therapy (13.9 percent); patient history of allergy to the same medication class (12.1 percent); use of the wrong drug name, dosage form, or abbreviation (11.4 percent); incorrect dosage calculations (11.1 percent); and atypical or unusual and critical dosage frequency considerations (10.8 percent) (Lesar et al., 1997). The factors most commonly associated with errors were found to be those related to knowledge and the application of knowledge regarding drug therapy (30 percent); knowledge and the use of knowledge regarding patient factors that affect drug therapy (29.2 percent); use of calculations, decimal points, or unit and rate expression factors (17.5 percent); and nomenclature, such as incorrect drug name, dosage form, or abbreviation (13.4 percent).

Many if not most errors might be prevented with better use of information technology to support care delivery. Many errors occur because clinicians do not have ready access to complete, accurate, and legible patient data; paper medical records are poorly organized, are dispersed in many different settings, contain illegible handwriting, and are difficult to locate (Institute of Medicine, 2001). Other errors occur because the health system relies on humans to remember large amounts of knowledge (e.g., contraindications and drug–drug interactions for numerous medications) and to make complex decisions that routinely exceed the bounds of the human mind (Masys, 2002). Finally, some errors occur because the health system relies on clinicians, who are often busy and sometimes tired, to perform simple calculations (e.g., determination of the proper drug dose for a small child) that can be performed more reliably by a computer (Lepage et al., 1992; Mekhjian et al., 2002; Sittig and Stead, 1994). Redesigning care processes to reduce the likelihood of most types of errors requires changes in the way health care workers perform their jobs, in particular greater use of information technology.

In 1991, the IOM created a new concept—computer-based patient record systems (CPRS)—to differentiate such systems from those that simply put the then-standard medical record into an electronic format (Institute of Medicine, 1997). CPRS included functions such as decision support and enabled other improvements that took advantage of computer capabilities not possible with paper-based systems. In particular, CPRS involved a more active focus on and involvement with the patient's care rather than being simply a record that held medical information.

More recently, these systems have been called electronic health record (EHR) systems to emphasize the point that health care not only involves care of people with illnesses but also includes activities that promote health and prevent illness. Because of the committee's focus on patient safety as the prevention of harm, we have adopted this newer term.

In the health care sector, a great deal of attention and resources are now being directed at the establishment of EHR systems. An EHR system encompasses (1) longitudinal collection of electronic health information, defined as information pertaining to the health of an individual or health care provided to an individual; (2) immediate electronic access to person- and population-level information by authorized, and only authorized, users;

(3) provision of knowledge and decision support that enhance the quality, safety, and efficiency of patient care; and (4) support for efficient processes of health care delivery (Institute of Medicine, 2003a). Investments in EHR systems will produce far greater gains in patient safety if such systems in all health care settings adhere to national data standards for the collection, coding, and sharing of patient data and possess the decision support capabilities (e.g., the ability to detect drug–drug interactions) necessary to provide safe and effective care. Accordingly, this committee was asked to provide guidance to DHHS on data standards; the committee was also asked to identify key capabilities of EHR systems that will promote patient safety.

STUDY CONTEXT

The work of this committee was undertaken within a broader context of health system change initiatives. For over a decade, the IOM and other expert bodies have issued reports addressing the need to build a communications and information technology infrastructure to support health care delivery and other national priorities, such as public health and homeland security. The work of this committee is in part an outgrowth of and where possible builds upon this earlier work.

As noted above, in 1991 the IOM issued a report concluding that CPRS is an essential technology for all health care and that electronic records should be the standard for medical and all other records related to health care. In 1997 the IOM issued a revised edition of this report noting the strides that had been made in the power and capacity of personal computers and other computer-based technologies, the growth in use of the Internet for research and some health applications, the increasing level of computer literacy among health professionals and the public, and the linkage of organizations and individuals through local and regional networks that were beginning to tackle the development of population databases (Institute of Medicine, 1997). Despite these advances, however, progress had been slow. The revised report also outlines the continuing challenges to the development and implementation of computer-based patient records, including resistance to change by the organizational culture, the lack of interoperability and data standards, security and privacy concerns, and financing and policy issues.

In March 2001, the IOM released *Crossing the Quality Chasm: A New Health System for the 21st Century*, which calls for fundamental change in the health care system to achieve improvement in six national quality aims: safety, effectiveness, patient centeredness, timeliness, efficiency, and equity

(Institute of Medicine, 2001). The report stresses the enormous potential of information technology to improve the quality of health care with regard to all of these aims and recommends a renewed national commitment to building an information infrastructure to support health care delivery, public accountability, clinical and health services research, and clinical education, leading ultimately to the elimination of most handwritten clinical data by the end of the decade (Institute of Medicine, 2001).

The *Quality Chasm* report also recommends that initial efforts to redesign the health care delivery system focus on a limited set of priority areas, mainly chronic conditions that account for the majority of health encounters and expenditures. In 2002, the IOM released *Priority Areas for National Action: Transforming Health Care Quality*, identifying 20 such priority areas (see Box 1-1) (Institute of Medicine, 2003b). Efforts are now under way to synthesize the evidence base pertaining to practice in each of these areas and to ensure that practice guidelines are available. The IOM has also recommended that sets of standardized performance measures be developed for each of these priority areas. As discussed below, the IOM committee that conducted the present study was asked to consider the types of standardized clinical data that will be needed by health care providers as they strive to redesign the care processes associated with one or more of the priority areas.

In recent years, numerous expert panels have called for the development of a national health information infrastructure (NHII) (National Committee on Vital and Health Statistics, 2001; President's Information Technology Advisory Committee, 2001). To this end, summits and workshops have been held by the DHHS (Department of Health and Human Services, 2003a), the National Quality Forum (National Quality Forum, 2003), and the Kaiser Permanente Institute for Health Policy (Raymond and Dold, 2002).

Components of an NHII include national data standards for the collection, coding, and exchange of patient and other information; computer-based patient records with decision support; and a secure platform for the exchange of patient health information. It will not be enough for individual providers making independent decisions to invest in information technology because patients often receive services from many different providers and in a variety of settings. In addition to supporting the delivery of high-quality and efficient patient care, the NHII must meet the nation's needs for public health, homeland security, and research. Several IOM reports have recommended that the federal government provide financial support for the NHII, including financial incentives to providers to encourage investment in EHRs (Institute of Medicine, 2001, 2002a, b). The IOM has also recom-

BOX 1-1
Priority Areas for National Action

1. Care coordination (cross-cutting)
2. Self-management/health literacy (cross-cutting)
3. Asthma—appropriate care for persons with mild/moderate persistent asthma
4. Cancer screening that is evidence based—focus on colorectal and cervical cancer
5. Children with special needs
6. Diabetes—focus on appropriate management of early disease
7. End of life with advanced organ system failure—focus on congestive heart failure and chronic obstructive pulmonary disease
8. Frailty associated with old age—preventing falls and pressure ulcers, maximizing function, and developing advanced care plans
9. Hypertension—focus on appropriate management of early disease
10. Immunization—children and adults
11. Ischemic heart disease—prevention, reduction of recurring events, and optimizing of functional capacity
12. Major depression—screening and treatment
13. Medication management—preventing medication errors and overuse of antibiotics
14. Nosocomial infections—prevention and surveillance
15. Pain control in advanced cancer
16. Pregnancy and childbirth—appropriate prenatal and intrapartum care
17. Severe and persistent mental illness—focus on treatment in the public sector
18. Stroke—early intervention and rehabilitation
19. Tobacco dependence treatment in adults
20. Obesity (emerging area)

SOURCE: Institute of Medicine (2003b).

mended that the federal government, working in partnership with the private sector, establish national data standards (Institute of Medicine, 2002a).

In recent years, important progress has been made toward establishing national data standards in the health care domain. In 1996, Congress passed the Health Insurance Portability and Accountability Act (Public Law 104-191), which mandated standardization of administrative and financial transactions. In 2001, the Consolidated Health Informatics (CHI) initiative, an interagency effort, was established as part of the Office of Management and Budget's eGOV initiative to streamline and consolidate government programs among like sectors (Office of Management and Budget, 2003). The CHI initiative played an important role in the recent decision by the federal government that programs of DHHS, the Veterans Administration, and the Department of Defense would incorporate certain data standards and terminologies (Department of Health and Human Services, 2003b). The efforts of the Markle Foundation's Connecting for Health initiative have also helped focus national attention on the data standards issue and forge public and private collaboration in this regard.

Efforts are now under way to establish standards for EHRs. In response to a request from DHHS, this IOM committee released a letter report in July 2003 identifying key capabilities of an EHR (Institute of Medicine, 2003a) (see Appendix E). That report identifies EHR capabilities in eight areas important for patient safety: health information and data, results management, order entry/management, decision support, electronic communication and connectivity, patient support, administrative processes, and reporting and population health management. Many of these capabilities relate to the availability of certain patient information and the provision of key decision support functions (e.g., the ability to alert providers to potential drug–drug interactions). Health Level 7, a leading private-sector standards-setting body, is now building on this work to develop a functional model of an EHR. A common set of expectations will assist providers in acquiring and vendors in developing the necessary software. A functional model will also assist public- and private-sector stakeholders in their efforts to encourage investment in EHRs through regulatory and purchasing policies.

Although progress has been made in setting national standards for health data, migration from paper to electronic records has been slow. Many hospitals have computerized the reporting of results in laboratory, imaging, and other ancillary areas, but only a fraction have comprehensive EHR systems (Brailer, 2003). Rates of adoption of EHRs in ambulatory settings are estimated to range between 5 and 10 percent.

Furthermore, only a handful of communities have established secure platforms for the exchange of data, so access to patient data by authorized users is limited (CareScience, 2003; Kolodner and Douglas, 1997; Markle Foundation, 2003; New England Healthcare EDI Network, 2002; Overhage, 2003). In a recently released report, *Fostering Rapid Advances in Health Care: Learning from System Demonstrations*, a bottom-up approach to establishing the NHII is recommended (Institute of Medicine, 2002a). Although data standards are set at the national level, the report recommends demonstration projects to establish state-of-the-art health care information technology infrastructure in a limited number of states, communities, or multistate regions by 2005. Steps would then be taken to replicate successful efforts or expand the geographic reach of these nodes to cover the entire United States. This infrastructure would include a secure platform for data exchange, computer-based patient records, and decision support systems. The IOM report was produced in response to a request from the Secretary of Health and Human Services that the National Academies identify bold ideas that might change conventional thinking about serious challenges facing the health care system.

CHARGE TO THE COMMITTEE

In this context, DHHS, through AHRQ, requested that the IOM conduct a study:

- To produce a detailed plan to facilitate the development of data standards applicable to the collection, coding, and classification of patient safety information.
- To identify key standardization issues pertaining to the "priority areas" recommended by the Priority Areas for Quality Improvement Project (Institute of Medicine, 2003b) and develop an action plan for addressing them.
- To provide guidance to DHHS on a set of "basic functionalities" that computer-based clinical records (i.e., EHRs) should possess to promote patient safety. The IOM committee will consider functions such as the types of data that should be available to providers when making clinical decisions (e.g., diagnoses, allergies, laboratory results) and the types of decision support capabilities that should be present (e.g., the capability to alert providers to potential drug-to-drug interactions).

As discussed above, the committee responded to the third part of this charge in July 2003 when it released its letter report on key capabilities of an EHR (see Appendix E). The present report addresses the first and second parts of the committee's charge. Its focus is on *data standards for patient safety*, i.e., standardized representations of clinical data important to systems that promote patient safety. In general, these standards fall into two categories:

- **Patient safety data standards**—formally accepted or endorsed definitions and rules regarding the format (e.g., structure), meaning (e.g., terminology), and encoding (e.g., interchange specifications) for transmission of patient data and scientific knowledge.
- **Patient safety reporting standards**—formally accepted or endorsed definitions and rules regarding the types of events reported to patient safety reporting systems, the data and information collected on these events, and the reporting formats used.

Patient safety data standards are critical to the development of the NHII, but they are not the only standards needed. For example, the continued development and application of standards to protect the privacy and security of personally identifiable data are also critical but are outside the scope of the present study. It is also important to note that data standards are not the only barrier to the implementation of an NHII. Other barriers include the lack of incentives to invest in information technology systems, the lack of a culture of safety in many health care organizations, unwillingness to share patient data for business reasons, and uncertainties about legal liability and privacy issues. As noted, the primary focus of this report is patient safety data standards. Other barriers are acknowledged and discussed briefly, but detailed analysis in those areas is beyond the scope of this report.

OVERVIEW OF THE REPORT

The remainder of this report is divided into three main parts:

- Part I: Building the National Health Information Infrastructure
- Part II: Establishing Comprehensive Patient Safety Programs
- Part III: Streamlining Patient Safety Reporting

Part I focuses on the NHII that is needed to make patient safety a standard of care. **Chapter 2** provides an overview of the components of an NHII. **Chapter 3** addresses the need for strong federal leadership to establish a public–private partnership for the ongoing promulgation of national data standards. **Chapter 4** reviews the types of data standards that are needed and provides an action plan for their establishment.

Part II focuses on patient safety programs in health care organizations. **Chapter 5** presents a general discussion of patient safety programs from the perspective of a health care provider organization and is intended to place reporting activities within a broader context. This is followed by detailed discussion of the functional requirements and data standards applicable to the prevention, detection, and reporting of adverse events (**Chapter 6**) and near misses (**Chapter 7**).

Part III of the report is devoted to patient safety reporting programs. **Chapter 8** provides an overview of the various types of reporting systems, from reporting for accountability purposes to reporting for system redesign. Finally, **Chapter 9** reviews the types of patient safety reporting standards that are needed to enable aggregation of data and reduce the reporting burden and to support the establishment of the national patient safety database first called for in *To Err Is Human*.

In addition, seven appendixes are provided. Appendix A contains biographical sketches of the committee members; Appendix B is a list of terms and acronyms used in the report; Appendix C presents examples of federal, state, and private-sector patient safety reporting systems; Appendix D provides a listing of those clinical domains important for patient safety and for which appropriate terminology should be developed; Appendix E is the committee's letter report on the key capabilities of an EHR system; Appendix F is a paper commissioned for this study on quality improvement and proactive hazard analysis models; and Appendix G outlines the Health Incident Type event taxonomy of the Australian Incident Monitoring System.

REFERENCES

Australian Council for Safety and Quality in Health Care. 2001. *Safety in Numbers: A Technical Options Paper for a National Approach to the Use of Data for Safer Health Care (Work in Progress)*. Online. Available: http://sq.netspeed.com.au/articles/Publications/numbers.pdf [accessed March 4, 2002].

Brailer, D. J. January 23, 2003. *Use and Adoption of Computer-Based Patient Records in the United States: A Review and Update*. PowerPoint presentation to the Institute of Medicine Committee on Data Standards for Patient Safety. Irvine, CA.

Brennan, T. A. 2000. The Institute of Medicine report on medical errors: Could it do harm? *N Engl J Med* 342 (15):1123–1125.

CareScience. 2003. *Santa Barbara County Care Data Exchange*. Online. Available: http://www.carescience.com/healthcare_providers/cde/care_data_exchange_santabarbara_cde.shtml [accessed May 30, 2003].

Cullen, D. J., D. W. Bates, S. D. Small, J. B. Cooper, A. R. Nemeskal, and L. L. Leape. 1995. The incident reporting system does not detect adverse drug events: A problem for quality improvement. *Jt Comm J Qual Improv* 21 (10):541–548.

Department of Health and Human Services. 2003a. *National Health Information Infrastructure 2003: Developing a National Action Agenda for NHII*. Online. Available: http://www.nhii-03.s-3.net/welcome.htm [accessed May 30, 2003].

————. 2003b. *HHS Launches New Efforts to Promote Paperless Health Care System*. Online. Available: http://www.hhs.gov/news/press/2003pres/20030701.html [accessed July 7, 2003].

Gurwitz, J. H., T. S. Field, J. Avorn, D. McCormick, S. Jain, M. Eckler, M. Benser, A. C. Edmondson, and D. W. Bates. 2000. Incidence and preventability of adverse drug events in nursing homes. *Am J Med* 109 (2):87–94.

Gurwitz, J. H., T. S. Field, L. R. Harrold, J. Rothschild, K. Debellis, A. C. Seger, C. Cadoret, L. S. Fish, L. Garber, M. Kelleher, and D. W. Bates. 2003. Incidence and preventability of adverse drug events among older persons in the ambulatory setting. *JAMA* 289 (9):1107–1116.

Hayward, R. A., and T. P. Hofer. 2001. Estimating hospital deaths due to medical errors: Preventability is in the eye of the reviewer. *JAMA* 286 (4):415–420.

Institute of Medicine. 1997. *The Computer-Based Patient Record: An Essential Technology for Health Care.* Washington, DC: National Academy Press.

———. 2000. *To Err Is Human: Building a Safer Health System.* Washington, DC: National Academy Press.

———. 2001. *Crossing the Quality Chasm: A New Health System for the 21st Century.* Washington, DC: National Academy Press.

———. 2002a. *Fostering Rapid Advances in Health Care: Learning from System Demonstrations.* Washington, DC: The National Academies Press.

———. 2002b. *Leadership by Example: Coordinating Government Roles in Improving Health Care Quality.* Washington, DC: The National Academies Press.

———. 2003a. *Key Capabilities of an Electronic Health Record System.* Washington, DC: The National Academies Press.

———. 2003b. *Priority Areas for National Action: Transforming Health Care Quality.* Washington, DC: The National Academies Press.

Kolodner, R. M., and J. V. Douglas, eds. 1997. *Computerized Large Integrated Health Networks: The VA Success.* New York, NY: Springer-Verlag.

Leape, L. L., T. A. Brennan, N. M. Laird, A. G. Lawthers, A. R. Localio, B. A. Barnes, H. L. Newhouse, P. C. Weiler, H. Hiatt. 1991. Incidence of adverse events and negligence in hospitalized patients: Results of the Harvard Medical Practice Study II. *N Engl J Med* 324:377–384.

Lepage, E. F., R. M. Gardner, R. M. Laub, and O. K. Golubjatnikov. 1992. Improving blood transfusion practice: Role of a computerized hospital information system. *Transfusion* (Paris) 32 (3):253–359.

Lesar, T. S., L. Briceland, and D. S. Stein. 1997. Factors related to errors in medication prescribing. *JAMA* 277 (4):312–317.

Markle Foundation. 2003. *Connecting for Health—A Public-Private Collaborative: Key Themes and Guiding Principles.* New York, NY: Markle Foundation.

Masys, D. R. 2002. Effects of current and future information technologies on the health care workforce. *Health Aff* 21 (5):33–41.

McDonald, C. J., M. Weiner, and S. L. Hui. 2000. Deaths due to medical errors are exaggerated in Institute of Medicine report. *JAMA* 284 (1):93–95.

McGlynn, E. A., S. M. Asch, J. Adams, J. Keesey, J. Hicks, A. DeCristofaro, and E. A. Kerr. 2003. The quality of health care delivered to adults in the United States. *N Engl J Med* 348 (26):2635–2645.

Mekhjian, H. S., R. R. Kumar, L. Kuehn, T. D. Bentley, P. Teater, A. Thomas, B. Payne, and A. Ahmad. 2002. Immediate benefits realized following implementation of physician order entry at an academic medical center. *J Am Med Inform Assoc* 9 (5):529–539.

National Committee on Vital and Health Statistics. 2001. *Information for Health: A Strategy for Building the National Health Information Infrastructure.* Online. Available: http://ncvhs.hhs.gov/nhiilayo.pdf [accessed April 18, 2002].

National Patient Safety Agency, Department of Health, United Kingdom. 2001. *Doing Less Harm* (Version 1.0a). Online. Available: http://www.npsa.org.uk/admin/publications/docs/draft.pdf [accessed April 16, 2002].

National Quality Forum. 2003. *Information Technology and Healthcare Quality: A National Summit.* Washington, DC: National Quality Forum.

New England Healthcare EDI Network. 2002. *NEHEN About Us.* Online. Available: http://www.nehen.net/ [accessed May 30, 2003].

Office of Management and Budget. 2003. *Consolidated Health Informatics.* Online. Available: http://www.whitehouse.gov/omb/egov/gtob/health_informatics.htm [accessed April 21, 2003].

Overhage, J. M. April 1, 2003. *Improving Patient Safety in Chronic Diseases Using Electronic Medical Records.* PowerPoint presentation to the Institute of Medicine Committee on Data Standards for Patient Safety. Washington, DC.

President's Information Technology Advisory Committee. 2001. *Transforming Health Care Through Information Technology.* Online. Available: http://www.hpcc.gov/pubs/pitac/pitac-hc-9feb01.pdf [accessed May 7, 2003].

Quality Interagency Coordination Task Force. 2000. *Doing What Counts for Patient Safety: Federal Actions to Reduce Medical Errors and Their Impacts.* Online. Available: http://www.quic.gov/report/index.htm [accessed June 18, 2001].

Raymond, B., and C. Dold. 2002. *Clinical Information Systems: Achieving the Vision.* Oakland, CA: Kaiser Permanente Institute for Health Policy.

Rosenthal, J. 2003a. *List of States with Mandatory Reporting Systems.* Personal communication to Institute of Medicine's Committee on Data Standards for Patient Safety.

———. 2003b. *State Reporting Systems Collecting Information on Near Misses.* Personal communication to Institute of Medicine's Committee on Data Standards for Patient Safety.

Runciman, W. B., and J. Moller. 2001. *Iatrogenic Injury in Australia.* Adelaide, Australia: Australian Patient Safety Foundation, Inc.

Sittig, D. F., and W. W. Stead. 1994. Computer-based physician order entry: The state of the art. *J Am Med Inform Assoc* 1 (2):108–123.

Sox, H. C., and S. Woloshin. 2000. How many deaths are due to medical error? Getting the number right. *Eff Clin Pract* 6:277–283.

Thomas, E. J., D. M. Studdert, J. P. Newhouse, I. Brett, W. Zbar, K. M. Howard, E. J. Williams, and T. A. Brennan. 1999. Costs of medical injuries in Utah and Colorado. *Inquiry* 36:255–264.

———. 2000. Negligent care and malpractice claiming behavior in Utah and Colorado. *Med Care* 38 (3):250–260.

Vincent, C., G. Neale, and M. Woloshynowych. 2001. Adverse events in British hospitals: Preliminary retrospective record review. *BMJ* 322 (7285):517–519.

Wilson, R. M., W. B. Runciman, R. W. Gibberd, B. T. Harrison, L. Newby, and J. D. Hamilton. 1995. The Quality in Australian Health Care Study. *Med J Aust* 163 (9):458–471.

Part I

Building the National Health Information Infrastructure

Americans should be able to count on receiving health care that is safe. To this end, a new health care delivery system is needed—one that both prevents errors and incorporates lessons learned from those errors that do occur. Achieving such a health care system requires, first, a commitment by all stakeholders to a culture of safety and, second, improved information systems.

Recommendation 1. Americans expect and deserve safe care. Improved information and data systems are needed to support efforts to make patient safety a standard of care in hospitals, in doctors' offices, in nursing homes, and in every other health care setting. All health care organizations should establish comprehensive patient safety systems that:

- **Provide immediate access to complete patient information and decision support tools (e.g., alerts, reminders) for clinicians and their patients.**
- **Capture information on patient safety—including both adverse events and near misses—as a by-product of care and use this information to design even safer care delivery systems.**

COMPONENTS OF A NATIONAL HEALTH INFORMATION INFRASTRUCTURE

Achieving the goal set forth in Recommendation 1 can be accomplished in the United States only by building a national health information infrastructure (NHII). As defined by the National Committee on Vital and Health Statistics and discussed in Chapter 2 of this report, the NHII consists of a set of values, practices and relationships, laws and regulations, health data standards, technologies, and systems and applications that support all facets of individual health, health care delivery, and public health (National Committee on Vital and Health Statistics, 2001).

Building the NHII requires actions on the part of health care providers, as well as public- and private-sector leadership at the national level. Of primary importance, it is necessary for health care providers to invest in electronic health record (EHR) systems that can capture patient and other clinical data and interact with decision support applications that improve safety and quality of care. In August 2003, this committee released a letter report entitled *Key Capabilities of an Electronic Health Record System* (Institute of Medicine, 2003) (see Appendix E) which provides guidance on the functional capabilities such systems should possess. Actions by individual health care providers, however, will not be enough to create a safe health care delivery environment. Patients receive services from many different health care providers. A nationwide infrastructure is required to support the exchange of patient information and to facilitate communication among the members of the patient's care team and between clinicians and the patient.

At the national level, the federal government, working collaboratively with the private sector, will need to provide financial resources and establish national standards for the NHII. Other IOM committees have recommended that the federal government provide both capital resources for the development of key aspects of the NHII and financial incentives to health care providers to invest in EHRs (Institute of Medicine, 2001, 2002a, b). It is essential that the federal government act on these recommendations.

Also critically important to the development of the NHII is the need for the federal government to enhance its leadership role in the establishment of national data standards. In fact, the federal government has already taken the initiative to assume this leadership role in some key areas. The Health Insurance Portability and Accountability Act of 1996 (Public Law 104-191) led to the establishment of standards to protect the privacy and confidentiality of personally identifiable data, and the Department of Health and Human Services recently endorsed the use of certain messaging standards to facilitate the exchange of data and information among health care providers, vendors, and others. However, much more remains to be done, and that is the focus of this committee's work.

> **Recommendation 2. A national health information infrastructure—a foundation of systems, technology, applications, standards, and policies—is required to make patient safety a standard of care.**
>
> • **The federal government should facilitate deployment of the national health information infrastructure through the provision of targeted financial support and the ongoing promulgation and maintenance of standards for data that support patient safety.**
> • **Health care providers should invest in electronic health record systems that possess the key capabilities necessary to provide safe and effective care and to enable the continuous redesign of care processes to improve patient safety.**

A PUBLIC AND PRIVATE PARTNERSHIP TO SET STANDARDS

The development of standards for health care data in the United States often occurs as a series of independent, voluntary processes. Many of the important standards are developed by standards development organizations using a consensus process.

Despite efforts toward harmonization and cooperation among the various standards development organizations, the development of health data standards in the United States is essentially an entrepreneurial activity. As a result, standards development organizations sometimes create competing standards, and there is no guarantee that all the necessary standards will be developed. Indeed, the full range of needs for health care data standards have not yet been fulfilled. Currently, there is no oversight body in the United States tasked with reviewing the full portfolio of existing health care data standards, identifying gaps, and fostering efforts to fill those gaps. The committee believes that, as the largest purchaser of health care services and the most influential regulator, it is critical that the federal government assume a more active role in the establishment of the data standards necessary to protect patient safety (see Chapter 3).

> **Recommendation 3. Congress should provide clear direction, enabling authority, and financial support for the establishment of national standards for data that support patient safety. Various govern-**

ment agencies will need to assume major new responsibilities, and additional support will be required. Specifically:

- The Department of Health and Human Services (DHHS) should be given the lead role in establishing and maintaining a public–private partnership for the promulgation of standards for data that support patient safety.
- The Consolidated Health Informatics (CHI) initiative, in collaboration with the National Committee on Vital and Health Statistics (NCVHS), should identify data standards appropriate for national adoption and gaps in existing standards that need to be addressed. The membership of NCVHS should continue to be broad and diverse, with adequate representation of all stakeholders, including consumers, state governments, professional groups, and standards-setting bodies.
- The Agency for Healthcare Research and Quality (AHRQ), in collaboration with the National Library of Medicine and others, should (1) provide administrative and technical support for the CHI and NCVHS efforts; (2) ensure the development of implementation guides, certification procedures, and conformance testing for all data standards; (3) provide financial support and oversight for developmental activities to fill gaps in data standards; and (4) coordinate activities and maintain a clearinghouse of information in support of national data standards and their implementation to improve patient safety.
- The National Library of Medicine should be designated as the responsible entity for distributing all national clinical terminologies that relate to patient safety and for ensuring the quality of terminology mappings.

AN AGENDA FOR DATA STANDARDS

The committee's recommendations address data standards that support patient safety. Data standards are formally accepted or endorsed definitions and rules regarding the format, meaning, and transmission of data elements. Data elements are individual pieces of data, such as age, medication, or diagnosis. This report is concerned specifically with standards for the following:

- *Data interchange formats*—standard formats for electronically encoding the data elements (including sequencing and error handling). Interchange standards can also include document architectures for structuring data elements as they are exchanged and information models that define the relationships among data elements in a message.

• *Terminologies*—the medical terms and concepts used to describe, classify, and code the data elements, and data expression languages and syntax that describe the relationships among the terms/concepts.

• *Knowledge representation*—standard methods for electronically representing medical literature, clinical guidelines, and the like for decision support (Hammond, 2002).

Chapter 4 details the committee's recommendations on data interchange, terminology, and knowledge representation standards.

Recommendation 4. The lack of comprehensive standards for data to support patient safety impedes private-sector investment in information technology and other efforts to improve patient safety. The federal government should accelerate the adoption of standards for such data by pursuing the following efforts:

• *Clinical data interchange standards.* **The federal government should set an aggressive agenda for the establishment of standards for the interchange of clinical data to support patient safety. Federal financial support should be provided to accomplish this agenda.**

    – **After ample time for provider compliance, government health care programs should incorporate into their contractual and regulatory requirements standards already approved by the secretaries of DHHS, the Veterans Administration, and the Department of Defense (i.e., the HL7 version 2.x series for clinical data messaging, DICOM for medical imaging, IEEE 1073 for medical devices, LOINC for laboratory test results, and NCPDP Script for prescription data).[1]**

    – **AHRQ should provide support for (1) accelerated completion (within 2 years) of HL7 version 3.0; (2) specifications for the HL7 Clinical Document Architecture and implementation guides; and (3) analysis of alternative methods for addressing the need to support patient safety by instituting a unique health identifier for individuals, such as implementation of a voluntary unique health identifier program.**

---

[1]HL7—Health Level Seven; DICOM—Digital Imaging and Communications in Medicine; IEEE—Institute of Electrical and Electronics Engineers; LOINC—Logical Observation Identifiers, Names, and Codes; NCPDP—National Council for Prescription Drug Programs.

- *Clinical terminologies.* The federal government should move expeditiously to identify a core set of well-integrated, nonredundant clinical terminologies for clinical care, quality improvement, and patient safety reporting. Revisions, extensions, and additions to the codes should be compatible with, yet go beyond, the federal government's initiative to integrate all federal reporting systems.
  - AHRQ should undertake a study of the core terminologies, supplemental terminologies, and standards mandated by the Health Insurance Portability and Accountability Act to identify areas of overlap and gaps in the terminologies to address patient safety data requirements. The study should begin by convening domain experts to develop a process for ensuring comprehensive coverage of the terminologies for the 20 IOM priority areas.
  - The National Library of Medicine should provide support for the accelerated completion of RxNORM[2] for clinical drugs. The National Library of Medicine also should develop high-quality mappings among the core terminologies and supplemental terminologies identified by the CHI and NCVHS.
- *Knowledge representation.* The federal government should provide support for the accelerated development of knowledge representation standards to facilitate effective use of decision support in clinical information systems.
  - The National Library of Medicine should provide support for the development of standards for evidence-based knowledge representation.
  - AHRQ, in collaboration with the National Institutes of Health, the Food and Drug Administration, and other agencies, should provide support for the development of a generic guideline representation model for use in representing clinical guidelines in a computer-executable format that can be employed in decision support tools.

---

[2]RxNORM is a normalized (standard) form for representing clinical drugs and their components.

REFERENCES

Hammond, W. E. 2002. *Patient Safety Data Standards: View from a Standards Perspective.* PowerPoint Presentation to IOM Committee on Data Standards for Patient Safety on May 6, 2002. Online. Available: http://www.iom.edu/file.asp?id=9915 [accessed December 16, 2003].

Institute of Medicine. 2001. *Crossing the Quality Chasm: A New Health System for the 21st Century.* Washington, DC: National Academy Press.

————. 2002a. *Fostering Rapid Advances in Health Care: Learning from System Demonstrations.* Washington, DC: The National Academies Press.

————. 2002b. *Leadership by Example: Coordinating Government Roles in Improving Health Care Quality.* Washington, DC: The National Academies Press.

————. 2003. Committee on Data Standards for Patient Safety. Key Capabilities of an Electronic Health Record System: Letter Report. Washington, DC: The National Academies Press.

National Committee on Vital and Health Statistics. 2001. *Information for Health: A Strategy for Building the National Health Information Infrastructure.* Online. Available: http://ncvhs.hhs.gov/nhiilayo.pdf [accessed April 18, 2002].

2

Components of a National Health Information Infrastructure

CHAPTER SUMMARY

A comprehensive approach to patient safety requires the ability to anticipate and protect against circumstances that might lead to adverse events and implement corrective actions. Both adverse events and near misses require standard collection/reporting processes, datasets, definitions, and analytic approaches that can be achieved only by integrating patient safety reporting systems into the context of health information systems in both large institutions and office practices. These systems employ multiple detection methods and multiple reporting channels and involve a broad array of data elements. Establishing a national health information infrastructure is necessary to provide the backbone for such systems.

This chapter is divided into three sections: the first provides a general overview of the national health information infrastructure and a conceptual model of standards-based integrated data systems to support patient safety in institutional and office practice settings for all audiences; the second presents a technical review of the informatics components that support an information infrastructure for the technical reader; and the third provides a discussion of how standards-based clinical systems can be and have been implemented to support this endeavor for both audiences.

GENERAL OVERVIEW

Improving patient safety requires much more than systems for reporting and analyzing events; errors must be prevented from occurring in the first place. Several effective tools are available that can assist in the prevention of adverse events. Clinical decision support systems (CDSSs), such as those for medication order entry, can prevent many errors from occurring (Bates et al., 1997, 1998, 1999). Computer-based reminder systems can facilitate adherence to care protocols (Balas et al., 2000); computer-assisted diagnosis and management programs can improve clinical decision making at the point of care (Durieux et al., 2000; Evans et al., 1998); and immediate access to clinical information, such as results of laboratory and radiology tests, can reduce redundancy, allowing for more efficient decision making. Incorporation of new research findings into clinical practice is also important for improving patient safety. Balas and Boren found that it takes an average of 17 years for research to reach clinical practice, whereas newer technological innovations take an average of 4 to 6 years. Actionable knowledge representation through the use of information systems holds promise for better connecting clinical research and patient care practices (Balas and Boren, 2000). In addition, the Internet can be used for customized health education for patients, thereby promoting more effective self-management of chronic and other medical conditions (Cain et al., 2000; Goldsmith, 2002). The Internet can be used as well for communication among all authorized members of the care team (e.g., primary care providers, specialists, nurses, pharmacists, home health aides, the patient, and lay caregivers), a capability that is especially important for the chronically ill. The capabilities provided by these clinical information systems cannot be achieved, however, without standards-based interoperability founded on the national health information infrastructure (NHII).

The NHII is defined as a set of technologies, standards, applications, systems, values, and laws that support all facets of individual health, health care, and public health (National Committee on Vital and Health Statistics, 2001). It encompasses an information network based on Internet protocols, common standards, timely knowledge transfer, and transparent government processes with the capability for information flows across three dimensions: (1) *personal health*, to support individuals in their own wellness and health care decision making; (2) *health care providers*, to ensure access to complete and accurate patient data around the clock and to clinical decision support systems; and (3) *public health*, to address and track public health concerns and health education campaigns (National Committee on Vital and Health

Statistics, 2001). As shown in Figure 2-1, there are significant areas of overlap among these three dimensions in terms of functionality and applications.

With the NHII, information systems will be able to provide the right information, at the right time, and to the right individuals, enabling safe care and supporting robust safety reporting systems for cases in which adverse events and near misses do occur. The NHII also will yield many other benefits in terms of new opportunities for care access, efficiency, and effectiveness; public health; homeland security; and clinical and health services research. For example, electronic health records (EHRs), in conjunction with secure data exchange, may allow for early detection of and rapid response to infectious diseases. The NHII will also facilitate the organization and execution of large-scale inoculation programs, as well as the dissemination to clinicians and patients of up-to-date information and practice guidelines on the presentation and treatment of morbidity due to chemical and biological threats.

Standards-based information systems built on the foundation of the NHII will permit cross-organizational data sharing. Several promising

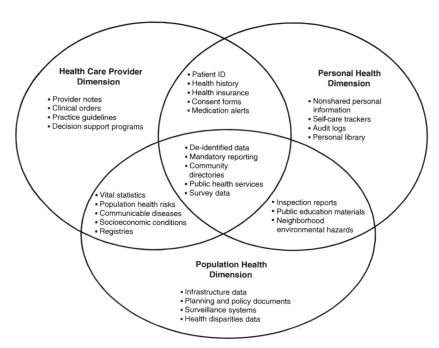

FIGURE 2-1 Examples of content for the three NHII dimensions and their overlap.
SOURCE: National Committee on Vital and Health Statistics, 2001.

public–private information technology demonstrations currently under way nationwide are exchanging data outside traditional organizational boundaries. One such project is the New England Healthcare Electronic Data Interchange (EDI) Network (NEHEN)—a consortium initiated in 1998 and led by Computer Science Corporation (New England Healthcare EDI Network, 2002). Membership is open to providers, health plans, and payers in Massachusetts and Rhode Island; there are currently 14 members, including most of the region's largest insurers and health plans. NEHEN provides its members, who pay a flat monthly fee, with access to a secure high-speed network for sending and receiving transactions. Members can either integrate NEHEN functions directly into their own management systems or access the NEHEN network using *NEHENLite*, a Web-based application.

A second promising project is the Indiana Network for Patient Care (INPC), initiated 10 years ago in Indianapolis by the Regenstrief Institute for Health Care. Currently, all 13 acute care hospitals in the city and approximately 20 percent of the metropolitan area's outpatient physician practices are participating (Overhage, 2003). Participating institutions pay a monthly fee for access to selected electronic information that forms the basis for an "operational community-wide electronic medical record" that includes reports from emergency room visits, laboratory results, admission notes/discharge summaries, operative reports, radiology reports, surgical pathology reports, inpatient medications, immunizations, and a tumor registry (Overhage, 2003). Each health care provider retains its patients' information in its organization's database; however, selected information in those datasets can be shared among organizations through use of a Global Patient Index (Overhage, 2003). INPC not only allows for the secure storage and exchange of clinical information but also provides clinical decision support and public health surveillance and reporting.

A third example of a regional data sharing network is the Santa Barbara County Care Data Exchange, initiated in 1998 through a partnership between CareScience and the California Healthcare Foundation (CareScience, 2003). More than 75 percent of the health care providers in Santa Barbara County are participating, including medical groups, hospitals, clinics, laboratories, pharmacies, and payers. The Care Data Exchange allows for rapid and secure delivery of patient data to authorized users who have informed consent.

While the above projects are all extremely promising, they remain isolated examples. Such efforts are unlikely to be replicated on a larger scale until the major technical, organizational, and financial impediments to the development of the NHII are addressed.

From a technical perspective, the NHII will require the construction of an information and communications infrastructure in much the same way as one builds an electrical power grid. The "materials" for constructing the infrastructure are the core informatics components required to generate data flows: data acquisition methods and user interfaces, health care data standards, data repositories and clinical event monitors, data mining techniques, digital sources of evidence or knowledge, communication technologies, and clinical information systems (each discussed in detail later in this chapter). To facilitate the development of the NHII, the Institute of Medicine (IOM) recently proposed several demonstration projects aimed at establishing state-of-the-art health care information and communications infrastructure at the community, state, and regional levels (Institute of Medicine, 2002a). That report suggests that information and communications infrastructure can contribute to improvements in four areas of relevance to patient safety: communication, access to patient information, knowledge management, and decision support.

At the organizational level, moving forward with a health information infrastructure requires the development of comprehensive, standards-based systems necessary for delivering clinical information at the point of care, facilitating communication for care coordination, and supporting patient safety systems for detection and prevention of adverse events and for detection and recovery from near misses. The first section of this chapter presents a conceptual model of a standards-based data system that draws on the above core informatics components of a national health information infrastructure; the second section provides a brief overview of each of those components. The results of a demonstration project to assess the current state of vendor information systems in attaining the conceptual model are then summarized. The next section presents several practical approaches to moving forward with integrated health data systems. Finally, we discuss how challenges to overcoming the implementation of information technology in the national health information infrastructure can be overcome.

CONCEPTUAL MODEL OF STANDARDS-BASED, INTEGRATED DATA SYSTEMS TO SUPPORT PATIENT SAFETY

A conceptual model for standards-based, integrated data systems to support patient safety is presented in Figure 2-2. This conceptual model encompasses several key principles of such systems:

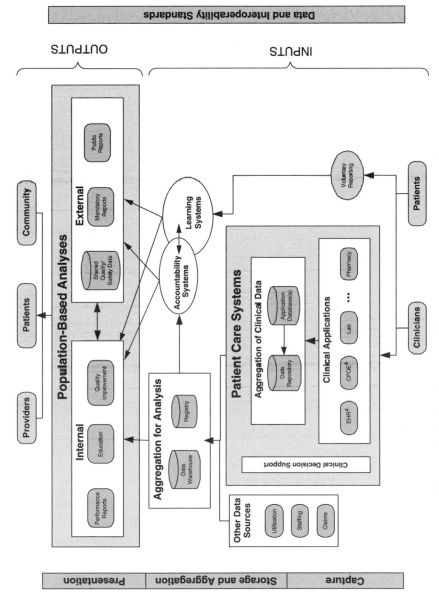

FIGURE 2-2 Conceptual model of standards-based, integrated data systems to support patient safety.
NOTE: [a]EHR = electronic health record; [b]CPOE = computerized physician order entry.

- Reuse of data
- Aggregation of data for learning and accountability
- Feedback from learning that results in improvement and system changes
  - Interoperability standards as essential glue
  - Parallel reporting pathway outside patient care systems
  - Usable by both providers and patients

Integrated Systems and Large Institutions

Under this model, patient data are captured in a variety of clinical applications, such as EHRs and computerized physician order entry systems, in a variety of inpatient and outpatient settings as part of the health care delivery process. Patients may also enter such data as symptoms and self-care behaviors directly into clinical systems and review aspects of their record, such as laboratory results.

In some organizations, patient data from different clinical applications are integrated in a clinical data repository; in other organizations, the EHR can be utilized for data integration. For patient safety purposes, data about adverse events and near misses also can be integrated and fed into the repository through CDSSs. Evidence-based care is enhanced over time with a constant infusion of new medical knowledge from the biomedical literature into decision support systems so that significant aspects of care are supported for such purposes as delivering preventive care reminders to clinicians.

Patient care data, along with other useful data sources, are aggregated for analysis in registries, analytic databases, and data warehouses. They can be used for analysis and reporting to support learning and accountability both within and outside individual health care organizations. These aggregated data resources can be used to generate insights into patient care processes and to monitor performance. Finally, while the majority of data for learning and accountability are reused from clinical care, it is essential that voluntary reports from patients and clinicians also feed into these systems— represented in Figure 2-2 as the "voluntary reporting" pathway.

While Figure 2-2 is the overall objective for integrated systems in the NHII, technology is currently at varying degrees of implementation across different health care settings. Thus, a strategy is needed to progressively increase the informatics capabilities, interoperability, and utilization of clinical systems and decision support applications. To begin the integration and data sharing process, local systems can establish interoperability by incorporating common standards for messaging formats, a generic information model, and terminology standards where appropriate. The primary systems that support most decision support applications—pharmacy, laboratory, radiology, and administrative databases—can also be linked so that computerized physician order entry, alert/reminder, and other such systems can be implemented. For patient safety, triggers can be implemented to identify potential adverse events or patient contraindications in laboratory and pharmacy systems, integrated with systems that can accept narrative patient safety reports.

Integrated Systems and Office Practice

A key result of the NHII will be to permit information exchange across institutional boundaries, providing more complete patient information and enabling better coordination of care. Traditionally, most data exchange has occurred within the boundaries of larger institutions or health systems. However, since most providers practice, at least in part, outside of large institutions, much of the anticipated benefit of the NHII may result from improved data linkages with and among smaller, office-based practices.

While large institutions and office practices require somewhat different information technology architectures, the informatics requirements to support systems integration and clinical decision support tools are the same. Instead of linking with internal departmental systems within larger organizations that account for the majority of patient data (e.g., pharmacy, laboratory, radiology), office practices will be able to use data exchange standards to send and receive important patient data (e.g., results of a laboratory test, a discharge summary) to/from external systems and retrieve information from knowledge sources (e.g., a medical literature database, disease registries).

Instead of the information technology architecture of distributed systems connected through a central data repository that would characterize a large institution, small office practices will use a simpler architecture, with the EHR and/or practice management system as the principal repository for information on their patients and general office operations. These systems will still link to external systems using common message and data standards. Patient safety systems will be connected to office practices by one of several means: (1) direct integration with the internal database of a practice as part of a quality improvement program, (2) linkage to an external patient safety organization, or (3) voluntary or mandatory participation in external public repositories. Common standards will allow the systems to exchange data that can be integrated into patient records and support tools in a manner that retains data comparability. Additionally, integrated systems and common data standards in clinical practice will yield the benefits of data reuse, lessening the burden of clinicians' regulatory obligations for reporting on quality measures, patient safety, accreditation, and the like.

Under this model, office practices will utilize the wide range of clinical information systems that make up the totality of the EHR. Information technology systems may include computers, personal digital assistants (PDAs), and/or voice recognition devices. These systems will be available in every examining room and clinician's office, offering the promise of greater convenience, accessibility, integration, and accuracy in information about patients and their health conditions (Bodenheimer and Grumbach, 2003). Electronic communications will enhance efficiency in patient–physician and physician–physician communications. For example, it will be possible to handle many interactions—such as reporting test results, arranging specialty referrals, receiving data on home glucose levels, and adjusting medication doses—by e-mail (Bodenheimer and Grumbach, 2003). Using electronic devices or computers, physicians will be able to store or electronically access vital knowledge bases, such as directories of pharmacies and specialists, descriptions of medications and drug interactions, reference texts, practice guidelines, and evidence-based abstracts (Bodenheimer and Grumbach, 2003).

To date, much discussion related to the use of technology in office practices has focused on administrative and financial transactions defined under the Health Insurance Portability and Accountability Act (HIPAA) and on the incorporation of the EHR. By 2002, however, only 17 percent of U.S. primary care physicians were using an EHR system, compared with 58 percent in the United Kingdom and 90 percent in Sweden. The lag in U.S. adoption of the EHR has been the result of several factors that are now being addressed: the cost of investing in health information technologies, inertia and a lack of incentives for change, the quality of medical information available on the Web, incompatibility of software programs, privacy concerns, lack of reimbursement, and concern about compromising the personal interaction between physician and patient (Bodenheimer and Grumbach, 2003). To move forward with the implementation of clinical information technology systems, a central focus of initiatives to implement the NHII must be on providing small practices with support comparable to that extended to large health care institutions. Public–private partnerships will be required that provide opportunities for financial incentives, technical assistance, and the development of a migration strategy that addresses the special needs of small practice physicians.

The process for creating integrated systems requires consideration and incorporation of the functionalities associated with the primary informatics components that support an information infrastructure. A more technical discussion of these components is provided in the next section.

TECHNICAL CONSIDERATIONS: INFORMATICS COMPONENTS OF THE INFORMATION INFRASTRUCTURE

The informatics components of the NHII provide a foundation for a comprehensive standards-based system and a migration strategy for its implementation. This section briefly describes the key components of a health information infrastructure that supports patient safety.

Data Acquisition Methods and User Interfaces

Data become available to learning or accountability systems by various means, including abstraction from paper records; direct entry into a computer system (keyboard entry, voice, touch screen, pen); and reuse of data collected by other systems, such as those used for clinical care or administrative purposes. Information capture per se takes many forms, including speech, free text, document imaging, clinical imaging (e.g., x-rays), motion video, binary electronic data representation (e.g., laboratory values, device settings, operational status, measurements), waveforms (e.g., electrocardiograms), graphical codes (e.g., digital ink), and indexing/clinical encoding (e.g., extensible markup language [XML], International Classification of Diseases [ICD]) (Waegemann et al., 2002). Regardless of entry mode, data that are captured in standardized terminologies are more accessible for reuse than narrative text. As discussed later in this chapter, however, significant advances have been made in the use of natural language processing of narrative text for the detection and prevention of adverse events.

Methods of acquiring data may also vary by domain. For example, speech input works well in radiology, where the reporting is structured. On the other hand, pen-based data entry using a wireless tablet computer suits the task of documentation associated with home health care nursing. Laboratory and pharmacy data that are essential to the detection and prevention of adverse events and near misses are typically available from department-level information systems and can be reused for patient safety and quality management purposes. Given variations in levels of technology adoption and the needs of different clinical domains, organizations should maintain the ability to accommodate various methods of data acquisition and styles of documentation in progressing toward fully automated learning and accountability systems.

Waegemann et al. (2002) have developed a set of essential overall principles for optimal information capture and report generation with information technologies. According to these principles, such technologies should provide for unique identification of the patient, accuracy of information capture through the use of standards-based terminologies, completeness of information and minimization of duplication, timeliness such that data can be captured at the point of care, interoperability with any clinical information system, retrievability so that information can be found efficiently, authentication and accountability so that all data can be attributed to its source, auditability for ongoing assessments of quality, and confidentiality and security features to protect the data.

An intuitive and efficient user interface, that part of the computer system that communicates with the user, is utilized for interactive data entry, and controls the execution and flow of data (van Bemmel and Musen, 1997); it is another key component of clinical information systems (Shortliffe et al., 2001). User interface tools to facilitate data acquisition are still in the early stages of development, and a number of research projects are now under way to resolve associated impediments to the widespread implementation of clinical information systems. Much is being learned from the ubiquity of Web interfaces (Shortliffe et al., 2001). Current research integrates a number of methodologies from both engineering and cognitive science to evaluate and design systems from the perspective of terminology use (e.g., coded data entry) and navigation (Cimino et al., 2001); customization for the intended users and their unique requirements related to data structure, collection, and display (e.g., physician, nurse, patient) (Kinzie et al., 2002); and integration with emerging advanced technologies, such as speech recognition, multimedia, hypermedia (documents that contain links to various media), and virtual reality (van Bemmel and Musen, 1997). Core guidelines for the successful design of user interfaces identify several approaches to facilitate usability, including grouping of information, minimization of information overload, consistent and standards-based information display, information highlighting relative to importance, use of graphics, optimal text presentation, and use of icons (van Bemmel and Musen, 1997). Additional information on standards for user interfaces is provided in Chapter 4.

Health Care Data Standards

Health care data standards are the foundation for any learning and accountability system, regardless of whether the system involves abstraction of paper charts with entry into a stand-alone database or is part of an integrated information system. As shown in Table 2-1, the types of interchange, content, and measurement standards discussed elsewhere in this report are necessary regardless of the technology base of the system. The representation of terms related to patient safety in computer-based systems in a manner that renders them machine processable and available for reuse for patient safety accountability and learning systems is essential for both stand-alone databases and integrated systems.

Data exchange standards, such as reference information models, message definition frameworks, and clinical document architectures, support semantic interoperability (i.e., the ability to receive and understand data from another system) among the heterogeneous computer-based systems that form an integrated information system. Data exchange standards provide the technical specifications for the functioning of application programs, equipment and media systems, decision support systems, and other technologies. The status of various types of health care data standards and the gaps that need to be addressed are described in detail in Chapter 4.

TABLE 2-1 Data Standards of Relevance to the Structure of Patient Safety Systems

Standard	Stand-alone Database	Integrated Information System
Data element definitions, including standardized measures	•	•
Datasets representing clinical practice measures	•	•
Standardized terminology	•	•
Knowledge representation (concepts, guidelines)		•
Health identifiers		•
Reference information model		•
Message structure		•
Clinical document architecture		•

The ability to utilize, process, analyze, and reuse information, whether for patient safety or clinical care purposes, depends directly on the ability to organize the information into meaningful domains with hierarchies of specificity. Structured *terminologies* support information management for all levels of technology integration. Standardized terminologies exist for the core phenomena of clinical practice: (1) patient problems (e.g., medical diagnoses, nursing diagnoses, signs and symptoms; (2) interventions, including those focused on prevention and health promotion; and (3) health outcomes (e.g., disability, functional status, symptom status, quality of life). Several authors have identified characteristics of a computer-processible terminology that would define health care concepts nonamibiguously and promote data reuse (Campbell, 1998; Chute et al., 1998; Cimino, 1998). These criteria form the basis for the recommendations of the National Committee on Vital and Health Statistics (NCVHS) regarding core terminologies to support the EHR. Terminologies are discussed in greater detail in Chapter 4.

Knowledge representation standards address the acquisition and maintenance of medical knowledge in databases (called knowledge bases) that systematically organize the information collected to facilitate decision making or help solve problems. Because the information collected combines both scientific knowledge from the medical literature and systemic reviews based on experiential knowledge from patient databases or validated clinical guidelines (van Bemmel and Musen, 1997), modeling of cognitive deductive and inductive processes requires standards for such matters as logic, decision trees, rule-based reasoning, frames (concepts and their defining attributes), and semantic networks, as well as the capability to represent the data at multiple levels of granularity. Knowledge representation is the foundation for the standardized data utilized in clinical decision support systems and other digital sources of evidence.

Data Repositories and Clinical Event Monitors

A clinical data repository is a database that collects and stores patient care information from diverse data sources. It is typically optimized for storage and retrieval of information on individual patients and used to support health care delivery, surveillance, and clinical decision support (e.g., drug–drug interactions at the time of order entry, reminders about preventive care). Further, such broad repositories are essential to patient safety because the clinical context usually cuts across multiple data sources. For example, determining a drug–laboratory value interaction requires information from the pharmacy and the clinical laboratory. Currently, most inpatient and outpatient specialty care organizations use "departmental" systems for limited functions to serve administrative, research, archiving, pharmacy, physiological function laboratory (e.g., electrocardiogram), clinical laboratory, radiology, and other purposes (van Bemmel and Musen, 1997). However, most such systems operate as silos as a result of the nature of older legacy systems and past nonuse of interoperability standards. Lack of information access and integration across the enterprise frequently results in issues of quality of care and safety.

Clinical event monitors work together with clinical data repositories, supporting real-time error prevention. They are usually triggered by clinical events (e.g., patient visit, medication order, new laboratory result), either when data representing the event enter a repository or when a provider uses a clinical information system. The event monitor uses clinical rules, the triggering event, and information present in the repository to generate alerts, reminders, and other messages of prime importance in preventing errors of both commission and omission. These messages are routed to the appropriate provider(s) using a variety of communication technologies and are also stored in the repository. A recent comprehensive review of studies in which information technology was used to detect adverse events documented the utility of clinical event monitors for preventing adverse drug events, nosocomial infections, and injurious falls (Bates et al., 2003). Another type of data repository that is useful for patient safety and quality management is a clinical data warehouse that contains information similar to that in the clinical data repository but optimized for long-term storage, retrieval, and analysis of records aggregated across patient populations. Consequently, the data warehouse is a core resource for data mining (discussed below), benchmarking, and other types of safety- and quality-related analysis. Data warehouses may be institution specific, regional, national, or even international. The systems implementation section of this chapter describes warehousing activities in greater detail and provides an example of a proprietary data warehouse to which more than 500 institutions subscribe.

Data Mining Techniques

Data mining is a method for obtaining useful information from large databases and includes data collection, extraction, manipulation, and summarization, as well as analysis (Berson, 1997; Fayyad et al., 1996; Mitchell, 1999). Data mining techniques have been used primarily with abstracted clinical data and less frequently with narrative clinical data. Uses of data mining relevant to learning and accountability systems for patient safety include surveillance (Brossette, 2000; Brossette et al., 1998), case-based reasoning (Aha et al., 2001), and rule induction for expert systems (Goodwin, 1997; Tsumoto and Tanaka, 1997).

Because health care data are often narrative, natural language processing (NLP) is another important technique for mining data for quality improvement and patient safety purposes (Bates et al., 2003). Sophisticated NLP techniques can extract information and structure from machine-readable narrative text. Consequently, the structured data are available for such purposes as triggering alerts and reminders (e.g., preventive care guidelines) and detecting potential adverse events. However, natural language extraction is currently a difficult and knowledge-intensive task.

To date, only a few NLP systems have been integrated with clinical information systems and used for improved quality of care and patient safety, including error detection and prevention, but the results of such efforts are encouraging (Fiszman and Haug, 2000; Friedman et al., 1995; Haug et al., 1990). One such system, MedLEE, a rule-based NLP system (Friedman et al., 1995), resulted in a significant decrease in respiratory isolation errors for patients with tuberculosis (Knirsch et al., 1998). In another study, NLP was performed on 889,921 radiological reports (Hripscak et al., 2002), and correlations between findings and changes over time were computed. Results showed that the NLP encoded output was more accurate than ICD-9 codes. A lexically based system for NLP has shown promise as a means of detecting adverse events in outpatient visit notes (Honigman et al., 2001).

Although the potential uses of NLP to promote quality and safety are broad, its wider implementation is hampered by a lack of standards. Of prime importance are standards related to the clinical document architecture (CDA), markup language, and a comprehensive standardized clinical vocabulary. A CDA is a critical step in the standardization of clinical reports and is essential to pave the way for widespread deployment of NLP systems. A standard CDA would make it possible to write simple NLP routines that could be based on regularities in the structure of the reports. For example, if all discharge summaries had a diagnosis section with the same tags and the same structure, it would be possible to write a relatively simple program to extract the diagnoses automatically from the reports. Increased functionality would be possible if the naming of clinical domains were standardized. Efforts are currently under way to establish a standardized ontology for documents through the Document Ontology Task Force at Health Level Seven. Subsequent efforts would be invaluable if the CDA were integrated with standardized clinical terminology and a standard way of expressing complex clinical conditions.

Data mining techniques, including NLP, are essential to both learning and accountability systems; however, many health care institutions lack the infrastructure, tools, and expertise to take advantage of those techniques. In addition, there is a need for studies that compare informatics approaches and develop methods for deploying such approaches more widely, particularly to rural and community hospitals (Bates et al., 2003).

Digital Sources of Evidence or Knowledge

Digital sources of evidence (i.e., health care knowledge) are another key component of a health information infrastructure and are essential for evidence-based practice. Sources of evidence, including bibliographic references, evidence-based clinical guidelines, and comparative databases, must be integrated with clinical expertise as practitioners make decisions (Bakken, 2001). Table 2-2 provides examples of digital sources of evidence. To sup-

TABLE 2-2 Digital Sources of Evidence or Knowledge: Examples

Type	Sources
Bibliographic	
Primary literature	
Traditional	MEDLINE, Cumulative Index of Nursing and Allied Literature
Full Text	OVID database; individual journals (e.g., *British Medical Journal*)
Structured reporting	Trial Bank Project (clinical trials)
Synthesized	
Electronic textbooks	Harrison's *Principles of Medicine*
Systematic reviews	Cochrane Collaboration
Practice parameters	
Standards of care	American Association of Critical Care Nurses
Practice guidelines	National Guideline Clearinghouse
Disease management plans	American Diabetes Association
Comparative databases	Health Plan Employer Data and Information Set (HEDIS)
Knowledge bases	
Diagnostic decision support	DXplain, Iliad
Pharmacy	National Drug File, Micromedex
Genomic	Genbank, Molecular Modeling database

SOURCE: Bakken, 2001.

port the redesign of care processes, the health information infrastructure must also facilitate the incorporation of new evidence derived from clinical practice (Bakken, 2001).

Many digital sources of evidence have applicability to management systems for patient safety and quality of care and play an important role in detection, analysis, recovery, and prevention for adverse events and near misses, as well as in quality management (Balas, 1998; Balas et al., 1998b). For example, within the context of a system to support patient safety and quality of care that is integrated with clinical care processes, digital sources of evidence would include, among others, guidelines related to the 20 priority health areas identified by the IOM, access to context-specific bibliographic retrieval, diagnostic decision support systems to assist with difficult diagnoses, and alerts and reminders of relevance to errors of omission and commission. Informatics techniques have the potential to decrease the amount of time from discovery to application of evidence in practice, as well as to deliver the evidence in a context-specific manner (Balas et al., 1998a).

A key challenge that is amenable to standards development is translating clinical practice guidelines into a format that can be shared across applications and organizations. This capability has significant potential to impact safety and quality care and will be a major contributor to the functionality of the EHR. Presenting guidelines on a computer monitor is the first stage in digitizing; the next level of automation occurs when the computer is able to make use of the patient's clinical data, follow its own algorithm internally, and present only information relevant to the current state (Maviglia et al., 2003). Models and tools for extracting and organizing knowledge, representation models for publishing and sharing guidelines, and computational models for implementing guidelines are in various stages of development (Maviglia et al., 2003). The range of possible applications for computer-based guidelines is very broad and includes disease management, encounter workflow facilitation, reminders/alerts, design and conduct of clinical trials, care plan/critical path support, appropriateness determination, risk assessment, demand management, education and training, and reference (Greenes et al., 2001).

Comparative databases (e.g., health plan utilization, disease registries, quality indicator databases) and knowledge bases (e.g., for pharmacy) are useful for benchmarking. Such databases associated with the priority areas identified by the IOM have the potential to provide a valuable source of evidence to support the attainment of national goals for quality improvement and patient safety. Many health care–related comparative databases are associated with specific quality measures for regulatory purposes, such as those of the Diabetes Quality Improvement Project (DQIP) developed through the Centers for Medicare and Medicaid Services. The addition of data related to errors of omission and commission associated with the DQIP measures would further facilitate redesign of care processes and improve safety and quality.

With the exception of guideline knowledge integrated into CDSSs, most digital sources of evidence operate as stand-alone systems, lacking true integration with clinical information systems. One approach to providing for retrieval of context-specific information during use of clinical information systems is the "infobutton" at New York Presbyterian Hospital. Infobuttons link digital sources of evidence to a particular section in the clinical information system. For example, a laboratory test for a drug level could be mapped to a National Drug Code or a drug trade name to search Micromedex for prescribing information (Cimino, 2000).

Leveraging the vast quantities of health care data and enterprise-wide knowledge requires the development of health information resource networks at the regional or national level. These networks must have the functionality and standards to acquire, share, and operationalize the various modalities of knowledge that exist in the health care domain (Abidi and Yu-N, 2000).

Communication Technologies

A number of authors have documented the importance of excellent communication in ensuring patient safety and providing quality care (Coiera, 2000; Covell et al., 1985; McKnight et al., 2001). More recently, investigators have turned their attention to the use of technologies that can enhance communication among members of multidisciplinary health care teams and between clinicians and patients (Coiera, 2000; McKnight et al., 2001; van Bemmel and Musen, 1997). Within the NHII, the primary mode of data exchange between organizations will be through the Internet and e-mail, while that within an organization will be through an Intranet or virtual private networks. Browser software developed for the Internet has made it easy to connect to, search, browse, and download information from anywhere on the network as if it were located on the user's personal computer (Institute of Medicine, 1997). In addition, this software has graphical, intuitive, and common interfaces to functions that locate and interact with remote data on the broader Internet without requiring the user to have technical knowledge (Institute of Medicine, 1997). Such features and their ease of use should contribute significantly to the facility of information transfer envisioned with the NHII. Whether the Internet will be adopted more widely for this purpose given the potential benefits will depend on the technical capabilities it can provide compared with other networking alternatives (National Research Council, 2000) and the development of clearly defined and enforced parameters for online health care communications.

Five technical factors have been identified that need to be considered when planning for the implementation of communication technologies: bandwidth needed and available, latency in transmission across the network, availability of the network on a continuous basis, confidentiality and security of data, and ubiquity of access to the network (National Research Council, 2000). From the communications perspective, it is necessary to resolve a number of parameters related to the primary types of health care–related data exchange:

- physician–physician communications,
- physician–patient communications,
- patient–patient support communications,
- interactive media and communication campaigns, and
- public availability of medical literature.

The credibility of online health information must also be addressed (Rice and Katz, 2001). Now that organizations are in the process of implementing the security protocols mandated in the Final HIPAA Security Rule, it is expected that integration of clinical information systems and use of the Internet will gain momentum.

Despite the flurry of interest in utilizing the Internet among many in the health sector, the incorporation of potential applications has yet to be fully realized. Of those organizations that do utilize communications technologies, many continue to rely on private networks (National Research Council, 2000). Table 2-3 provides examples of network-based applications currently in use.

In addition to the Internet and private networks, mobile communication technologies, such as cellular telephones, digital pagers, and personal digital assistants, are increasingly being used to support safety and quality in point-of-care applications. These technologies have the potential for widespread adoption because of their greater flexibility, convenience, and mobility relative to wired network communication systems. Many physicians and other health care providers are already incorporating handheld devices into their day-to-day functioning to better manage the care of their patients while at the same time reduce medical errors, administrative burdens, and overall

TABLE 2-3 Representative Applications Conducted over the Internet and Private Networks

Functions Commonly Performed Today over the Internet	Functions Performed Today over Private Networks	Functions Not Commonly Performed Today over Either the Internet or Private Networks
• Search for consumer health information • Participate in chat/ support groups • Exchange electronic mail between patients and care providers (limited) • Access biomedical databases and medical literature • Find information about health plans, select physicians (limited) • Purchase pharmaceuticals and other health-related products	• Transfer medical records among affiliated health organizations • Transfer claims data to insurers and other payer organizations • Conduct remote medical consultations (limited) • Send medical images (X-rays, etc.) to remote site for interpretation (very limited) • Broadcast medical school classes over campus networks (limited)	• Videoconferencing among public health officials • Remote surgery or guidance of other procedures • Public health survelllance/incident reporting • Home-based remote medical consultations • In-home monitoring of patients

SOURCE: National Research Council, 2000.

health care expenditures. Handheld devices have been developed to serve such purposes as physician documentation in an EHR, results review, alert notification, bedside registration, e-prescribing, case management, pharmacy, and materials management. For handheld applications, data are exchanged through "synching" directly with land-based or wireless networks. With increased security features and integration with land-based information technologies, wireless local area networks will further transform hospital and clinical communication networks, allowing for radio wave transmission of important data from handheld devices and portable personal computers. Along with handheld devices, paging and telecommunication systems are vital to patient safety. However, use of such technologies will depend on data standards and other components of the NHII so that compatibility and interoperability within the health information system can be established.

Clinical Information Systems

The components of the informatics infrastructure are linked through clinical information systems that provide the mechanism for sharing data collected from the various systems, reducing or eliminating redundancies in data collection/documentation and increasing the reliability and comprehensiveness of patient data available to the clinician. Within the context of a comprehensive integrated system, clinical information systems can support patient safety and quality management through the use of decision support tools for the prevention and detection of adverse events and near misses.

Ideally, the NHII will rely on the EHR as the central integrating component for data acquisition, analysis, and storage. Key capabilities of an EHR system include core health information, results management, order management, decision support, communication, patient support, and reporting (Institute of Medicine, 2003). Technical issues related to the EHR structure, function, and data standards are being resolved by NCVHS and by private-sector standards development organizations (e.g., Health Level Seven).

Decision support systems are the key tools enabling clinicians to access health care knowledge at the point of care as they progress through the care continuum. For example, encoded medical knowledge about the meaning and significance of changing laboratory test results would allow a system to provide alerts, an active function, in addition to the passive data retrieval function (Institute of Medicine, 1997). Methodologies for decision support can take many forms—reminders and alerts, embedded controls, decision assistance, and/or risk prediction (Institute of Medicine, 1992)—all of which have significant potential to improve patient safety. CDSSs can be only as effective as the strength of the underlying evidence base (Sim et al., 2001). Therefore, CDSSs must be designed to be evidence adaptive such that the clinical knowledge base is derived from and continually reflects the most up-to-date evidence from the research literature and practice-based resources (Sim et al., 2001).

IMPLEMENTING THE SYSTEMS

The IOM–Health Level Seven Demonstration Project: Where Are We Now?

The committee participated in the Health Level Seven (HL7) Interoperability Demonstration project at the Annual Conference of the Health Information Management Systems Society (HIMSS), held February 10–13,

2003, in San Diego, California, as an assessment of where the majority of the industry stands in relation to information systems and associated data standards for data interchange. The Interoperability Demonstration Project was a series of live technology demonstrations, conducted in partnership with the Centers for Disease Control and Prevention (CDC), the Food and Drug Administration (FDA), the Markle Foundation/Connecting for Health initiative, and 19 participating member organizations. The project presented real-world scenarios and clinical cases focused on the prevention and reporting of potential adverse drug events (ADEs), public health reporting of notifiable diseases, and continuity of care. It was intended to highlight several HL7 standards and show how they currently address these critical health care issues, as well as to explore the gaps between what is available today and what is needed to meet a set of increasingly complex demands on the health care system.

The basis for one of the interoperability demonstrations was a patient scenario describing an ADE as well as a near miss. The events in this scenario were characterized by the need to coordinate care across multiple providers in different settings; thus the demonstration was focused in particular on exploring the potential for using interoperability standards to improve care coordination. From the committee's perspective, the goals of participating in this demonstration were to:

• Highlight how interoperability standards can improve communication and coordination of clinical data among care settings (inpatient, outpatient, pharmacy).
• Identify limitations of existing systems and emerging standards with regard to patient safety.

The participants in the demonstration worked together over several months to define what functions would be demonstrated and how they would be implemented. The scenario was modified to reflect the available vendor participants and corresponding system functionality (see Box 2-1).

Participants learned several lessons in preparing for the demonstration. They spent considerable time making decisions, compromising, and agreeing on how to capture and share data, in part because there were several potential approaches and no clearly established standard for implementing particular functions. In the scenario, for example, the clinicians treating the patient in the emergency department and in the hospital must discover what medications she is taking; as it turns out, medication recently prescribed for hypertension may have resulted in an ADE. This information may be requested from and retrieved from the family physician's electronic records in several ways: as an order or prescription, from a medication list, or from a progress note. In this case, the demonstration participants chose to use the HL7 CDA to retrieve the prescription information, which was then used to drive clinical decision support (drug–laboratory interaction) and to inform the clinicians of the potential ADE.

During the demonstration, it became clear that while an ADE can be recorded as an allergy or as a problem on a problem list, current data standards do not support the documentation of an ADE as such. An ADE is not an allergy, although some individuals do have allergies to certain medications. This observation prompted HL7 to define a specification for representing ADEs. Finally, patients should be able to authorize release/transmission of their data. The demonstration showed that this functionality is not possible with the current systems and standards. Box 2-2 presents the results of the demonstration in terms of a report card summarizing progress to date on interoperability standards in health information management systems.

From the data standards perspective, the assessment of systems functionality was based on whether a standard exists and was/was not used in the demonstration, whether there are nonstandard methods for executing the task, or whether no technology exists to solve this interoperability issue.

BOX 2-1
Final ADE Scenario for
Interoperability Demonstration

- A 78-year-old woman sees her family physician at a small office practice. She is diagnosed with hypertension. A prescription is generated and sent to the pharmacy.
- A few days later, she is taken to the emergency room and admitted to the hospital with symptoms of diarrhea, disorientation, and a rash. The physician orders a complete blood count and electrolyte replenishment.
- Laboratory results indicate hyponatremia. Is the rash a new adverse event associated with losartan/hydrochlorothiazide (Hyzaar)?
- An adverse event message is sent to the FDA.
- Decision support prevents prescription of a second counterindicated drug (triamterine-hydrochlorothiazide). A different medicine (metoprolol) is prescribed instead. The patient improves and is discharged.
- The patient's family physician reviews the inpatient laboratory results and the discharge summary.

BOX 2-2
Interoperability Demonstration Project: Report Card

As part of the demonstration process, HL7 presented a report card delineating progress with regard to interoperability standards. Key findings in this assessment include the following:

- A certain level of systems integration is routine within the enterprise, but with few exceptions, stops at the enterprise boundary.
- We are only beginning to understand how to mine the information contained in narrative and to encode and make use of discrete findings.
- Strengths include admission–discharge–transfer information and laboratory results reports.
- Emerging strengths include a common approach to documenting metadata and to producing readable, transferable documents; findings-based reporting; and decision support.
- Weaknesses include lack of a business and technical infrastructure for distributed access.

More information about the Interoperability Demonstration project can be found at http://www.hl7.org/library/himss/2003SanDiego/HL72003DemoPress Overview.zip.

Table 2-4 provides an outline of the functions executed for the scenario and the standards utilized. The scenario demonstrated that even with the current state of relatively disparate data standards and interaction of multiple vendors, use of available data standards[1] allowed for a level of interoperability to support cross-organizational data flows and care coordination.

The committee found participation in the demonstration to be a useful experience. This project revealed some of the potential of interoperability standards. It also highlighted current gaps in standards supporting the communication of patient information between systems and revealed areas in which additional standards—e.g., for documenting ADEs—are needed. Based on these capabilities, and with effort in linking vendors through exist-

---

[1]Standards used in the demonstration include: HL7 context management for the user interface, HL7 data interchange formats and clinical document architecture, clinical terminology SNOMED CT (Systemized Nomenclature of Human and Veterinary Medicine, Clinical Terms), clinical drug notations of RxNORM, and laboratory terminology of LOINC (Logical Observation Identifiers, Names, and Codes) for the patient's data.

TABLE 2-4 IOM–HL7 Demonstration Project—Patient Scenario Data Standards

Scenario Event	Location
78-year-old woman sees her family doctor at a small office practice. She is diagnosed with hypertension.	Doctor's office
A blood pressure medication is prescribed.	Doctor's office
Prescription is sent to the pharmacy.	Doctor's office
The patient calls her physician and is referred to a hospital emergency department. She is admitted with symptoms of diarrhea, disorientation, and rash.	Emergency Department
The patient is admitted. The admitting physician views the outpatient progress note.	Hospital
Physician orders complete blood count and blood chemistries.	Hospital
Lab results indicate low sodium (hyponatremia). The patient is treated. A review of the patient's inpatient chart verifies an ADE due to a preadmission-prescribed diuretic. An ADE report is sent to the FDA.	Hospital
The physician prescribes a second drug to treat the patient's hypertension. The EHR alerts the physician that this drug may also cause an adverse reaction. An alternative drug is recommended and prescribed.	Hospital
The patient is discharged back to the care of her family physician. The family physician wants the hospitalization records and discharge medications.	Doctor's office
Practice manager can track the patient's status, but confidentiality rules prevent access to the body of clinical documents.	Doctor's office
The family physician and hospital submit claims but are asked for further information.	Hospital and doctor's office (billing)

Standards-Based Actions	Applications
CDA progress note created. Findings are SNOMED encoded through a call to a remote vocabulary server.	XML forms editor, terminology server
Medication is documented in the "plan" portion of the CDA progress note. RxNorm code is inserted by call to a remote server. An HL7 Version 3 prescription order is created automatically from the information in the CDA note and presented to the physician for review.	XML forms editor, terminology server
HL7 Java parser. Java Refined Message Information Model graph.	HL7 RIM application programming interface
HL7 Version 2 ADE message created from CDA header. Admission diagnosis, signs/symptoms coded with SNOMED and ICD9CM and sent to hospital.	Interface engine, EHR
Outpatient CDA note is retrieved via Web services call to repository.	Clinical document repository (CDR), EHR
HL7 Version 3 lab order is sent and translated by router from Version 3 to Version 2. Version 2 order is received by lab. Results are translated back to Version 3. LOINC codes are used for orders and test results.	HL7 toolkit and server
Using CDA as the data source, a draft HL7 Version 3 ADE report message is created and sent to the FDA. Report uses RxNorm and FDA-specified codes and terms.	EHR
Drug–allergy interaction checking between the EHR and decision support system is performed via HL7 CCOW. Data are communicated via RxNORM. Alert is sent via HL7 Version 2 OBX.	EHR, decision support
Repository is queried. ADE message, medications, and CDA discharge summary are retrieved. Discharge summary is human readable but not coded for automated decision support (it does not encode symptom data or diagnosis).	Portal, CDR
CDA confidentiality codes (user-defined) indicate which portions should be accessible.	Portal
Information is supplied by hybrid X12/HL7 electronic claims attachment. ICD9CM and LOINC codes used for clinical data.	Claim attachments, EHR, server

ing data standards, health care organizations can immediately begin to aggregate information on patient safety events using several well-developed terminologies that are currently in use or are planned for implementation, including the HIPAA-mandated code sets and the NCVHS core terminology group.

PRACTICAL APPROACHES TO MOVING FORWARD WITH STANDARDS-BASED DATA SYSTEMS

The development of integrated, standards-based data systems to improve patient safety can be perceived as a daunting task. Fortunately, many paths can lead to the optimal automation environment encompassed by the conceptual model presented earlier. This section describes several different practical approaches and effective interim solutions for moving forward with the integration of standards-based systems.

The committee believes the optimum means of implementing the systems that make up the conceptual model is to pursue a progressive migration plan for the implementation of EHRs, with appropriate adaptation to the various health care settings. Specific patient safety systems and data requirements are part of the overall strategy for institution of the NHII. Several health care organizations in the public and private sectors have already started to integrate the informatics components discussed above and can serve as successful models for progressing toward the envisioned infrastructure. Despite the operating differences that exist among large institutions and small office practices, a well-designed organizational strategy that aligns business and information technology goals can ease the transition and overcome challenges to implementation of the many applications that make up the EHR.

The committee's letter report on key capabilities of an EHR provides guidance on such a strategy, including considerations for inpatient care, ambulatory care, nursing homes, and personal health/self-care (Institute of Medicine, 2003) (see Appendix E). The committee's recommendations in that report encompass those CDSSs of high value to patient safety, as well as reporting formats. Building comprehensive systems to support both EHRs and patient safety systems must begin with a solid infrastructure based on the essential informatics components discussed in this chapter. Early adopters of EHRs are already using many of the data standards recommended in this report. As standards continually evolve and the integration of clinical systems gains momentum, early adopters can be expected to be prepared for a full transition to the data standards identified by NCVHS. In addition, the implementation guides to be developed and made publicly available will address issues associated with both transitioning from other local standards and adopting information technology for the first time.

To date, a number of organizations have successfully integrated the EHR employed by the Nicholas E. Davies award winners listed in Box 2-3. This award is given to those organizations that have demonstrated a favorable impact on health care quality, costs, and access to care through the use of computerized patient records (CPRs). Among the institutions that have received the award, some have implemented commercial software offerings, and some have developed their own systems. Some of these institutions have

---

BOX 2-3
Nicholas E. Davies Award Winners

1995 Intermountain Health Care, Salt Lake City, Utah
Columbia Presbyterian Medical Center, New York, New York
Department of Veterans Affairs

1996 Brigham and Women's Hospital, Boston, Massachusetts

1997 Kaiser Permanente of Ohio, Cleveland, Ohio
North Mississippi Health Services, Inc., Tupelo, Missouri
Regenstrief Institute for Health Care, Indianapolis, Indiana

1998 Northwestern Memorial Hospital, Chicago, Illinois
Kaiser Permanente Northwest, Portland, Oregon

1999 Kaiser Permanente of Colorado
Queens Medical Center, Honolulu, Hawaii

2000 Harvard Vanguard Medical Associates, Boston, Massachusetts
Veterans Administration Puget Sound Health Care System, Washington
St. Vincent's Hospital, Westchester County, New York, and New York,
New York

2001 University of Illinois at Chicago Medical Center, Chicago, Illinois
The Ohio State Medical Center, Columbus, Ohio

2002 Maimonides Medical Center, Brooklyn, New York
Queens Health Network, Queens, New York

SOURCE: Wise, 2003.

been at the forefront of the clinical information systems movement, and some have quietly assembled highly effective infrastructure systems and services in relative obscurity. To illustrate the variety of effective systems possible, we provide below a review of some very different but successful approaches utilizing commercially available CPR software.

In the history of the Davies award, several institutions have been recognized for CPR achievements utilizing commercially available software. Such software is capable of supplying many of the basic components necessary to begin the process of building integrated data systems to support patient safety. We provide detailed overviews of two Davies Award winners—Kaiser Permanente of Ohio and North Mississippi Health Services. Both have employed relatively low-technology approaches that have yielded high value. The approach of Kaiser Permanente (see Figure 2-3 and Box 2-4) illustrates how a network of ambulatory care sites associated with a single provider organization can use computer systems to simplify office practice and support the physician with important clinical reminders. The Kaiser Permanente system allows clinicians to use both paper and technology without requiring a complete shift to a paperless system. North Mississippi Health Services exemplifies how providers that work in rural environments or areas of low resources can develop basic computer systems for administrative and clinical information (see Box 2-5). This achievement is particularly impressive given that the technology integration involved was accomplished during the early stages of implementation of information technology, before its incorporation into the mainstream of daily life.

In the public sector, the Veteran's Health Administration (VHA) and the Military Health System (MHS) have developed and implemented models for quality improvement through the integration of comprehensive health information systems. In general terms, their information systems evolved from automated systems for administrative and financial transactions to gradually incorporate modified off-the-shelf technology and specially designed middleware for integrating disparate and legacy systems (Institute of Medicine, 2002b). As integration of clinical systems progressed, a foundation for the EHR was established that enables electronic documentation of health data, real-time access to important clinical information at the point of care (e.g., radiological images and laboratory test results), and linkages to facilitate administrative and financial processing. VHA and MHS also have implemented a consumer-oriented, Internet-based e-health model to support their patient population's communication and information needs (Institute of Medicine, 2002b). Other applications, such as those for reporting adverse events, are spearheading the use of health information systems to

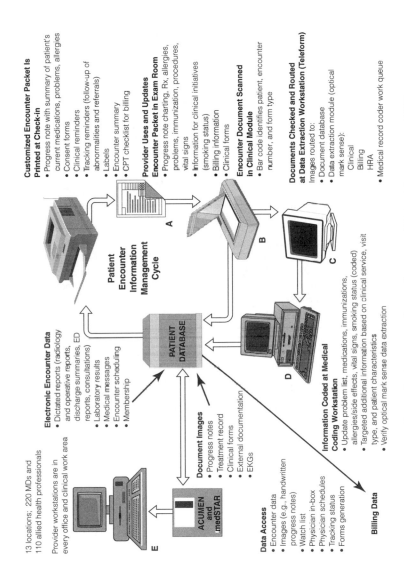

FIGURE 2-3 Information management in the medical automated record system of Kaiser Permanente of Ohio.

NOTE: ACUMEN = Ambulatory Clinical User Meaningful Enterprise Navigation; CPT = common procedure terminology; ED = emergency department; EKG = electrocardiogram; HRA = health risk assessment; Rx = prescription.

SOURCE: Khoury, 1998.

BOX 2-4
Kaiser Permanente of Ohio

Kaiser Permanente of Ohio has developed a Medical Automated Record System that has been fully implemented in 13 ambulatory care locations in Cleveland and surrounding communities, linking 220 physicians and 110 allied health professionals. The system was designed to meet the needs of providers—require minimal training and minor changes to physician documentation (e.g., physician's record of diagnoses, medications, allergies, and immunizations), capture information from external sources (e.g., reports, consults), and be implementable without affecting physician productivity. The approach selected utilizes personal computers that provide access to patient information in all physician offices and work areas, a paper intermediary to provide patient information and document clinical encounter information, and document imaging to capture nonelectronic information. Figure 2-3 provides a conceptual view of the system.

In the ambulatory setting, when a patient checks in, a customized information packet is printed that includes a summary of current problems, medications, allergies, etc.; a summary of diagnoses and vital signs from past visits; laboratory test results from the previous month; patient-specific clinical reminders generated from the organization's quality initiatives; standardized forms to collect coded information (e.g., billing, clinical interventions); and other forms (e.g., consent). The packet also serves as a charting document for physician notes. The use of clinical reminders in targeted clinical areas has led to increased physician compliance with guidelines and substantial improvement of the health care provided to Kaiser patients in the treatment of coronary artery disease, congestive heart failure, asthma, diabetes, and hypertension. Reminders also address other clinical areas, such as mammography and smoking cessation. The reminders have made a significant contribution to Kaiser's quality improvement initiatives and could do the same for patient safety. Patient safety reminders, such as those related to drug–drug interactions and comorbidities, could easily be added to Kaiser's information system and generated for the patient's clinical information packet. Further, several spaces on the clinician documentation sheet could be added for documentation of any adverse events or near misses that might occur during the treatment process. More comprehensive documentation of the event could follow, whereby the clinician could provide details either through direct use of the electronic system or on paper for input by a designated patient safety officer.

SOURCE: Khoury, 1998.

improve patient safety. The success of the VHA and MHS systems is rooted in a commitment to standardizing the information processing of the organization's architecture with off-the-shelf technology, specially developed applications, and medical vocabulary for describing clinical phenomena. In addition, the success of these systems is rooted in a philosophy that is patient centered and strives to achieve ongoing quality improvement. The system architectures are built around these important concepts.

Those organizations not planning to build large data repositories in the short term but seeking to improve patient safety reporting capabilities can participate in external comparative clinical performance offerings. One such offering, which is also an example of a public–private partnership to test the

---

BOX 2-5
North Mississippi Health Services

North Mississippi Health Services (NMHS) is a rural-based health system that serves patients in a 22-county region with five acute care hospitals, six dialysis centers, three nursing homes, and 12 offices for home care services. Over a 20-year period, NMHS progressively developed its integrated information systems, producing an EHR with automated input of the following information: medications, intake/output, vital signs, nurses' notes, histories and physicals, operative reports, consult reports, and cardiology results. The online records can be accessed on an as-needed basis in 100 different buildings in a two-state area.

NMHS understood that building an EHR was a complex process requiring a significant level of planning. In assessing the technology capabilities of all the sites to be linked in the network, NMHS found that many of the ancillary systems were at different stages of automation, requiring equipment upgrades and investment to establish the backbone of the network for interconnectivity. NMHS first initiated its system integration by automating and integrating the financial systems as the foundation for expansion to clinical and operational areas. Services and capabilities were added to the information systems on an annual basis as the need arose or as the technology became available. Given technology innovations and advances over the past decades, a migration strategy to an integrated health network is attainable in an accelerated time frame by 2010.

Of particular note, the NMHS EHR incorporates real-time decision support tools to screen patients at risk for adverse events and provide caregivers with individualized clinical information. NMHS's long-standing programs encompass drug–drug and drug–food interactions and drug allergy checks. If a problem exists, a notice is printed at the nursing unit and pharmacy. In addition, the adverse drug reaction monitoring program is designed so that each day the computer searches for the use of certain drugs. The pharmacist reviews this information daily and, based on guidelines for determining whether an ADE has occurred, contacts the physician. Another highly effective patient safety program is the dosage screening program for two sets of high-risk patients—pediatric and chemotherapy patients. A pediatric dosage screen was established that checks a patient's dose against preestablished dosing guidelines for milligrams per kilograms. Regardless of the way the patient's weight is entered, the computer converts it to kilograms and then performs a calculation to determine the dosage range for that patient. The same method of dosage calculation is applied to those receiving chemotherapy. As with the Kaiser Permanente of Ohio system (see Box 2-4), an application for generating patient safety reports could simply be added to the existing clinical information systems.

SOURCE: Bozeman et al., 1997.

effectiveness of a Medicare reimbursement premium for quality, is Perspective Online from Premier, Inc., a clinical data program used to illustrate the functions and processes associated with such systems. Premier collects and aggregates the data elements, subjecting each facility's raw data to various data management procedures that result in reliable comparative information. Premier currently manages clinical and administrative data for more than 500 facilities using several data management methodologies: data cleaning and editing procedures, patient de-identification methods, and procedures for capturing missing or incomplete data. Specific procedures are summarized in Box 2-6. Premier uses software controls to block access to specific data elements. For its hospital customers, the tool is used to limit access to patient-identifiable information from facilities other than their own, thus preventing unauthorized access to the data and downloading of any data elements. The extensive data management procedures employed suggest not only that there is ample opportunity to simplify data collection and submission for hospitals but also that there is considerable room for streamlining data management if data standards are adopted.

Other approaches taken by some organizations employ systems that directly target patient safety. Two systems in particular are gaining popularity in efforts to minimize medication events—computerized physician order entry systems and barcode medication administration systems. The order entry systems utilize data from pharmacy, laboratory, radiology, and patient monitoring systems to relay the physician's or nurse practitioner's diagnostic and therapeutic plans and alert the provider to any allergy or contraindication the patient may have so that the order can be revised immediately at the point of entry (Metzger et al., 2003) before being forwarded electronically for the targeted medical action. This is a critical step in the care process, a point at which intervention through the use of clinical information systems can have a high impact on preventing adverse events and improving adherence to care guidelines (Metzger et al., 2003). In fact, one study found that 50 percent of all ADEs originate with errors during medication ordering (Bates et al., 1995). Because the essence of computerized provider order entry is managing orders, these systems impact not only the physician or nurse practitioner but also their decision making and care planning, the pharmacist's decision making and work flow, the nurse's work flow and documentation, and communication with ancillary services (e.g., laboratory, radiology) (Metzger et al., 2003). While such a system requires computer workstations and/or wireless devices to function, a fast, highly responsive ordering interface is necessary to win the clinician's acceptance (Metzger et al., 2003). Also, because computerized provider order entry systems are de-

BOX 2-6
Perspective Online: Data Management Procedures

- *Data verification*—As data are received from each hospital, operations staff check for correct file formats and record counts. Staff calculate total discharges, charges, and costs from the records and compare them with the totals submitted by the hospital. Should there be any discrepancy at this point, the entire file is returned to the hospital for correction and resubmission.
- *Initial reconciliation*—At this point, the totals on the discharge data file are compared with financial data submitted separately by the hospital. This comparison allows for a limited variance between the totals; for example, discharges from both sources cannot vary by more than 0.5 percent. If the variance exceeds the threshold, the entire file is returned to the hospital for correction and resubmission.
- *Data validation*—Data in each record are compared with acceptable values and ranges. Codes are compared with code master tables. Records that appear to be in error are returned to the facility for correction.
- *Final reconciliation*—Once data have been corrected, the reconciliation process is repeated to ensure that there is no further discrepancy between the discharge records and the financial data.
- *Clinical resource consumption quality assurance*—Data are reviewed to determine whether the values are consistent with what would be expected from a clinical perspective; for example, anesthesia time and operating room time must be within a certain range of each other. Records failing this review are returned to the facility for correction.
- *Manual data audit*—A final review of the data is performed manually. This review checks for errors that cannot be found through automated processes, for example, whether the outlier percentage is consistent with other values.
- *Warehouse audit*—Once data are in the warehouse, one more check is performed. The current data file is compared with historical patterns to see whether the number of cases with specific characteristics differs from the hospital's historical experience.
- *De-identification methods*—Full compliance with all privacy and security requirements of the Health Insurance Portability and Accountability Act (HIPAA) is essential. De-identification policies and practices are reviewed, documented, and modified as necessary to ensure that the vendor meets or exceeds all such requirements.

pendent on data from departmental systems, they necessitate upgrading of legacy systems for interoperability and the use of common data standards to allow sharing of data.

VHA has implemented a bar-code medication administration system for inpatient care, in which all products in the pharmacy are bar coded in single dosage units. The patient also is provided with a bar-coded wristband upon admission to the hospital. The VHA system links such data as demographic data, medical history, medication history, drug terminology, drug reference data, drug interaction data, and drug–laboratory correlations. The system is used at the point of care to validate that the medication ordered, timing of administration, and dosage are correct and to maintain a medication administration history (Department of Veterans Affairs, 2001). For patient safety and quality research, reports can be generated for medication log, missed medications by patient or ward, missing dose request, follow-up and report, medication due list, medication administration history, drug inquiry, and other information (Department of Veterans Affairs, 2001).

OVERCOMING CHALLENGES TO IMPLEMENTATION OF INFORMATION TECHNOLOGY FOR THE NATIONAL HEALTH INFORMATION INFRASTRUCTURE

Organizational Leadership

Traditionally, a lack of organizational commitment to information technology and organizational culture have been significant barriers to the development of an informatics infrastructure within health care organizations. Leaders of health care organizations struggle with their organizations' use of and commitment to information technology (Glaser, 2002), and the health sector as a whole continues to lag significantly behind other industries in this regard. Achieving the vision described in this chapter requires commitment, leadership, and strategy.

Aligning information technology strategy with business strategy requires adjustment of the organizational structure to provide strong leadership and strategic support at the highest levels of management, adequate resources and incentives to support the required cultural change, and front-line decision making and feedback regarding the development and maintenance of patient safety and quality improvement systems. While structures, strategies, and approaches vary among organizations, certain fundamental principles correlate directly with successful integration of information technology and business strategies:

- A high-level, long-term commitment to information technology that starts at the level of the board of directors and senior management
- An integrated vision for the building of an information technology infrastructure
- Direct linkage between the information technology division and users, creating a feedback loop that provides for input and adjustment of the system to ensure that its functionality meets user needs

- Implementation of an adoption strategy for information technology systems and active support by senior medical staff for the cultural change necessary for effective adoption
- Systematic implementation (within an integrated vision) to build experience and confidence, to uncover unexpected problems, and to spread the cost out over time
- Continual adaptation and modification of systems and processes to reflect current medical science and technological advancements

The cultural change that is inherent in the deployment of information technology is dependent on organizational drivers from both the top down and the bottom up. An example to illustrate this point is offered by the success of the Latter Day Saints (LDS) Hospital in Salt Lake City, Utah, in creating a culture for both innovative clinical systems automation and quality improvement. Top management made its support known through planning, providing the necessary resources, and encouraging an attitude of willingness to change and experiment. Simultaneously, clinical department leadership undertook with zeal the effort to achieve continuous improvement. When the clinical information system and clinical improvement processes were transferred from LDS Hospital to other institutions, one of the greatest challenges was to transfer the continuous improvement mind-set (e.g., emerging deficiencies in information technology systems were often viewed as "works in progress" rather than failures). Careful attention to both the product being developed, whether information technology systems or patient safety reporting, and the culture in which they reside is essential to success.

Comprehensive systems such as the NHII develop over time. Because of the dynamic nature of medical practice and information systems, one of the most important principles for organizational leadership to embrace is the need for constant adaptation and modifications to reflect science and technological innovation and advancement. Strategic planning with forethought to incorporate this need for continued evolution can assist organizations in achieving greater business value for their information technology investments as the horizon continually shifts (Glaser, 2002). The organization's culture and leadership should also encourage innovation through creativity and experimentation in addressing business problems, crises, and opportunities for better meeting the needs of those interacting with the systems (Glaser, 2002). For example, an area of expected high-growth opportunity that would require system expansion could include personal health records for consumers. The personal health record includes a subset of the data in the individual's EHR and information recorded by them to support their care, disease management, and clinical communication (Markle Foundation, 2003). The personal health record could be made available to consumers through a link to a health care organization's secure Web-based portal that utilized HIPAA standards for authentication.

Another area for organizational expansion is the establishment of global health networks of population-based information. Organizational leadership should also pursue a more global perspective in aligning the organization's evolutionary adaptations and modifications with accepted international standards and technologies that can support the development of and linkage to a global health network. Global health networks based on common data standards can facilitate information access for health care providers on important concerns related to public health, such as infectious disease surveillance and the effects of bioterrorism that may directly affect their patients. The recent emergence of severe acute respiratory syndrome–SARS–is a prime example of this critical need. At the time the disease presented, each country was utilizing different standards to define and store salient information. It was not possible to share electronically vital information that could have eased the burden of tracking and monitoring the spread of the disease or facilitated a global research database.

Financial Incentives

The committee recognizes that building the NHII is an enormous undertaking with sizable costs in terms of human, organizational, financial, and governmental resources. The committee also understands that the majority of the effort for developing and implementing the information systems and data standards of the NHII will fall to the private sector. Estimating the costs to build the NHII is a major endeavor and one that was outside the scope of this study. However, the primary areas where costs are expected to arise include those related to the NHII (e.g., architecture, consumer health, homeland security, research, and population health), data standards (e.g., data interchange, terminologies, and knowledge representation), and patient safety reporting systems (e.g., organizational, state, national). These areas of significant cost can best be evaluated by those organizations that are directly involved in their respective areas. Those organizations should initiate large-scale studies of the costs and resources required to fulfill the goal of building the NHII.

To date, there has also been some broader-scale progress in addressing the challenges to the development of the NHII. In particular, the NHII

Conference, convened in July 2003 by the Department of Health and Human Services, brought stakeholders together to develop a consensus on a national action agenda to guide the development of the NHII (Department of Health and Human Services, 2003). The conference focused on several key topics, including data standards and vocabulary, as well as financial incentives.

Private-sector investments, such as those discussed earlier, will likely account for a good deal of the capital required to build the NHII, but the federal government also has an important role in providing financial support. To achieve the greatest gains, federal financial support should be targeted toward three areas. First, federal resources should support the development of critical building blocks of the NHII that are unlikely to receive adequate support through the combined investments of individual private-sector stakeholders. On the regional level, this support should come in the form of start-up funds to public–private partnership organizations to develop secure platforms for exchanging patient and other data and for carrying out transactions, along with the necessary technical assistance to enable providers to begin using the platform. Nationally, the federal government should provide the financial support and leadership needed for the establishment and ongoing maintenance of national data standards.

Second, the federal government should provide financial incentives to stimulate private-sector investments in the necessary information technology. Multiple approaches should be taken to this end and then evaluated to identify those that are most effective. These approaches might include revolving loans, differential payments to providers with certain information technology capabilities (e.g., inclusion of fees in the Medicare fee schedule for the provision of information technology services to patients, such as e-mail communications), or one-time-only payments to small physician offices to offset the costs and loss of productivity associated with the transition from paper to computer-based records.

Third, in the absence of considerable help from the federal government, safety net providers will likely fall behind in the transition to a safer health care delivery system. The federal government should provide grants, in-kind contributions, and technical assistance to such providers. This support might include offering one-time-only grants through the Health Resources and Services Administration to federally qualified health centers or VHA making its Veterans Health Integration System and Technology Architecture—VISTA available in the public domain and facilitating its use by safety net providers.

The federal government should thoroughly evaluate the various possibilities for providing incentives and investment support to facilitate the adoption of information technology in health care, with a special focus on office practice providers. Specific criteria for participation in each incentive and/or investment support program should be determined, along with parameters for analysis of program effectiveness.

Technical Assistance

A significant amount of technical assistance will be needed to support those implementing the clinical systems and EHRs associated with the NHII. Because the United States has a private-sector–based health care delivery system, many companies have already been established specifically for the purpose of providing technical assistance and support for the implementation of information technology systems in health care organizations. These companies will play an important role in bringing the conceptual model presented earlier to fruition. Likewise, there is an important role for the Agency for Healthcare Research and Quality (AHRQ) in providing assistance to safety net providers and in leveraging and/or expanding existing educational programs for small group providers in office practice settings.

Enforcement of Privacy and Security

Enforcement of privacy provisions and security protocols will be essential to build the confidence of providers and patients utilizing the networks and information systems of the NHII. Consequently, the federal government will play a particularly important leadership role in the enforcement of HIPAA standards for privacy and security. Penalties for violations must be strongly enforced. Likewise, from a technology perspective, the federal government, through AHRQ, should develop strong application certification requirements for health-sector technologies to minimize potential threats to information systems that compose the NHII. For example, a requirement could be established that all application programs used in health care be certified as defect-free such that all known "holes" in software programming that could be exploited have been appropriately corrected. Given recent events and the current climate, moreover, the federal government may have an interest in extending its scope as a resource in handling sensitive situations and Internet-related problems that may affect health information systems.

CONCLUSIONS

Because patient safety is an integral part of delivering quality health care, the committee believes that ensuring patient safety requires multiple measures throughout the continuum of care that can be accomplished through the establishment of an NHII. The key to the development of the NHII is threefold: (1) the implementation of a strategic plan for progressive migration from the current state to the comprehensive integrated network incorporating the principal informatics components outlined earlier in this chapter, (2) the provision of financial incentives by the federal government to support investments in information technologies, and (3) the implementation of common data standards for interoperability and comparability of health information.

Although a health information infrastructure that supports learning and accountability systems for patient safety has not been implemented in most organizations to date, the barriers involved are not primarily technological. The technologies needed for building the integrated systems described in this chapter exist today. Rather, the lack of technology implementation and the failure to use common data standards have been the principal barriers. This chapter has explicitly highlighted the need for standards for (1) a concept-oriented terminology that supports nonambiguous definitions of concepts and data reuse for safety and quality purposes; (2) a CDA that will improve the utility of using NLP techniques for extracting the data required for learning and accountability systems from textual documents, such as clinical notes and voluntary reporting systems; (3) messaging standards that enable data integration across disparate computer-based systems, including those that cut cross organizations; and (4) knowledge representation standards that support the development of computable guidelines for evidence-based practice and decision support rules that are shared among organizations. The accelerated adoption of such standards in turn requires public–private partnerships and sufficient incentives, rather than technical innovation, as discussed in the next chapter.

REFERENCES

Abidi, S. S. R., and C. Yu-N. 2000. *A Convergence of Knowledge Management and Data Mining: Towards 'Knowledge-Driven' Strategic Services.* Proceedings from the Third International Conference on the Practical Applications of Knowledge Management, Manchester.

Aha, D. W., L. A. Breslow, and H. Munoz-Avila. 2001. Conversational case-based reasoning. *Appl Intel* 14 (1):9–32.

Bakken, S. 2001. An informatics infrastructure is essential for evidence-based practice. *J Am Med Inform Assoc* 8 (3):199–201.

Balas, E. A. 1998. From appropriate care to evidence-based medicine. *Pediatr Ann* 27 (9):581–584.

Balas, E. A., and S. A. Boren. 2000. Managing clinical knowledge for health care improvement. *Yearbook of Medical Informatics* 65–70.

Balas, E. A., S. A. Boren, L. L. Hicks, A. M. Chonko, and K. Stephenson. 1998a. Effect of linking practice data to published evidence: A randomized controlled trial of clinical direct reports. *Med Care* 36 (1):79–87.

Balas, E. A., K. C. Solem, J. F. Su, Z. R. Li, and G. Brown. 1998b. Upgrading clinical decision support with published evidence: What can make the biggest difference? *Medinfo* 9 (2):845–848.

Balas, E. A., S. Weingarten, C. T. Garb, D. Blumenthal, S. A. Boren, and G. D. Brown. 2000. Improving preventive care by prompting physicians. *Arch Intern Med* 160 (3):301–308.

Bates, D. W., D. J. Cullen, N. Laird, L. A. Petersen, S. D. Small, D. Servi, G. Laffel, B. J. Sweitzer, B. F. Shea, R. Hallisey, M. Vander Vliet, R. Nemeskal, and L. L. Leape. 1995. Incidence of adverse drug events and potential adverse drug events: Implications for prevention. *JAMA* 274 (1):29–34.

Bates, D. W., N. Spell, D. J. Cullen, E. Burdick, N. Laird, L. A. Petersen, S. D. Small, B. J. Sweitzer, and L. L. Leape. 1997. The costs of adverse drug events in hospitalized patients: Adverse drug events prevention study group. *JAMA* 277 (4):307–311.

Bates, D. W., L. L. Leape, D. J. Cullen, N. Laird, L. A. Petersen, J. M. Teich, E. Burdick, M. Hickey, S. Kleefield, B. Shea, M. Vander Vliet, and D. L. Seger. 1998. Effect of computerized physician order entry and a team intervention on prevention of serious medication errors. *JAMA* 280 (15):1311–1316.

Bates, D. W., J. M. Teich, J. Lee, D. Seger, G. J. Kuperman, N. Ma'Luf, D. Boyle, and L. Leape. 1999. The impact of computerized physician order entry on medication error prevention. *J Am Med Inform Assoc* 6 (4):313–321.

Bates, D. W., S. Murff, H. Evans, P. D. Stetson, L. Pizziferri, and G. Hripcsak. 2003. Policy and the future of adverse event detection using information technology. *J Am Med Inform Assoc* 10 (2):226–228.

Berson, A. 1997. *Data Warehousing, Data Mining, and OLAP.* New York, NY: McGraw-Hill.

Bodenheimer, T., and K. Grumbach. 2003. Electronic technology: A spark to revitalize primary care. *JAMA* 290 (2):259–264.

Bozeman, T. E., K. Harvey, I. Jarrell, W. Jones, K. Kock, L. Morgan, G. Parada, F. Perry, K. Robinson, and G. Wages. 1997. *The Development and Implementation of a Computer-Based Patient Record in a Rural Integrated Health System.* Proceedings from the Third Annual Nicholas E. Davies CPR Recognition Symposium. Chicago, IL: Health Information Management Systems Society.

Brossette, S. E. 2000. A data mining system for infection control surveillance. *Meth Inform Med* 39 (4):303–310.

Brossette, S. E., A. P. Sprague, J. M. Hardin, K. B. Waites, W. T. Jones, and S. A. Moser. 1998. Association rules and data mining in hospital infection control and public health surveillance. *J Am Med Inform Assoc* 5 (4):373–381.

Cain, M. M., R. Mittman, J. Sarasohn-Kahn, and J. C. Wayne. 2000. *Health E-People: The Online Consumer Experience.* Oakland, CA: Institute for the Future, California Health Care Foundation.

Campbell, K. E., D. E. Oliver, K. A. Spackman, and E. H. Shortliffe. 1998. Representing thoughts, words, and things in the UMLS. *J Am Med Inform Assoc* 5 (5):421–431.

CareScience. 2003. *Santa Barbara County Care Data Exchange.* Online. Available: http://www.carescience.com/healthcare_providers/cde/care_data_exchange_santabarbara_cde.shtml [accessed May 30, 2003].

Chute, C. G., S. P. Cohn, and J. R. Campbell. 1998. A framework for comprehensive terminology systems in the United States: Developmental guidelines, criteria for selection, and public policy. *J Am Med Inform Assoc* 5 (6):503–510.

Cimino, J. J. 1998. Desiderata for controlled medical vocabularies in the twenty-first century. *Methods Inf Med* 37 (4–5):394–403.

———. 2000. From data to knowledge through concept-oriented terminologies. *J Am Med Inform Assoc* 7 (3):288–297.

Cimino, J. J., V. L. Patel, and A. W. Kushniruk. 2001. Studying the human-computer-terminology interface. *J Am Med Inform Assoc* 8 (2):163–173.

Coiera, E. 2000. When conversation is better than computation. *J Am Med Inform Assoc* 7 (3):277–286.

Covell, D., G. Uman, and P. Manning. 1985. Information needs in office practice: Are they being met? *Ann Intern Med* 103:596–599.

Department of Health and Human Services. 2003. *Federal Government Announces First Federal EGov Health Information Exchange Standards.* Online. Available: http://www.dhhs.gov/news/press/2003pres/20030321a.html [accessed May 29, 2003].

Department of Veterans Affairs. 2001. *VISTA Monograph.* Washington, DC: Department of Veterans Affairs.

Durieux, P., R. Nizard, P. Ravaud, N. Mounier, and E. Lepage. 2000. A clinical decision support system for prevention of venous thromboembolism: Effect on physician behavior. *JAMA* 283 (21):2816–2821.

Evans, R. S., S. L. Pestotnik, D. C. Classen, T. P. Clemmer, L. K. Weaver, J. F. Orme Jr., J. F. Lloyd, and J. P. Burke. 1998. A computer-assisted management program for antibiotics and other anti-infective agents. *N Engl J Med* 338 (4):232–238.

Fayyad, U. M., G. Piatetsky-Shapiro, P. Smyth, and R. Uthurusamy. 1996. *Advances in Knowledge Discovery and Data Mining.* Menlo Park, CA: AAAI Press.

Fiszman, M., and P. J. Haug. 2000. *Using Medical Language Processing to Support Real-Time Evaluation of Pneumonia Guidelines.* Proceedings of the Annual American Medical Informatics Association Symposium. Philadelphia, PA: Hanley and Belfus, 235–239.

Friedman, C., G. Hripcsak, W. DuMouchel, S. B. Johnson, and P. D. Clayton. 1995. Natural language processing in an operational clinical information system. *Natural Language Engineering* 1:83–108.

Glaser, J. P. 2002. *The Strategic Application of Information Technology in Health Care Organizations (Second Edition).* San Francisco, CA: Jossey-Bass.

Goldsmith, J. 2002. The Internet and managed care: A new wave of innovation. *Health Aff (Millwood)* 19 (6):42–56.

Goodwin, L. 1997. Data mining issues for improved birth outcomes. *Biomed Sci Instrumentation* 34:291–296.

Greenes, R. A., M. Peleg, A. T. S. Boxwala, V. Patel, and E. H. Shortliffe. 2001. Sharable computer-based clinical practice guidelines: Rationale, obstacles, approaches, and prospects. *Medinfo* 10 (Pt 1):201–205.

Haug, P., D. Ranum, and P. Frederick. 1990. Computerized extraction of coded findings from free-text radiologic reports (work in progress). *Radiology* 174 (2):543–548.

Honigman, B., P. Light, R. M. Pulling, and D. W. Bates. 2001. A computerized method for identifying incidents associated with adverse drug events in outpatients. *Int J Med Inf* 61 (1):21–32.

Hripscak, G., J. H. Austin, P. O. Alderson, and C. Friedman. 2002. Use of natural language processing to translate clinical information from a database of 889,921 chest radiographic reports. *Radiology* 224:157–163.

Institute of Medicine. 1992. *Guidelines for Clinical Practice: From Development to Use.* Washington, DC: National Academy Press.

———. 1997. *The Computer-Based Patient Record: An Essential Technology for Health Care.* Washington, DC: National Academy Press.

———. 2002a. *Fostering Rapid Advances in Health Care: Learning from System Demonstrations.* Washington, DC.: The National Academies Press.

———. 2002b. *Leadership by Example: Coordinating Government Roles in Improving Health Care Quality.* Washington, DC: The National Academies Press.

———. 2003. Key Capabilities of an Electronic Health Record System: Letter Report. Washington, DC: The National Academies Press.

Khoury, A. T. 1998. Support of quality and business goals by an ambulatory automated medical record system in Kaiser Permanente of Ohio. *American College of Physicians: Effective Clinical Practice* 1:73–82.

Kinzie, M. B., W. F. Cohn, M. F. Julian, and W. A. Knaus. 2002. A user-centered model for Web site design. *J Am Med Inform Assoc* 9 (4):320–330.

Knirsch, C. A., N. Jain, A. Pablos-Mendez, C. Friedman, and G. Hripcsak. 1998. Respiratory isolation of tuberculosis patients using clinical guidelines and an automated clinical decision support system. *Infect Cont Hosp Epi* 19 (2):94–100.

Markle Foundation. 2003. *Connecting for Health—A Public–Private Collaborative: Key Themes and Guiding Principles.* New York, NY: Markle Foundation.

Maviglia, S. M., R. D. Zielstorff, M. Paterno, J. M. Teich, D. W. Bates, and G. J. Kuperman. 2003. Automating complex guidelines for chronic disease: Lessons learned. *J Am Med Inform Assoc* 10:154–165.

McKnight, L. K., P. D. Stetson, S. Bakken, C. Curran, and J. J. Cimino. 2001. *Perceived Information Needs and Communication Difficulties of Inpatient Physicians and Nurses.* S. Bakken, ed. Proceedings of the Annual American Medical Informatics Association. Philadelphia, PA: Hanley and Belfus, 596–599.

Metzger, J., J. Fortin, and California Health Care Foundation. 2003. *Computerized Physician Order Entry in Community Hospitals.* Online. Available at http://www.fcg.com/healthcare/ps-cpoe-research-and-publications.asp [accessed Apr., 2003].

Mitchell, T. 1999. Machine learning and data mining. *Com ACM* 42 (11):31–36.

National Committee on Vital and Health Statistics. 2001. *Information for Health: A Strategy for Building the National Health Information Infrastructure.* Online. Available: http://ncvhs.hhs.gov/nhiilayo.pdf [accessed April 18, 2002].

National Research Council. 2000. *Networking Health: Prescriptions for the Internet.* Washington, DC: National Academy Press.

New England Healthcare EDI Network. 2002. *NEHEN About Us.* Online. Available: http://www.nehen.net/ [accessed May 30, 2003].

Overhage, M. June 7, 2003. *Enhancing Public Health, Healthcare System, and Clinician Preparedness: Strategies to Promote Coordination and Communication.* The Indiana Network for Patient Care. PowerPoint presentation to the Institute of Medicine Committee on Data Standards for Patient Safety.

Rice, R. E., and J. E. Katz. 2001. *The Internet and Health Communication: Experiences and Expectations.* Thousand Oaks, CA: Sage Publications, Inc.

Shortliffe, E. H., L. E. Perreault, G. Wiederhold, and L. M. Fagan. 2001. *Medical Informatics: Computer Applications in Healthcare and Biomedicine.* New York, NY: Springer-Verlag.

Sim, I., P. Gorman, R. A. Greenes, R. B. Haynes, B. Kaplan, H. Lehmann, and P. C. Tang. 2001. Clinical decision support systems for the practice of evidence-based medicine. *J Am Med Inform Assoc* 8 (6):527–534.

Tsumoto, S., and H. Tanaka. 1997. *Incremental Learning of Probabilistic Rules from Clinical Databases Based on Rough Set Theory.* Proceedings of the Annual American Medical Informatics Association 198–202. Bethesda, MD: American Medical Informatics Association.

van Bemmel, J. H., and M. A. Musen. 1997. *Handbook of Medical Informatics.* Heidelberg, Germany: Springer-Verlag.

Waegemann, C. P., C. Tessier, A. Barbash, B. H. Blumenfeld, J. Borden, R. M. Brinson, T. Cooper, E. L. Elkin, J. M. Fitzmaurice, S. Helbig, K. M. Hunter, B. Hurley, B. Jackson, J. M. Maisel, D. Mohr, K. Rockel, J. H. Schenieder, T. Sullivan, and J. Weber. 2002. *Healthcare Documentation: A Report on Information Capture and Report Generation.* Newton, MA: Medical Records Institute.

Wise, P. July 2, 2003. *Healthcare Information and Management Systems Society List of Davies Winners.* Personal communication to Institute of Medicine's Committee on Data Standards for Patient Safety.

3

Federal Leadership and Public–Private Partnerships

CHAPTER SUMMARY

Common clinical data standards are critical to establishing a national health information infrastructure that can support patient safety. While progress is being made in selecting core groups of these clinical data standards for national adoption, issues remain with the different standards development, approval, and maintenance processes currently employed by the multitude of organizations that produce data interchange and terminology standards. Delays in the ability of health care organizations to implement data standards will likely slow investment in information technology and necessitate sizable reworking of the information technology systems that currently exist to enable connectivity. Successful transition to and operation of the national health information infrastructure will require a more efficient, streamlined mechanism for standards development and implementation processes that can be achieved only through strong federal leadership and effective public–private partnerships. This chapter reviews current standards development and implementation processes and presents the committee's recommendations for leveraging existing organizations and standards initiatives to build and sustain the informatics infrastructure envisioned in this report.

Development and implementation of data standards for the national health information infrastructure (NHII) will require the participation of both industry and government to create an optimal set of specifications that meet compatibility and interoperability needs, enable regulatory requirements, and allow for continued innovation and technology advancement by a variety of vendors. The organizations associated with the development of the three types of standards required—data interchange, terminologies, and knowledge representation—have differing methods for developing and implementing those standards. Both standards and methods have remained rather uncoordinated to date, resulting in overlaps and gaps in the comprehensive set of data standards needed for full operation of the national health information infrastructure. This chapter describes current processes for setting each type of standard; reviews current standards activities in the federal and private sectors; and presents the committee's recommendations for how the standards development, implementation, and dissemination process can be streamlined and coordinated for greater usefulness and efficiency.

CURRENT STANDARDS-SETTING PROCESSING

Data Interchange Standards

Data interchange standards are developed by three means—*federal mandate* by legislation or regulation, *voluntary consensus* through balloting of an industry professional group or sector, or *de facto* as the result of dominance in the commercial marketplace (see Figure 3-1). Once standards have been developed and approved, an integral part of their utilization is the conformity assessment process used to evaluate the compliance of products and processes with particular standards.

Most technical standards in the health sector and other industries are developed at the national and international levels through the voluntary consensus process, with the participation of industry members of standards development organizations (SDOs) and government representatives having an interest in the use of the standard. More recently, these three pathways have converged, primarily as a result of the administrative simplification provisions of the Health Insurance Portability and Accountability Act (HIPAA), which require that standards for transactions be selected from those developed through the voluntary consensus process and/or those available because of marketplace dominance, rather than from government-unique standards.

The American National Standards Institute (ANSI) bears the responsibility for endorsing consensus standards in the United States and for representing U.S. interests internationally in the International Organization for

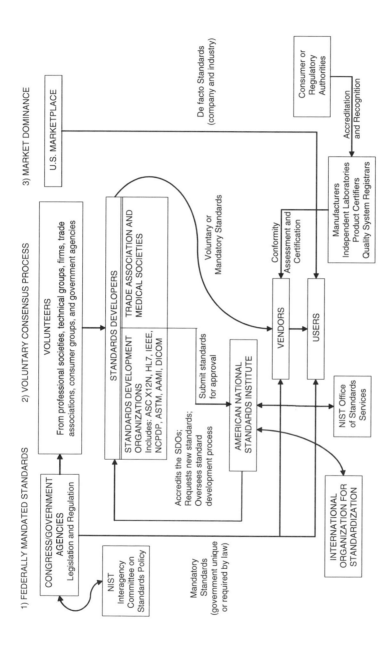

FIGURE 3-1 Overview of processes used to set standards for the exchange of health care data in the United States.

NOTE: AAMI = American Association of Medical Instrumentation; ASC = Accredited Standards Committee; ASTM = American Society for Testing and Materials; DICOM = Digital Imaging and Communication in Medicine; HL7 = Health Level Seven; IEEE = Institute for Electrical and Electronics Engineers; NCPDP = National Council for Prescription Drug Programs; NIST = National Institute of Standards and Technology.

Standardization (ISO). ANSI does not produce standards itself but functions as an accreditor of SDOs through its Accredited Standards Committee (ASC). ANSI primarily ensures that SDOs adhere to the principles of openness, balance of interests, due process, and an appeals process and approves standards that could become U.S. national standards. ANSI does not perform quality checks on the data interchange standards developed or distribute standards interpretation and implementation guides for consistency. Several primary SDOs in the United States develop the various types of data interchange standards required for health care data (see Box 3-1).

Other independent groups are involved indirectly. They include the National Uniform Billing Committee, which develops a single billing form and standard dataset to be used nationwide by institutional providers and payers for handling health care claims, and the National Uniform Claims Committee, which develops a standardized dataset for use by the noninstitutional health care community in transmitting claim and encounter information to and from all third-party payers.

BOX 3-1
Primary Standards Development Organizations Setting Standards for Data Interchange in the United States

ASC X12N—the ANSI committee responsible for developing health care–related electronic data interchange (EDI) standards for administrative and financial transactions.

Health Level Seven (HL7)—chief developer of clinical data exchange, vocabulary, and document architecture standards.

Institute for Electrical and Electronics Engineers (IEEE)—developer of medical device transmission and vocabulary specifications.

American Society for Testing and Materials (ASTM)—developer of standards for medical and surgical materials and devices, emergency medical services, and health information systems.

Digital Imaging and Communication in Medicine (DICOM)—developer of transmission and vocabulary standards for radiological images; created jointly by the American College of Radiology and the National Equipment Manufacturers Association and now is an international organization.

American Dental Association (ADA)—developer of all standards relating to dentistry.

National Council for Prescription Drug Programs (NCPDP)—developer of transmission standards for documents related to prescription drugs.

TABLE 3-1 Overlap of Work by the Major Standards Development Organizations

Category	ASTM	DICOM	HL7	NCPDP	X12N	IEEE	CEN	ISO[a]
Clinical laboratory	X		X				X	X
Data interchange	X	X	X	X	X	X		X
Vocabulary	X	X	X	X	X	X	X	X
Object modeling	X	X	X		X		X	X
Security	X	X	X	X	X		X	
Patient information	X	X	X	X	X		X	X
Accounting			X	X	X			
XML[b]	X		X		X		X	X
Electronic health records (EHR)	X		X				X	X
Medical devices						X		X
Templates	X	X	X				X	

[a]ISO documents are generally derived from standards originally developed by CEN, DICOM, HL7, and/or IEEE.
[b]Extensible markup language.

standards exist, terminologies have not been agreed upon for all the important domain areas (e.g., laboratory, devices). The committee believes that stronger leadership and coordination can position the ANSI HISB to address these issues.

Another important issue in standards development and implementation is financial support. Producing a standard is expensive in terms of both time and money. In the United States, vendors and users must be willing to support the hours of work involved (usually on "company time"), the travel expenses, and the costs of documentation and distribution. In contrast, most European and Asian (e.g., Japanese, Australian, and Korean) standards are developed and entirely funded by a government agency, then designated for widespread adoption.

Terminologies

The process for developing and updating terminologies is highly variable. Currently, there are well over 150 terminology systems in use to describe various medical domains. Other than the HIPAA-mandated standards, there has been little agreement on or implementation of common clinical terminologies across institutions and settings. Many of the terminologies that are used are either locally developed and maintained and exchangeable with other entities only at great effort; developed by proprietary vendors for specific system implementations; or broad international termi-nologies (e.g., the International Classification of Diseases [ICD]) that are often modified at the local level. Thus, one laboratory system has not been able to communicate with another without great difficulty. This "custom" approach incurs high costs and inhibits efforts to reuse clinical data to un-derstand and prevent patient safety events. For computer interoperability, data must be recorded in a terminology that is recognized and understood by the receiving computer; local terms are not interoperable. Adoption of a set of core terminologies for use in clinical information systems will accom-plish this task, and such terminologies are in the process of being selected through public–private partnerships. Vendor compliance with the standards will ensure the interoperability of products for buyers, users, and regulators. Box 3-2 and the following subsections provide a brief overview of the pro-cesses used by these organizations to develop their terminology data stan-dards.

International Organizations

Some international organizations (i.e., World Health Organization [WHO] for ICD codes and International Classification of Functioning, Dis-ability and Health [ICF], and the World Organization of National Colleges, Academies and Academic General Practice and Family Physicians for the International Classification of Primary Care [ICPC]) engage in terminology development through a relatively formalized consensus process that requires approval by a governing oversight or steering committee (Institute of Elec-trical and Electronics Engineers, 2001; World Health Organization, 1999). For WHO terminologies, submissions for changes are accepted by the heads of the WHO collaborating centers established around the world. If accepted by the WHO regional office, they are then circulated to the other centers no later than 6 months in advance of the official WHO annual meeting, where they may receive final approval upon consensus of the group.

Federal Government

Development of clinical modifications for the ICD codes is accom-plished through the National Center for Health Statistics at the Centers for Disease Control and Prevention (CDC) using an open and formal process that accepts suggestions by the public and private sectors and is managed by the Coordination and Maintenance Committee. Proposals for a new code must include a description of the code, why it is needed, and supporting

BOX 3-2
Types of Terminology Development Organizations and Examples of Specific Terminology Developers

1. International Organizations
- World Health Organization (WHO)—developed the International Classification of Diseases (ICD)-9; ICD-10; the International Classification of Functioning, Disability, and Health (ICF); and ICD-O for oncology.
- International Conference on Harmonization (ICH)—developed the Medical Dictionary for Drug Regulatory Affairs (MedDRA).
- World Organization of National Colleges, Academies and Academic Associations of General Practitioners/Family Physicians (WONCA)—developed the International Classification of Primary Care (ICPC).

2. Federal Government
- Department of Health and Human Services (DHHS)
  - Centers for Medicare and Medicaid Services (CMS)—developed the ICD-9 Clinical Modifications (CM) Volume 3 (procedures) and the ICD-10 Procedure Coding System (PCS) and the Healthcare Financing Administration Common Procedure Coding System (HCPCS).
  - National Committee for Health Statistics—developed the ICD-9 CM Volumes 1 and 2 (diagnoses) and ICD-10 CM (diagnoses).
  - Food and Drug Administration (FDA)—responsible for National Drug Codes (NDCs) and developed the Orange Book.
- Joint effort by the Veterans Health Administration (VHA), National Library of Medicine (NLM), and Health Level Seven (HL7) to develop the clinical drug terminology RxNORM.

3. Professional Associations/Academic Institutions
- Nursing groups, including professional associations and academic research-

references and literature. Final decisions are made by the director of the National Committee on Health Statistics and the administrator of the Coordination and Maintenance Committee (National Center for Health Statistics and Centers for Disease Control and Prevention, 2003).

The Food and Drug Administration's (FDA) process for incorporating new National Drug Codes (NDCs) has been highly informal; new codes are

ers—developed many terminologies;[1] other efforts focus on integrating nursing terminologies into the Systemized Nomenclature of Human and Veterinary Medicine (SNOMED) Clinical Terms (CT) and Logical Observation Identifiers, Names, and Codes (LOINC).

- College of American Pathologists (CAP)—developed SNOMED (RT—reference terminology); developed SNOMED CT through a collaboration with the National Health Service of the United Kingdom.
- Regenstrief Institute—developed LOINC.
- American Medical Association (AMA)—developed Current Procedural Terminology (CPT).
- American Psychiatric Association (APA)—developed the Diagnostic and Statistical Manual of Mental Disorders (DSM).
- Emergency Care Research Institute (ECRI)—developed the Universal Medical Device Nomenclature System (UMDNS).
- National Cancer Institute (NCI)—developed genetics-related terminologies

4. Standards Development Organizations
- Health Level Seven (HL7)—registers existing controlled terminologies and defines required terminologies for which no controlled terminologies exist.
- Institute of Electrical and Electronics Engineers (IEEE)—developed medical device terminologies.

5. Other Private Entities
- Medicomp Systems Incorporated—developed Medcin®, which is not a standard terminology but a vendor-developed set of coordinated terms used locally by some health care organizations.

6. Standardized Mappings of Terminologies
- National Library of Medicine (NLM)—developed the Unified Medical Language System (UMLS), which can store and cross-reference existing terminologies, and the Medical Subject Headings (MeSH)

[1]Nursing terminologies include: HHCC—Home Health Care Classification; ICNP—International Classification of Nursing Practice; NANDA—North American Nursing Diagnosis Association classification; NIC—Nursing Intervention Classifications; NOC—Nursing Outcomes Classifications; Omaha System; PCDS—Patient Care Data Set; and PNDS—Perioperative Nursing Data Set.

submitted by the manufacturer, reviewed by the FDA for redundancy or overlap, and added to the set of codes. However, this procedure has been associated with several issues. One such issue is that drug codes for pharmaceuticals that are considered obsolete are often reused by the manufacturer, a practice that contributes to problems in tracking medication usage and potential drug interactions or contraindications. A second issue is the lack of a single standard for chemical names, ingredient listings, and dosage sizes associated with NDCs, resulting in variation from one organization to another.

Professional Associations and Academic Institutions

Many terminologies in use are developed by professional associations and academic institutions. The processes for terminology development vary, generally depending on the size of the organization and the purpose of the standard. Organizations such as the College of American Pathologists (which produces the Systemized Nomenclature of Human and Veterinary Medicine [SNOMED]) and the American Medical Association (which produces Current Procedural Terminology [CPT]) have relatively formal sets of processes for developing and refining terminology concepts that rely on an editorial board for final approval. SNOMED technical subgroups evaluate and model terminology and then advise the editorial board regarding scope of coverage, creation of hierarchies, semantic definitions, and scientific accuracy (SNOMED International, 2000). Because CPT codes are used for reimbursement, new codes are not based on technical criteria but on the need to code new medical procedures. These updates are incorporated quarterly once approved by the American Medical Association editorial board. Processes used by other terminology development organizations, such as nursing groups, are very informal, with general group approval occurring annually.

Standards Development Organizations and Other Private Entities

IEEE has a highly formal approach to developing standards based on due process, openness, consensus, balance, and right of appeal. The membership of working groups is defined. Three-quarters of the members of a group must vote on ballots of official documents, and of those who vote, three-quarters must support the document for it to be accepted.

The HL7 process for obtaining consensus on terminologies is not as formal as that for data interchange standards since HL7 is not actually a terminology developer per se but maps registered terminologies for encoding in its messaging formats. Participants in the HL7 terminology special interest group agree to the additions, mappings, and technical specifications. However, sign-off by the HL7 steering committee is still required.

Private companies developing terminologies, such as Medicomp, create new terms at will without a formal or open process and as required by clients for the integration of clinical information systems. Vendors of laboratory systems also have historically developed and maintained terminologies that are modified locally for use within their systems.

Standardized Mappings of Terminologies

In addition to the terminology developers, two organizations have undertaken the development of standardized mappings among the different terminologies to facilitate data interchange—the National Library of Medicine (NLM) and HL7. While not a terminology developer, NLM has created a single database of the various terminologies—the Unified Medical Language System (UMLS). NLM has played a unique role in the development of the standardized mappings and cross-references from one terminology to another, and the UMLS is now considered the global reference database for linking disparate terminologies (National Library of Medicine, 2002). The UMLS cross-referencing function unifies terminologies that may have different content, structure, or semantics (National Library of Medicine, 2002), making it the key database for the development and maintenance of terminology extensions and/or new terminologies to represent medical concepts.

The UMLS is the result of a major collaboration among terminology developers and NLM (National Library of Medicine, 2002), which will be even more important to the evolution and maintenance of the National Committee on Vital and Health Statistics (NCVHS)–Consolidated Health Informatics (CHI) core terminology group for the electronic health records (EHR). To date, NLM has also collaborated with HL7 and pharmacy knowledge vendors, among others, to develop a common representation for clinical drugs as well as a comprehensive clinical drug reference terminology (Nelson et al., 2002). For example, NLM and several other federal agencies (i.e., Veterans Health Administration [VHA], CDC, FDA, National Aeronautics and Space Administration [NASA], and National Cancer Institute [NCI]) have contracted with Apelon, a private software and informatics company, to develop a set of integrated terminologies for clinical information (Apelon, 2003). In addition, terminology developers themselves are engaging in more collaborative relationships to establish terminology coverage for all medical domain areas and the multiplicity of uses defined for the NHII (e.g., College of American Pathologists and the United Kingdom's National Health Service collaborated to create SNOMED Clinical Terms [CT]) (Bakken et al., 2000; Ozbolt, 2000; Wang et al., 2002). The College of American Pathologists also recently licensed SNOMED CT to the public sector through the UMLS, as announced in July 2003 by the secretary of the

Department of Health and Human Services (DHHS) (Department of Health and Human Services, 2003).

Because the UMLS has the informatics infrastructure to cross-reference many different terminology systems and provides its services in the public domain, NLM is ideally positioned to lead the oversight and maintenance of the core terminology group to be determined by the CHI initiative and associated patient safety data standards. Thus it is highly important that the UMLS be capable of adapting and constantly evolving to reflect current thinking in medicine and informatics (Campbell et al., 1998). To support the data standards initiatives of the NHII, NLM should establish a more formalized process for working in collaboration with terminology developers on the evolution and maintenance of the necessary data standards.

Knowledge Representation Standards

The establishment and maintenance of data standards are integrally linked to the advancement of clinical knowledge. The discovery of new knowledge leads to the redefinition of what constitutes best practices in a specific clinical area. Changes in best practices have implications for the design of care processes specifically for the clinical data requirements to support care delivery. For example, in 1981 new scientific evidence became available indicating that early diagnosis of certain eye conditions leads to improved outcomes in diabetes care (Diabetic Retinopathy Study Research Group, 1981). To ensure that this new evidence is applied consistently in practice, it must be translated into a practice guideline, and in 1988 the American Diabetes Association published eye care guidelines for patients with diabetes mellitus that included a recommended annual eye exam (American Diabetes Association, 1988).

Once a guideline has been issued, hospitals, physicians, and other providers must modify their care processes to be consistent with the new best practice. Likewise, information systems must be modified to capture the new information. However, the current health care delivery system lacks well-defined processes for translating new knowledge into consistent practice. For example, according to a 1997 report by the National Committee on Quality Assurance, the national rate for an annual diabetic eye exam (38.4 percent) was still below the recommended level (National Committee for Quality Assurance, 1997). Similar examples can be found in virtually every area of clinical practice (Balas and Boren, 2000; Chassin, 1997). Indeed, another recent study found that patients receive only about half (55 percent) of the recommended care interventions (McGlynn et al., 2003). Overall, the toll in terms of lost lives, pain and suffering, and wasted resources is staggering. The Agency for Healthcare Research and Quality (AHRQ) has established a track record in funding the synthesis and dissemination of clinical knowledge and best practices through its work with the evidence-based practice centers (EPCs), primary care practice-based research networks (PBRNs), and the Integrated Delivery System Research Network (IDSRN). There are currently 13 EPCs developing evidence-based reports and technology assessments based on rigorous analysis of the scientific literature on clinical, social science/behavioral, economic, and other health care and delivery issues (Agency for Healthcare Research and Quality, 2003a). The EPCs and their partners, including federal and state agencies, private-sector professional societies, health delivery systems, providers, payers, and others, are expected to translate the findings into practice guidelines or other implementation tools to improve the quality of care within their organizations. To date, most of the EPCs have focused on selected chronic conditions, such as diabetes, epilepsy, stroke, congestive heart failure, and cancer.

Putting these evidence-based guidelines into a computer-readable format that can be used with decision support systems during clinical encounters is the objective of the informatics community. Many groups have been undertaking applied research on various approaches to modeling the guidelines (Peleg et al., 2003); however, none of these approaches are providing optimum performance in clinical practice (Maviglia et al., 2003). Another issue that impacts the development of computer-readable guidelines is the need for interoperability with a number of information systems operating in the context of the NHII. Therefore, several of the research groups are banding together to use the best from research to date and develop a generic model intended to serve as the baseline standard guideline format (Peleg et al., 2003). Chapter 9 provides a detailed discussion of these efforts.

Since 1993, AHRQ has supported important research through PBRNs. A PBRN is a group of ambulatory practices devoted to the primary care of patients, formed to investigate research questions related to community-based clinical practice (Agency for Healthcare Research and Quality, 2001). Typically, PBRNs draw on the experience and insight of practicing clinicians to identify and frame research questions that can be investigated with rigorous research methods to produce findings that can improve primary care practice (Agency for Healthcare Research and Quality, 2001). To date, the PBRNs have studied such topics as the role of antibiotics in improving outcomes in children with acute otitis media, the referral process in pediatric care, and primary and secondary prevention of coronary artery disease and stroke (Agency for Healthcare Research and Quality, 2001). Nineteen networks are established across the United States, providing an outstanding resource on which AHRQ can draw to assist in the implementation of the clinical information systems, data standards, patient safety reporting systems, and other components of the NHII.

The IDSRN was initiated by AHRQ in September 2000 with the purpose of linking researchers and large health care delivery systems. It is made up of nine partners, selected because they provide health care services to large populations in a variety of organizational settings. Each partner is working with several collaborators, including other health care systems, research institutions, and managed care organizations, to conduct research within their integrated delivery systems and then disseminate the scientific evidence obtained (i.e., organizational best practices related to care delivery) to the entire network. The ISDRN also includes researchers and sites that are testing ways to adapt and apply existing knowledge to care delivery. To date, 44 IDSRN projects have been funded covering a wide range of topics, including quality measurement and improvement, bioterrorism, information technology, organization and financing, and disparities in access to care. The efforts of the EPCs, IDSRN, and others, including the Cochrane Collaboration (Cochrane Collaboration, 2003) and the *ACP Journal Club* (American College of Physicians, 2003), are excellent models and provide the building blocks for a more comprehensive effort to address the 20 priority areas identified by the Institute of Medicine (IOM) that account for the bulk of health care services (Institute of Medicine, 2003).

AHRQ's Centers for Education and Research on Therapeutics (CERTs) program is a national initiative to conduct research and provide education on the benefits and risks of new, existing, or combined uses of therapeutics (drugs, medical devices, biologics) (Agency for Healthcare Research and Quality, 2002). The CERTs program has three primary aims: (1) to increase awareness of both the uses and risks of new drugs and drug combinations, biological products, and devices, as well as of mechanisms to improve their safe and effective use; (2) to provide clinical information to patients and consumers, health care providers, pharmacists and pharmacy benefit managers and purchasers, health maintenance organizations and health care delivery systems, insurers, and government agencies; and (3) to improve quality while reducing cost of care by increasing the appropriate use of drugs, medical devices, and biological products and by preventing their adverse effects and the consequences of those effects (such as unnecessary hospitalizations) (Agency for Healthcare Research and Quality, 2002). Because adverse drug events (ADEs) are one of the most common types of patient safety event, use of AHRQ's expertise in evaluating information and disseminating it to the public should prove very helpful and may contribute greatly to the number of ADE reports that are submitted.

Another recent promising initiative in this area of linking the evidence base to care is MedBiquitous, a consortium of professional medical associations and related organizations that is creating an extensible markup language (XML) framework for professional medicine, with a focus on medical education and credentialing (MedBiquitous Consortium, 2003). The XML standards allow providers to search the literature more easily to locate specific types of content related to particular medical conditions and also permit professional societies to verify board certifications of providers automatically.

Reporting Standards

The health care sector also currently lacks standardized measurement and reporting mechanisms for routinely monitoring the extent to which health care is safe and effective. In designing and building information technology systems, it is helpful to know in advance the reporting specifications that must be satisfied. As noted earlier in this report, many safety and quality measurement and improvement efforts are sponsored by health care providers, public and private purchasers, federal and state agencies, and accreditors. Some focus on near misses or adverse events, while others assess compliance with best practices through medical care performance and outcome measures. However, as noted by a previous IOM committee, too many resources are spent on health care measures that are either duplicative or ineffective, and little comparative quality information is made available in the public domain for use by beneficiaries, health professionals, or other stakeholders (Institute of Medicine, 2002). In addition, users of the available measures are hindered by the lack of reporting standards and consistent methodologies (Eddy, 1998; Rhew et al., 2001).

Standardized measurement and reporting mechanisms not only will facilitate the building of effective information technology systems and reduce confusion over reporting requirements but also could drive quality improvement in other ways, such as assisting efforts to reward quality care through payment or other means. For example, the Centers for Medicare and Medicaid Services (CMS), in partnership with Premier, Inc., a private alliance of more than 200 hospitals and health care systems, is currently conducting a demonstration project to evaluate the linking of standard performance measurements to differential hospital reimbursement (McGinley, 2003; Premier, 2003). Over the course of this 3-year project, those hospitals identified as top performers will receive an additional 1 to 2 percent reimbursement over current diagnosis-related group levels for a subset of conditions. Another program linking payment to quality has been proposed in House Resolution 2033, the Medicare Equity and Access Act (Government Printing Office, 2003). This proposal would award financial incentives to Medicare+Choice organizations that demonstrate superior-quality health care, based on their Health Plan Employer Data and Information Set (HEDIS) and Consumer Assessment of Health Plans data. Other ways in which standardized reporting and measurement could drive improvement include aiding in the development of national benchmarks that could be used to identify regional differences, enabling the research community to identify the factors that promote or hinder quality health care, and assisting in linking patient outcomes with those responsible for those outcomes (Institute of Medicine, 2002).

Recently, some noteworthy efforts have been made to encourage standardization of reporting requirements. In terms of event reporting, the Patient Safety Task Force is beginning to standardize the reporting mechanisms among DHHS agencies. This task force, which began functioning in 2000 and was rechartered in 2001 by the secretary of DHHS, includes representatives from AHRQ, CDC, FDA, and CMS. Their primary activity has been a project to integrate the patient safety reporting systems within DHHS through a contract awarded to the Kevric Corporation. This integration will result in user-friendly reporting formats, cross-matching and electronic analysis of data, and more rapid responses to patient safety problems. The identification of standards for coding the content of reports made to these systems is a primary task of the project. While the project is initially integrating six of the DHHS systems, all patient safety reporting systems under the jurisdiction of the department will eventually be incorporated. (For further information on federal patient safety reporting systems, see Appendix C.)

In the area of best practices, the Quality Interagency Coordination Task Force (QuIC) was established in 1998 with representation from all of the federal agencies involved in purchasing, providing, studying, or regulating health care services.[2] QuIC has worked to address tasks that are key to the use of quality performance measures, such as developing an inventory of all

---

[2]QuIC membership includes the Departments of Defense, Veterans Affairs, Labor, Commerce, and Health and Human Services; the Office of Management and Budget; the Coast Guard; the Bureau of Prisons; the Federal Trade Commission; and the National Highway Transportation Safety Administration.

the measures and risk adjustment methods being used by federal agencies; documenting their uses, strengths, and weaknesses; and examining how to institute appropriate risk adjustment methods (Quality Interagency Coordination Task Force, 2001). QuIC has also made considerable progress in establishing standardized safety and quality measures and tools, such as the Diabetes Quality Improvement Project measures, which have been incorporated into multiple government health care programs.

Several private-sector groups are also working in this area. For example, the National Quality Forum (NQF), an organization created to develop and implement a national strategy for health care quality measurement and reporting, has established standardized reporting requirements for a set of 27 preventable adverse events called "never" or serious reportable adverse events (National Quality Forum, 2002).

On the performance and outcome measurement side, a large part of the work of the National Committee for Quality Assurance (NCQA), the accreditation program for managed care organizations, is reporting on a set of performance measurements in selected areas using HEDIS (National Committee for Quality Assurance, 2003). The set is updated annually and allows for comparison of the quality of commercial, Medicaid, and Medicare managed care plans. It measures the quality of care for many common health conditions and incorporates other established measure sets, including the Consumer Assessment of Health Plans, the Diabetes Quality Improvement Project, and the Health Outcomes Survey. Another private-sector group working in the area of standardization of performance measures is the Joint Commission on Accreditation of Healthcare Organizations (JCAHO), which accredits hospitals, ambulatory clinics and surgical centers, clinical laboratories, home health agencies, assisted living and long-term care facilities, behavioral health services, hospices, integrated delivery systems, health maintenance organizations, and preferred provider organizations. JCAHO initiated the ORYX initiative in 1997, under which accredited hospitals must contract with listed performance measurement vendors, who work to aggregate the organizations' patient-level data and report on a set of core performance measures in a standardized manner to JCAHO (Joint Commission on Accreditation of Healthcare Organizations, 2003). The Foundation for Accountability (FACCT), an organization of health care purchasers and consumer groups, has also been working toward more standardized performance measurement. Beginning in 1997, under a project initially funded by the Health Care Financing Administration (now CMS) for Medicare beneficiaries, FACCT created a "consumer information framework" that consists of a set of standard measures in five major categories:

the basics, staying healthy, getting better, living with illness, and changing needs (Foundation for Accountability, 1999). FACCT selected measures from multiple sources and is continuing to develop new measures to fill perceived gaps.

Despite all of these efforts, work on standardizing event reporting and performance measurement activities has been slow. In 2002, the IOM recommended that QuIC be given the statutory authority and adequate resources to coordinate and standardize the government's activities in the area of quality performance reporting (Institute of Medicine, 2002). This committee endorses that recommendation and agrees with the previous IOM committee that QuIC should coordinate its efforts with private-sector groups—including NQF, NCQA, JCAHO, and FACCT—involved in the promulgation of standardized event reporting and performance and outcome measures.

CURRENT STANDARDS ACTIVITIES IN THE FEDERAL AND PRIVATE SECTORS

As noted earlier, the efforts of both the public and private sectors to invest in information technology are hampered by the lack of national standards for the collection, coding, classification, and exchange of clinical, administrative, and reporting and quality assurance data. The role of the federal government in the promulgation of standards is one that is well developed in other sectors of the economy. For example, the Securities and Exchange Commission has statutory authority to establish financial accounting and reporting standards for all publicly held companies under the Securities and Exchange Act of 1934 (University of Cincinnati College of Law, 2003). Despite some well-publicized recent failures, these standards are meant to require credible, transparent, and comparable financial information that can be used by investors, creditors, and auditors. The commission often authorizes private-sector entities, such as the Financial Accounting Standards Board, to conduct this work and then officially recognizes the standards these entities develop as authoritative. In the health care sector, however, there has been a historical lack of federal coordination in the establishment of national standards. With the exception of morbidity and mortality codes for public health reporting (i.e., ICD-9 codes) and code sets for reimbursement (i.e., ICD-9, CPT, and the Healthcare Financing Administration Common Procedure Coding System), each agency has determined any additional data interchange, reporting, and terminology standards for its own system.

This trend is changing, and efforts are currently under way that constitute important building blocks toward a national infrastructure for the promulgation of health care reporting requirements and standards. These efforts include AHRQ's EPCs and the work of QuIC, discussed earlier in this chapter, as well as the partnership between NCVHS and the CHI initiative.

National Committee on Vital and Health Statistics

A significant effort to establish common data standards is in progress under the leadership of NCVHS (National Committee on Vital and Health Statistics, 2000). NCVHS, first established in 1949 as a federal advisory committee on heath statistics issues, is made up of 18 members from the private sector. Its role was broadened by HIPAA to include identifying and recommending standards for administrative simplification and for the privacy and security of health care information, as well as to "study the issues related to the adoption of uniform data standards for patient medical record information (PMRI) and the electronic exchange of such information." While NCVHS has the lead in identifying and recommending clinical data standards, it has only an advisory role to DHHS and has not been empowered to designate or mandate standards.

Specifically, the HIPAA standards accomplished the following:

* Designated specific SDOs for the development and maintenance of HIPAA standards.
* Approved the ANSI ASC X12N standard as the EDI messaging format standard for eight administrative/financial transactions and NCPDP as the messaging standard for pharmacy billing transactions.
* Selected code sets for diagnoses and procedures for administrative/financial transactions, i.e., ICD-9 Clinical Modification (CM); Healthcare Financing Administration Common Procedure Coding System (HCPCS); CPT-4; NDCs; and Common Dental Terminology, Second Edition (CDT-2).
* Mandated identifiers for employers.
* Established privacy rules and security safeguards for the protection of personal health information.

Compliance deadlines have been established for all of the above HIPAA standards. In addition, the use of unique identifiers for health care providers has undergone the Notice of Proposed Rulemaking process and is awaiting announcement of the final rule. The HIPAA standard for claims attachments is being developed.

Consolidated Health Informatics Initiative

NCVHS is also serving as the primary advisory body to the CHI initiative, established in October 2001 as the first of the 24 Office of Management and Budget eGOV initiatives to streamline and consolidate government programs among like sectors (Office of Management and Budget, 2003). DHHS was designated as the managing partner for the CHI initiative, with CMS in the lead. Other members of CHI include the VHA, the Department of Defense, the Indian Health Service, the U.S. Department of Agriculture, Environmental Protection Agency, and the FDA. CHI's mission is to articulate and execute a coherent vision and strategy for the adoption of federal interoperability standards for health care information while providing technical support to selected projects. As noted earlier in this report, in March 2003 the secretary of DHHS announced that DHHS, the Department of Defense, and VHA would be adopting an initial set of clinical data interchange standards recommended to the secretary by NCVHS, including HL7, NCPDP, IEEE 1073, DICOM, and the Logical Observation Identifiers, Names, and Codes (LOINC) for laboratory tests and results (usually referred to as Laboratory LOINC). This announcement was based directly on the recommendations of CHI for standards that should be adopted government-wide. CHI is also continuing to identify standardized terminologies for the clinical domain areas associated with the EHR for use among federal agencies. The organizations are expected to announce their selection of the core group of standard terminologies in fall 2003. Given the sizable purchasing power (more than 40 percent of health care expenditures) and regulatory authority of the federal government, incorporation of these data standards into government programs is a powerful and effective approach to establishing national standards. However, CHI still lacks a clear mandate to establish standards that will be applied by all government programs. The CHI initiative also would benefit from greater participation of private-sector stakeholders and standards-setting bodies and from more clearly defined linkages with AHRQ's evidence synthesis program and QuIC's performance measurements standardization program.

Public Health Data Standards Consortium

In the public sector, in addition to CHI's activities, an organization that is involved in the promotion of national data standards is the Public Health Data Standards Consortium, which is coordinated by the National Center for Health Statistics. It was developed to organize the public health and health services research communities on data standards issues. This consortium serves as a mechanism for ongoing representation of public health and health services research interests in HIPAA implementation and other data standards–setting processes. Its membership comprises a variety of state-based public health data organizations, health services research organizations, federal public health representatives (e.g., CDC, AHRQ, and CMS), managed care organizations, business coalitions, and consumer groups. The consortium's tasks have included an ad hoc work group on External Causes of Injury Codes (E-Codes), which will evaluate current practices in E-Codes collection and propose next steps to improve E-Codes reporting in discharge data systems and electronic reporting standards. Two other consortium work groups recently developed a standardized format as a guide for reporting health care service data. This guide is compatible with the health claim transaction set standards identified by HIPAA. It is intended to provide assistance in developing and executing the electronic transfer of health care systems data for reporting purposes to local, state, and federal agencies that use the data for monitoring utilization rates, assessing patterns of health care quality and access, and other purposes required by legislative and regulatory mandates. Given the past difficulties and financial constraints of state-based public health organizations, the consortium could serve as one of the key facilitators helping states to implement national data standards for the NHII and guiding implementation of the common format for reporting to the AHRQ national patient safety database.

In addition to the efforts of NCVHS, other activities to promotion and implement data standards are being conducted in the private sector. The Markle Foundation's Connecting for Health initiative is focusing on building consensus around and accelerating the development of clinical data standards. In June 2003, this initiative released the results of a 9-month collaborative effort focused on key aspects of the adoption of clinical data standards, which included identifying strategies and solutions for the secure and private transmission of medical information and actively working to understand what consumers will need and expect from an interconnected electronic health system.

National Alliance for Health Information Technology

Another recent private-sector effort in the area of promotion and implementation of data standards is the National Alliance for Health Information Technology, founded in June 2002 by the American Hospital Association and other interested organizations (The National Alliance for Health Information Technology, 2002). Its membership currently includes provider organizations, such as hospitals, health systems, medical groups, and professional associations; technology companies and vendors; and other stakeholders, such as standards groups, the government, and payers. The purpose of the alliance is to develop and promote interoperability standards for health care information technology systems in order to improve patient outcomes and increase patient safety. In the near term, the alliance is focusing on standardized bar codes for products used by health care organizations. Plans for the longer term are to focus on connectivity and communications technology, automated order entry, electronic medical records, and standardized nomenclatures.

Integrating the Healthcare Enterprise

A third effort in the private sector was initiated by the Healthcare Information and Management Systems Society and the Radiological Society of North America in November 1998. The Integrating the Healthcare Enterprise initiative is working to facilitate the adoption of existing standards for communicating clinical and operational data by specifying how to apply such standards to real-world scenarios and integration problems (HIMSS, 2003). The initiative process consists of four steps: (1) identification of common integration problems and needs by clinicians and information technology experts, represented by their professional societies; (2) specification of the existing health care or other general information technology standards that address the identified needs; (3) participation by vendors in an open testing process; and (4) publication of Initiative Integration Statements documenting the integration profiles, which can be accessed by users to assist in the vendor selection process (HIMSS, 2003). To date, Integrating the Healthcare Enterprise has introduced several integration profiles—12 for radiology and 5 for information technology infrastructure—which were published in August 2003 (HIMSS, 2003). Despite these activities, the absence of national leadership in the establishment of standards for the collection, coding, and classification of data means that the information and communications systems built over the coming decade will provide inadequate support for the delivery of safe and effective care, will be unable to share information among all of a patient's caregivers, and will require costly rework to respond to external reporting requirements.

NEED FOR MORE FORMALIZED LEADERSHIP

If the NHII is to be realized, more formalized leadership in the establishment of data standards will be required. The committee's recommendations to this end center on a principal partnership among CHI, NCVHS, and NLM; overarching coordination; and strengthened leadership on the part of DHHS.

Principal Partnership: Consolidated Health Informatics, National Committee on Vital and Health Statistics, and National Library of Medicine

It is critical that Congress provide clear direction, enabling authority, and financial support for the establishment of national data standards to support patient safety. DHHS should be given the lead role in establishing and maintaining a public–private partnership for the promulgation of national standards for data interchange, terminologies, knowledge representation, and reporting (see Figure 3-2). Central to this public–private partnership is the CHI initiative, which should work collaboratively with NCVHS to identify data standards appropriate for national adoption as well as gaps in existing standards that need to be filled. Although NCVHS has already become a primary advisory body to CHI, this relationship needs to be formalized to ensure adequate representation of all stakeholders in the decision-making process. As a federal body that is subject to the Federal Advisory Committee Act, CHI cannot have private-sector members, but the viewpoints of many interested parties outside of the federal government should be considered. NCVHS is in a strong position to provide that input, as it is already designated as a private-sector advisory body to DHHS. The current membership of NCVHS includes individuals from health plans, universities, and other private organizations and associations with backgrounds in health statistics, electronic interchange of health care information, privacy and security of electronic information, population-based public health, purchasing or financing of health care services, integrated computerized health information systems, health services research, consumer interests in health information, health data standards, epidemiology, and the provision of health services (National Committee on Vital and Health Statistics, 2001). The membership of NCVHS should continue to be broad and diverse with adequate representation of all stakeholders, including consumers, state governments, professional groups, and standards-setting bodies.

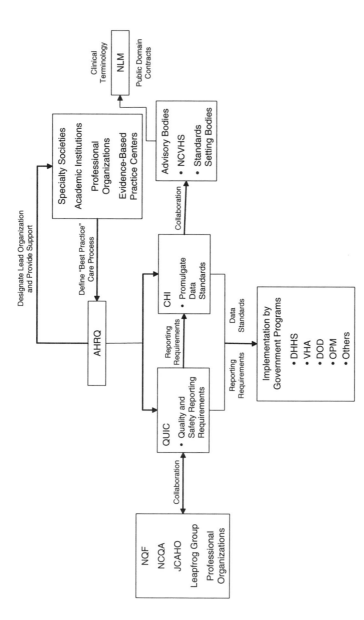

FIGURE 3-2 Proposed public-private partnership to establish national standards.

NOTE: AHRQ = Agency for Healthcare Research and Quality; CHI = Consolidated Health Informatics; DHHS = Department of Health and Human Services; DOD = Department of Defense; JCAHO = Joint Commission on Accreditation of Healthcare Organizations; NCQA = National Committee for Quality Assurance; NCVHS = National Committee on Vital and Health Statistics; NLM = National Library of Medicine; NQF = National Quality Forum; OPM = Office of Personnel Management; QuIC = Quality Interagency Coordinating Task Force; VHA = Veterans Health Administration.

One of the most powerful roles played by the federal government in the U.S. health care sector is that of regulator, and the government has historically used this role to address quality and patient safety concerns. Regulatory requirements (e.g., Medicare conditions of participation) generally focus on institutional providers, clinicians, and health plans that seek to receive payment from or deliver care under an identified program; however, these responsibilities can also be exercised by state governments that administer the programs. Therefore, once CHI and NCVHS have identified national data standards, those standards should be incorporated into the contractual and regulatory requirements of the major federal government health care programs, including those operated or sponsored by DHHS, VHA, and the Department of Defense. Broad stakeholder input into the data standards selection process should facilitate such incorporation, which will aid in rapid adoption of the identified data standards nationwide.

NLM also will need to assume new responsibilities for ensuring the establishment of national data standards for patient safety. As noted earlier in this chapter, NLM has worked to develop standardized mappings from one terminology to another through the UMLS and is therefore ideally positioned to become the primary oversight body for maintenance of the core terminology group to be established by CHI and associated patient safety data standards. The committee also recommends that NLM be designated as the responsible entity for the distribution of all national clinical terminologies related to patient safety and for assuring the quality of terminology mappings. NLM should work closely with the terminology developers to establish a more formalized development process and serve as a primary information source for CHI–NCVHS regarding available terminologies and areas in which terminologies are still needed.

Overarching Coordination

In addition to the need to strengthen the partnership and leadership of CHI, NCVHS, and NLM, the committee believes that AHRQ is an agency positioned to provide overarching coordination among all public- and private-sector organizations involved in the development, implementation, and dissemination of data standards, evidence-based guidelines, and patient safety and quality improvement programs. AHRQ is already the chief agency leading efforts in two of the three areas—evidence-based guidelines and patient safety and quality improvement programs—and as such has well-established core competencies in these areas, public–private networks, and relationships with the provider community that are critical to the successful development of the NHII. The committee believes it is important to build on AHRQ's expertise and capabilities by extending that agency's role in overarching coordination for the implementation and dissemination of data standards that support the agency's programs in clinical guidelines, patient safety data, and quality measures, as well as public health and the NHII. Additionally, AHRQ is playing a key role with providers and public health entities in addressing the challenges of building the NHII and has allocated $50 million of its $84 million fiscal year 2004 budget to support health information technology initiatives ($24 million for safety- and quality-related projects and $26 million for community and rural projects); $10 million of the budget has been allocated for standards adoption projects (Agency for Healthcare Research and Quality, 2003b). AHRQ also has the breadth and depth of resources to support the overarching coordination needed for widespread development of the NHII. The committee recognizes that the costs to support the corresponding programs and initiatives that would fall within the scope of AHRQ's coordinating activities would be significant. Because of AHRQ's historical, extensive experience in critical areas that directly relate to the NHII, it is best placed to provide a detailed cost estimate for development, implementation, and dissemination activities.

AHRQ can support the work of CHI–NCVHS in several ways. AHRQ should:

• Provide financial support for standards development activities as necessary to fill the standards gaps identified by CHI–NCVHS.
• Work with SDOs to ensure the development of implementation guides (which provide the specifications and instructions for how to implement a standard (*Federal Register*, 2000), certification procedures, and conformance testing for all data standards to facilitate their adoption by vendors and users. Additional information on the standards implementation process is presented in Chapter 4.
• Coordinate activities and maintain a clearinghouse of information in support of national data standards and their implementation to improve patient safety.
• Move forward with the establishment of a national patient safety database that utilizes a common report format and associated data standards as recommended by the IOM (2000).
• Take on a chief role in the development of a robust agenda for applied research in patient safety, focused on enhancing knowledge, developing information technology tools, and disseminating research findings as outlined in Chapter 5.

- Build on its track record in funding the synthesis and dissemination of clinical knowledge and assume a lead coordinating role in working with health professions leadership, specialty societies, academic institutions, and others to translate clinical knowledge into best-practice care processes, which in turn will inform the CHI–NCVHS decision-making process regarding national knowledge representation standards.

Strengthened Department of Health and Human Services Leadership for the National Health Information Infrastructure

The NCVHS report *Information for Health* provides a high-level strategy for building the NHII (National Committee on Vital and Health Statistics, 2001). It includes as one of its chief recommendations the establishment of a new and separate office to handle policy, coordination, and strategic oversight for NHII initiatives and projects, led by a senior officer reporting directly to the secretary of DHHS. Since the report was issued, the NHII office has been established in the Office of Science and Data Policy within the Office of the Assistant Secretary for Planning and Evaluation. The NCVHS recommendations empowered the Office of Science and Data Policy with broad responsibilities, including coordination with all relevant stakeholders, the strategic planning for NHII development, management of the NHII budget, promotion of effective training methods in health informatics, and assurance that all population groups will share in the activities and benefits of information technology integration. The office is now beginning to exercise leadership and held its first NHII conference to develop specific goals and a strategic plan for the key areas of the infrastructure's operation: architecture, standards and vocabulary, safety and quality, financial incentives, consumer health, homeland security, privacy and security, and research and population health. The committee fully supports the NCVHS recommendations and the NHII activities conducted to date. At the same time, the committee believes that the NHII office must step forward more aggressively with stronger leadership and an accelerated approach to the integration of information technology into the health care delivery system.

REFERENCES

Agency for Healthcare Research and Quality. 2001. *Primary Care Practice-Based Research Networks: Fact Sheet.* Online. Available: http://www.ahcpr.gov/research/pbrnfact. htm [accessed September 5, 2003].

————. 2002. *Centers for Education and Research on Therapeutics: Overview.* Online. Available: http://www.ahcpr.gov/clinic/certsovr.htm [accessed September 15, 2003].

————. 2003a. *AHRQ—Evidence-Based Practice.* Online. Available: http://www. ahrq.gov/clinic/epcix.htm [accessed April 25, 2003a].

————. 2003b. *U.S. Department of Health and Human Services FY 2004 Budget in Brief.* Online. Available: http://www.hhs.gov/budget/04budget/fy2004bib.pdf [accessed November 10, 2003].

American College of Physicians. 2003. *About ACP Journal Club.* Online. Available: http://www.acpjc.org/shared/purpose_and_procedure.htm [accessed July 14, 2003].

American Diabetes Association. 1988. Eye care guidelines for patients with diabetes mellitus. *Diabetes Care* 11 (9):745–746.

American National Standards Institute. 2002. *ANSI Procedures for the Development and Coordination of American National Standards.* Online. Available: http://public. ansi.org/ansionline/Documents/Standards%20Activities/American% 20National%20Standards/Procedures,%20Guides,%20and%20Forms/ anspro2002r.doc [accessed June 1, 2003].

Apelon. 2003. *Apelon Awarded $4.7 Million Contract to Assist VA with Enterprise Terminology Development.* Online. Available: http://www.apelon.com/news/ press_040803.htm [accessed July 28, 2003].

Bakken, S., K. E. Campbell, J. J. Cimino, S. M. Huff, and W. E. Hammond. 2000. Toward vocabulary domain specifications for Health Level 7-coded data elements. *J Am Med Inform Assoc* 7 (4):333–342.

Balas, E. A., and S. A. Boren. 2000. Managing clinical knowledge for health care improvement. *Yearbook of Medical Informatics* 65–70.

Campbell, K. E., D. E. Oliver, and E. H. Shortliffe. 1998. The unified medical language system: Toward a collaborative approach for solving terminologic problems. *J Am Med Inform Assoc* 5 (1):12–16.

Chassin, M. R. 1997. Assessing strategies for quality improvement. *Health Aff (Millwood)* 16 (3):151–161.

Cochrane Collaboration. 2003. *Cochrane Collaboration Brochure.* Online. Available: http://www.cochrane.org/software/docs/newbroch.pdf [accessed July 14, 2003].

Department of Health and Human Services. 2003. *HHS Launches New Efforts to Promote Paperless Health Care System.* Online. Available: http://www.hhs.gov/news/press/ 2003pres/20030701.html [accessed July 7, 2003].

Diabetic Retinopathy Study Research Group. 1981. Photocoagulation treatment of proliferative diabetic retinopathy. Clinical application of Diabetic Retinopathy Study (DRS) findings, DRS report number 8: The diabetic retinopathy study research group. *Ophthalmology* 88 (7):583–600.

Eddy, D. M. 1998. Performance measurement: Problems and solutions. *Health Aff (Millwood)* 17 (4):7–25.

Federal Register. 2000. Rules and regulations—Part 160: General administrative requirements. *Fed Regist* 65 (160):50365–50367.

Foundation for Accountability. 1999. *The FACCT Consumer Information Framework.* Online. Available: http://www.facct.org/facct/doclibFiles/documentFile_203.doc [accessed July 30, 2003].

Government Printing Office. 2003. *H.R. 2033: Medicare Equity and Access Act.* Online. Available: http://frwebgate.access.gpo.gov/cgi-bin/getdoc.cgi?dbname=108_cong_ bills&docid=f:h2033ih.txt.pdf [accessed July 30, 2003].

Health Level Seven. 2002. *Bylaws of Health Level Seven, Inc.* Online. Available: http://www.hl7.org/about/bylaw.htm [accessed June 1, 2003].

HIMSS. 2003. *Integrating the Healthcare Enterprise (IHE) Fact Sheet.* Online. Available: http://www.himss.org/content/files/IHE_FactSheet.pdf [accessed July 30, 2003].

Institute of Electrical and Electronics Engineers. 2001. *About IEEE 1073.* Online. Available: http://www.ieee1073.org/info/about-contacts.html [accessed February 12, 2002].

Institute of Medicine. 2000. *To Err Is Human: Building a Safer Health System.* Washington, DC: National Academy Press.

———. 2002. *Leadership by Example: Coordinating Government Roles in Improving Health Care Quality.* Washington, DC: The National Academies Press.

———. 2003. *Priority Areas for National Action: Transforming Health Care Quality.* Washington, DC: The National Academies Press.

Joint Commission on Accreditation of Healthcare Organizations. 2003. *Performance Measurement.* Online. Available: http://www.jcaho.org/pms/index.htm [accessed July 30, 2003].

Maviglia, S. M., R. D. Zielstorff, M. Paterno, J. M. Teich, D. W. Bates, and G. J. Kuperman. 2003. Automating complex guidelines for chronic disease: Lessons learned. *J Am Med Inform Assoc* 10:154–165.

McGinley, L. 2003, May 27. Medicare plan would give bonuses for superior care. *The Wall Street Journal.* Online. Available: http://online.wsj.com/article/0,,SB10539733 1989909600,00.html.

McGlynn, E. A., S. M. Asch, J. Adams, J. Keesey, J. Hicks, A. DeCristofaro, and E. A. Kerr. 2003. The quality of health care delivered to adults in the United States. *N Engl J Med* 348 (26):2635–2645.

MedBiquitous Consortium. 2003. *MedBiquitous Homepage.* Online. Available: http://www.medbiq.org [accessed May 13, 2003].

National Center for Health Statistics and CDC. 2003. *ICD 9 CM Coordination and Maintenance Committee.* Online. Available: http://www.cdc.gov/nchs/about/otheract/icd9/maint/maint.htm [accessed August 1, 2003].

National Committee for Quality Assurance. 1997. *Quality Compass 1997.* Annapolis Junction, MD: NCQA Publications Center.

———. 2003. *NCQA Overview.* Online. Available: http://www.ncqa.org/Communications/Publications/overviewncqa.pdf [accessed July 28, 2003].

National Committee on Vital and Health Statistics. 2000. *Uniform Data Standards for Patient Medical Record Information.* Online. Available: http://ncvhs.hhs.gov/hipaa000706.pdf [accessed April 15, 2002].

———. 2001. *Information for Health: A Strategy for Building the National Health Information Infrastructure.* Online. Available: http://ncvhs.hhs.gov/nhiilayo.pdf [accessed April 18, 2002].

National Library of Medicine. 2002. *UMLS Knowledge Sources.* January Release—13th Edition. Washington, DC: U.S. Department of Health and Human Services.

National Quality Forum. 2002. *Serious Reportable Events in Patient Safety: A National Quality Forum Consensus Report.* Washington, DC: National Quality Forum.

National Research Council. 1995. *Standards, Conformity Assessment, and Trade: Into the 21st Century.* Washington, DC: National Academy Press.

Nelson, S. J., S. H. Brown, M. S. Erlbaum, N. Olson, T. Powell, B. Carlsen, J. Carter, M. S. Hole, and W. T. Tuttle. 2002. A semantic normal form for clinical drugs in the UMLS: Early experiences with the VANDF. *J Am Med Inform Assoc* 557–561.

Office of Management and Budget. 2003. *Consolidated Health Informatics.* Online. Available: http://www.whitehouse.gov/omb/egov/gtob/health_informatics.htm [accessed April 21, 2003].

Ozbolt, J. 2000. Terminology standards for nursing: Collaboration at the summit. *J Am Med Inform Assoc* 7 (6):517–522.

Peleg, M., S. Tu, J. Bury, P. Ciccarese, J. Fox, R. Greenes, R. Hall, P. Johnson, N. Jones, A. Kumar, S. Miksch, S. Quaglini, A. Seyfang, E. Shortliffe, and M. Stefanelli. 2003. Comparing computer-interpretable guideline models: A case study approach. *J Am Med Inform Assoc* 10(1):52–68.

Premier, Inc. 2003. *HHS, Premier Announce New Initiative to Improve, Reward Healthcare Quality.* Online. Available: http://www.premierinc.com/all/newsroom/press-releases/03-jul/premier-cms.htm [accessed July 14, 2003].

Quality Interagency Coordination Task Force. 2001. *QuIC Fact Sheet.* Online. Available: http://www.quic.org/about/quicfact.htm [accessed April 28, 2003].

Rhew, D. C., M. B. Goetz, and P. G. Shekelle. 2001. Evaluating quality indicators for patients with community-acquired pneumonia. *Jt Comm J Qual Improv* 27 (11):575–590.

SNOMED International. 2000. *About SNOMED.* Online. Available: http://www.snomed.org/governance_txt.html [accessed August 1, 2003].

The National Alliance for Health Information Technology. 2002. *The National Alliance for Health Information Technology Prospectus.* Online. Available: http://www.hospitalconnect.com/nahit/content/prospectus.pdf [accessed May 30, 2003].

University of Cincinnati College of Law. 2003. *The Securities Lawyer's Deskbook: Securities Exchange Act of 1934.* Online. Available: http://www.law.uc.edu/CCL/34Act/index.html [accessed August 5, 2003].

Wang, A. Y., J. H. Sable, and K. A. Spackman. 2002. The SNOMED clinical terms development process: Refinement and analysis of content. *Proc AMIA Symp* 845–849.

World Health Organization. 1999. *Procedures for Updating ICD-10.* Online. Available: http://www.who.int/whosis/icd10/update.htm [accessed August 1, 2003].

4

Health Care Data Standards

CHAPTER SUMMARY

Data standards are the principal informatics component necessary for information flow through the national health information infrastructure. With common standards, clinical and patient safety systems can share an integrated information infrastructure whereby data are collected and reused for multiple purposes to meet more efficiently the broad scope of data collection and reporting requirements. Common data standards also support effective assimilation of new knowledge into decision support tools, such as an alert of a new drug contraindication, and refinements to the care process. This chapter provides both a short overview introducing data standards to the lay reader and a more technical review of the specific data standards required for the informatics-oriented professional. Please note that in the technical portion of the paper, once a standard is introduced it will be referred to in its acronym form due to the number of data standards involved. Readers may refer to the list of acronyms in Appendix B for assistance as needed.

OVERVIEW OF HEALTH CARE DATA STANDARDS

Although much of the data needed for clinical care, patient safety, and quality improvement resides on computers, there is as yet no means to trans-

127

fer these data easily and economically from one computer to another, despite the availability of the communications technologies to support such data exchange. The chief obstacle to achieving this capability has been the haphazard adoption of data standards for organizing, representing, and encoding clinical information so that the data can be understood and accepted by the receiving systems (Hammond, 2002). At the level of the health care organization, the lack of common data standards has prevented information sharing between commercial clinical laboratories and health care facilities, between pharmacies and health care providers regarding prescriptions, and between health care organizations and payers for reimbursement (Hammond, 2002). The lack of standards has also prevented the reuse of clinical data to meet the broad range of patient safety and quality reporting requirements, shown in Table 4-1. The first column of this table lists the data sources often associated with an electronic health record (EHR); the second, those associated with clinical information systems, decision support tools, and external data sources; the third, state, regulatory, and private-sector patient safety reporting systems; and the fourth, federal reporting systems. The fact that there is no standard means of representing the data for any of these datasets or requirements is astonishing and highlights the amount of unnecessary work performed by health care and regulatory organizations to prepare, transmit, and use what amount to custom reports. The federal government has recognized this problem and is moving forward with the integration of its safety-related systems. This study goes further by recommending common standards for the clinical and patient safety data that span the full range of data sources listed in Table 4-1. Many of the data standards required are already available; others need further development.

What Are Data Standards?

In the context of health care, the term *data standards* encompasses methods, protocols, terminologies, and specifications for the collection, exchange, storage, and retrieval of information associated with health care applications, including medical records, medications, radiological images, payment and reimbursement, medical devices and monitoring systems, and administrative processes (Washington Publishing Company, 1998). Standardizing health care data involves the following:

- *Definition of data elements*—determination of the data content to be collected and exchanged.
- *Data interchange formats*—standard formats for electronically encod-

ing the data elements (including sequencing and error handling) (Hammond, 2002). Interchange standards can also include document architectures for structuring data elements as they are exchanged and information models that define the relationships among data elements in a message.

- *Terminologies*—the medical terms and concepts used to describe, classify, and code the data elements and data expression languages and syntax that describe the relationships among the terms/concepts.
- *Knowledge Representation*—standard methods for electronically representing medical literature, clinical guidelines, and the like for decision support.

At the most basic level, data standards are about the standardization of data elements: (1) defining what to collect, (2) deciding how to represent what is collected (by designating data types or terminologies), and (3) determining how to encode the data for transmission. The first two points apply to both paper-based and computer-based systems; for example, a laboratory test report will have the same data elements whether paper or electronic. A data element is considered the basic unit of information, having a unique meaning and subcategories of distinct units or values (van Bemmel and Musen, 1997). In computer terms, data elements are objects that can be collected, used, and/or stored in clinical information systems and application programs, such as patient name, gender, and ethnicity; diagnosis; primary care provider; laboratory results; date of each encounter; and each medication. Data elements of specific clinical information, such as blood glucose level or cholesterol level, can be grouped together to form datasets for measuring outcomes, evaluating quality of care, and reporting on patient safety events.

Associated with data elements are data types that define their form. Simple data types include date, time, numeric, currency, or coded elements that rely on terminologies (Hammond, 2002). Examples of complex data types are names (a structure for names) and addresses. For comparability and interchange, data types must be universal and must be carried through all uses of the data. The designation of common scientific units is also necessary. Units (e.g., kilograms, pounds) must be specified as another measure to prevent adverse events such as those related to dosing errors. Until recently, each institution or organization defined independently the data it wished to collect and the units employed, did not use data types, and created local vocabularies, resulting in fragmentation that prevented reuse.

For data elements that rely on terminologies and their codes for definition, merely referencing a terminology alone does not provide enough speci-

TABLE 4-1 Comprehensive List of Health Care Data Sources and Reporting Requirements

Clinical Datasets	Other Data Sources for Patient Safety Information
Histories	Policies and procedures
Allergies	Human resources records
Immunizations	Materials management systems
Social histories	Time and attendance records
Vital signs	Census records
Physical examination	Decision support alert logs
• Physicians' notes	Coroners' datasets
• Nurses' notes	Claims attachments
Laboratory tests	Admissions data
Diagnostic tests	Disease registries
Radiology tests	Discharge data
Diagnoses	Malpractice data
Medications	Patient complaints and reports of adverse
Procedures	events
Clinical documentation	Reports to professional boards
Clinical measures for specific clinical	Trigger datasets (e.g., antidote drugs for
conditions	adverse drug events)
Patient instructions	Computerized physician order entry
Dispositions	systems
Health maintenance schedules	Bar-code medication administration systems
	Clinical trial data

Patient Safety Datasets and Taxonomies	Federal Reporting Systems Datasets

Patient Safety Datasets and Taxonomies

Eindhoven classification taxonomy
Near misses (development needed)
Adverse events (development needed)
Accreditation reporting dataset (Joint
Commission on Accreditation of
Healthcare Organizations [JCAHO])
Medical Specialty Society—such as
- Trauma/emergency
- Surgery
- Anesthesia
- Radiology
- Family practice
- Pediatrics
Private sector—subsets
- Medical Event Reporting System for
Transfusion Medicine (MERS TM)
- United States Pharmacopea (USP)
- National Coordinating Council for
Medication Error Reporting and
Prevention (NCC MERPS)
- MedMarx (by USP for medication
events)
- Emergency Care Research Institute
(ECRI)
States with mandatory reporting systems
- Colorado
- California
- Connecticut
- Florida
- Georgia
- Kansas
- Massachusetts
- Maine
- Minnesota
- New Jersey
- New York
- Nevada
- Ohio
- Pennsylvania
- Rhode Island
- South Carolina
- South Dakota
- Tennessee
- Texas
- Utah
- Washington
- Oregon (voluntary system)

Federal Reporting Systems Datasets

Agency for Healthcare Research and Quality
- Prevention Quality Indicators (PQI)
- Quality Indicators for Patient Safety
(QIPS)
Centers for Disease Control and Prevention
- National Electronic Disease
Surveillance System (NEDSS)
- Dialysis Surveillance Network (DSN)
- Vaccine Adverse Event Reporting
System (VAERS)
- Vaccine Safety Datalink (VSD)
- National Nosocomial Infection
Surveillance System (NNIS)
- National Center for Health Statistics
(NCHS)
Centers for Medicare and Medicaid Services
- Medicare Patient Safety Monitoring
System (MPSMS)
- Minimum Data Set (MDS) for Nursing
Home Care
- End-stage renal disease (ESRD)
- Outcome and Assessment Information
Set (OASIS) for Home Care
Food and Drug Administration
- Adverse Event Reporting System
(AERS)
- Manufacturer and User Data
Experience (MAUDE)
- Special Nutritionals Adverse Event
Monitoring System (SNAEMS)
- Biological Product Deviation Reporting
System (BPDR/BIODEV)
- Medical Product Surveillance Network
(MedSun)
- MedWatch (postmarket surveillance)
Nuclear Regulatory Commission
- Radiation events
Noncommunicable Diseases
- Cancer Registry

ficity. To ensure data comparability, specific codes must be identified within each terminology set to represent the data elements. This becomes a major issue for some of the larger clinical terminologies, which may have hundreds or thousands of terms. It is also a major issue given the amount of data that must be collected for the data sources and requirements listed in Table 4-1 and that will be encompassed by the national health information infrastructure (NHII). Common data standards are essential to simplify and streamline data requirements and allow the information systems that carry the data to function as an integrated enterprise.

TECHNICAL REVIEW OF HEALTH CARE DATA STANDARDS[1]

This section provides a detailed technical review of the three primary areas in which standards for health care data need to be developed: data interchange, terminologies, and knowledge representation. The final subsection addresses the implementation of these data standards.

Data Interchange Standards

In the area of data interchange, standards are needed for message format, document architecture, clinical templates, user interface, and patient data linkage.

Message Format Standards

Message format standards facilitate interoperability through the use of common encoding specifications, information models for defining relationships between data elements, document architectures, and clinical templates for structuring data as they are exchanged. In March 2003, the Consolidated Health Informatics (CHI) initiative announced its requirement that all federal health care services agencies adopt the primary clinical messaging format standards (i.e., the Health Level Seven [HL7] Version 2.x [V2.x] series for clinical data messaging, Digital Imaging and Communications in Medicine [DICOM] for medical images, National Council for Prescription Drug Programs [NCPDP] Script for retail pharmacy messaging, Institute of Elec-

---

[1]Numerous acronyms appear in the discussion in this section. We follow the convention of defining each upon its first appearance and using the acronym thereafter. All acronyms used here are defined in Appendix B.

trical and Electronics Engineers [IEEE] standards for medical devices, and Logical Observation Identifiers, Names and Codes [LOINC] for reporting of laboratory results) (Office of Management and Budget, 2003). It is worth noting that HL7, through its Laboratory Automated Point-of-Care Special Interest Group, has also developed messaging standards for the devices used in laboratory automation (e.g., robots and laboratory instruments) and point-of-care test devices (e.g., blood glucose monitors). These standards are in the process of being incorporated into IEEE standards and eventually will become standards at the International Organization for Standardization (ISO).

The HL7 V2.x series is the primary data interchange standard for clinical messaging and is presently adopted in 90 percent of large hospitals (American National Standards Institute, 2002). However, there have been a number of technical problems with the standard that have been difficult to resolve. For one, "conditional optionality" was built into the framework such that it permits a number of terminologies to represent a data element (e.g., Systemized Nomenclature of Human and Veterinary Medicine [SNOMED], LOINC) without being precise about the specific codes (i.e., allowable values) within the terminology (Hammond, 2002). The "openness" of the optionality has led to discrepancies in the application of the standard and misunderstanding of the specifications due to different vendor information models. Also, although V2.x does not support Web-based protocols (e.g., Simple Object Access Protocol [SOAP]), it can be sent over the Internet and expressed as an extensible markup language (XML) syntax standard (Hammond, 2002). However, V2.x does not incorporate an information model that is needed for more advanced messaging of clinical information.

Resolving these issues would be time consuming and labor intensive and could easily be accomplished by completion and implementation of HL7 Version 3.0 (V3), in which few of the data fields are open to interpretation. Currently, the scope of the V3 standard remains the same as that of V2.x; however, the initial release of V3 did not include the domains for patient referrals, patient care, or laboratory automation, all of which are important to patient safety (Health Level Seven, 2001). To move forward, the first step is to accelerate the completion of V3 and develop implementation guides for the use of both V2.x and V3 and interoperability between the two standards, with clear definition of the standard specifications. Both V2.x and V3 require a controlled terminology specified at the data element level to support interoperability. Additionally, since V2.x will probably continue to be widely used for some time, it is important that any difficulties with interoperability between this standard and others be resolved. For example,

V2.x is used for medication order messages in the inpatient and outpatient settings, while the NCPDP Script standard is used by retail pharmacies. Ensuring interoperability between these two standards is necessary for high-functioning systems.

HL7 V3 differs from V2.x in that it incorporates a Reference Information Model (RIM) for setting up the messaging format. The RIM is based on object-oriented modeling, expressing the classes of information required and the properties of those classes, including attributes, relationships, and states (Health Level Seven, 2001). The structured specifications of the information requirements minimize optionality by clearly defining each aspect of the RIM (Van Hentenryck, 2001). Data fields are populated with explicit controlled vocabulary, increasing semantic interoperability among various code sets (Van Hentenryck, 2001). Additionally, HL7 V3 messages are encoded using XML (as are Versions 2.4 and 2.5), which is easy to use, extensible, capable of representing complex data, and Internet compatible (Van Hentenryck, 2001). XML is used to exchange the data quickly and simply, but the RIM is needed to provide the necessary semantic interoperability.

At the core of the RIM are four high-level classes from which all other classes are derived—entity, role, participation, and act. Figure 4-1 is a simplified depiction of the structural relationships encompassed by the RIM that should aid in understanding the basis of the model.

Information modeling facilitates recognition of high-risk procedures having a direct impact on patient safety (Russler, 2002). Both safe active patient care and retrospective analysis for a patient safety event depend on proper information relationships (Russler, 2002). To this end, the information model must facilitate the process of care such that the link from entities to their intentional actions can support the information relationships used in analyzing patient safety issues, as well as larger issues of cost and quality improvement (Russler, 2002). Using an analogy from aviation, examination of the link between a precipitating event and an adverse event is as important as comparing the data from a flight data recorder with the data from the voice recording in the cockpit in the case of an airline accident (Russler, 2002).

HL7 V3 and the RIM are particularly important to the advancement of integrated clinical systems because they provide the backbone for the next set of standards needed for the EHR including those required for the use of concept-oriented terminologies, document architectures, clinical templates, alerts and reminders, and automated clinical guidelines, all of which would result in improved interoperability and structuring of clinical and patient data.

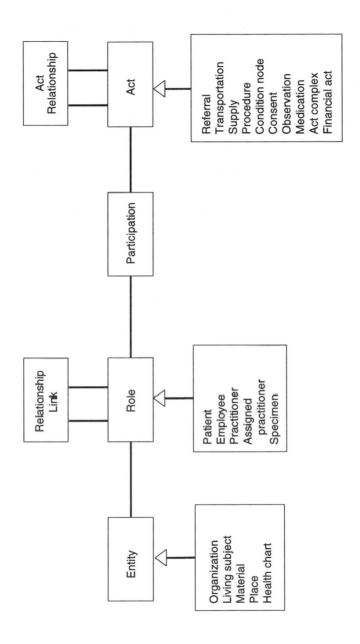

FIGURE 4-1 HL7 reference information model.
SOURCE: Hammond, 2002.

Document Architecture

A method for representing electronically clinical data such as discharge summaries or progress notes and patient safety reports requires a standardized document architecture. This need stems from the desire to access the considerable content currently stored in free-text clinical notes and to enable comparison of content from documents created on information systems of widely varying characteristics (Dolin et al., 2001). The architecture should be designed as a markup standard (Dolin et al., 2001) so that clinical documents can be revised as needed or appended to existing documents. It should also be able to accommodate the desire for rich narrative text that makes up a significant portion of patient safety information from voluntary and mandatory reports.

One example is the HL7 Clinical Document Architecture (CDA), a defined, complete information object that can include text, images, sounds, and other multimedia content (Dolin et al., 2001). The CDA provides a hierarchical set of specifications for the structure of clinical documents and derives its semantic content from the RIM (Dolin et al., 2001). Initial specifications define the document header in detail (i.e., identifying document name, type, source, author, date–time, and the like, including an area for narrative text), while the document body is structured to represent narrative clinical notes. This structure minimizes technical barriers to the adoption of the standard in that it intentionally lacks some of the complex semantics used in HL7 V3 messages. The initial specifications lay the foundation for future specifications that will incorporate clinical templates and additional RIM-derived markup, enabling the clinical content to be expressed more formally to the extent that it can be encompassed fully in the RIM or V3 message (Dolin et al., 2001). Again, because both HL7 V2.x and V3 will be in use for the short term and midterm, implementation protocols should include the ability of systems to translate CDA documents to and from V2.x and V3.

Clinical Templates

HL7 V3 provides the mechanism to specify further constraints on the optionality of the data elements through the use of templates that can be applied against a V3 message or document. The HL7 V3 messages maintain moderate optionality, although the RIM provides some constraints. For greater precision in standardization of clinical data, more targeted specifications of the allowable values for the data elements must be applied. A template in the broadest sense is simply a constraint on a more generic model that permits, among other things, the definition of a complex object, such as a blood chemistry measurement or a heart murmur (Hammond, 2002). For example, an HL7 message format for laboratory observations may specify that the data elements for a complete blood count test must include measurements for hemoglobin, hematocrit, and platelets. The design of constraints will be left to the discretion of health care organizations and providers, as HL7 provides the mechanisms and technical specifications for their use. Clinical templates will be important in the development of electronic structure for the collection and analysis of clinical and patient safety data, particularly those related to the 20 priority areas identified by the Institute of Medicine (2003).

User Interface

The medical device industry is well versed in developing user interfaces that make devices safer, more effective, and easier to use by employing a voluntary standard for human factors design established by the Association for the Advancement of Medical Instrumentation (AAMI) and approved by the American National Standards Institute (ANSI) (Association for the Advancement of Medical Instrumentation, 2001). This standard—the ANSI/AAMI HE74 Human Factors Design Process for Medical Devices—establishes tools and techniques to support the analysis, design, testing, and evaluation of both simple and complex systems; these tools and techniques have been applied for many years in the engineering of consumer products, military applications, aviation equipment, and nuclear power systems. Consideration of the HE74 standard may provide insight into the processes employed for designing and developing user-friendly clinical information systems, including electronic patient safety reporting systems.

An overview of the human factors engineering process that governs HE74 is provided in Figure 4-2. The specific activities at each step in the cycle vary with the particular development effort (Association for the Advancement of Medical Instrumentation, 2001). The cycle in Figure 4-2 emphasizes the iterative nature of the development process, whereby the outcomes (i.e., outputs) of one step provide input to the next step, but also, as needed, the output of some steps feeds back to previous steps. Although entry into the cycle can begin at any step, involving users at the early stages of development is critical. Once user needs and the consequent concept for the device (system) have been well defined, it becomes possible to address the design criteria/requirements that define the operating conditions, user

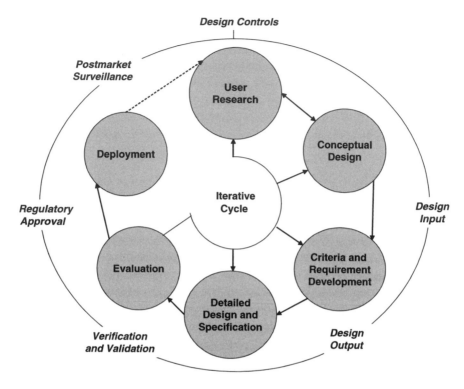

FIGURE 4-2 Human factors engineering process governing the HE74 standard.
SOURCE: Association for the Advancement of Medical Instrumentation, 2001.

characteristics, functions, and potential hazards of the device/system. The
hardware and software designers can then craft the necessary technical requirements and specifications. Next, structured evaluation of the resulting
device/system can ensure that the design is technically sound (i.e., verification) and that it also meets the user's needs and intended uses (i.e., validation). The last step—implementation and deployment—is related to the
manufacturing, marketing, sales, and regulatory aspects of the device/sys-
tem, including postmarket surveillance and vigilance reporting that provide
critical data on design strengths and shortcomings (Association for the Advancement of Medical Instrumentation, 2001). Whether this model or another is developed, the committee urges further research on the development of user interfaces for integrated systems.

HL7 has taken an approach to data integration at the visual level by way of the user interface. These applications and standards facilitate the integration of multiple independent applications from many different systems through interface standards (Van Hentenryck, 2001). An example is the ANSI-certified HL7 Context Manager standard, illustrated in Figure 4-3. The context manager standard establishes the primary architecture, a core set of data definitions, rules for application user interfaces, security specifications, and translation of the architecture for interoperability with applications in a way that is technology neutral (Van Hentenryck, 2001). With the Context Manager, an organization can give providers a single sign-on capability so they do not have to log on for each separate clinical application program they need (Seliger, 2003). Likewise, the Context Manager provides a single patient selection that, similar to a single clinician sign-on, allows all patient data in multiple applications to be readily available for use as needed by the clinician (Seliger, 2003). This context management gives users the experience of using a single system, when in fact they are accessing multiple applications simultaneously (Seliger and Royer, 2001).

For example, to review patients of immediate importance, a physician might inspect a patient list in a scheduling application. To further the understanding of each patient, the physician might also wish to view laboratory test results via a laboratory application, view computed axial tomography (CAT) scans via a picture archiving and communications system (PACS) application, and order new tests or medications via an order entry application (Seliger and Royer, 2001). The physician's selection of patient Jane Smith via the scheduling application would cause the other applications to tune into the same. In this way, the laboratory application, the PACS application, and the order entry application would all be synchronized with the physician's clinical context, in this case, Jane Smith as the patient currently of interest (Seliger and Royer, 2001).

Along with identifying users and patients, the Context Manager can identify concepts for unifying the availability of clinical data across applications. Two concepts for which the Context Manager specifications have been developed are the clinical encounter and clinical observation (Seliger, 2003). Thus a clinician can use an encounter or observation identifier to access multiple applications for information related to that encounter or observation.

User interface standards such as the Context Manager provide a mechanism to begin the process of achieving interoperability at the level of the user interface. Data linkage allows the users to create tiles of the different applications and compose them into a single visual window utilizing the

140

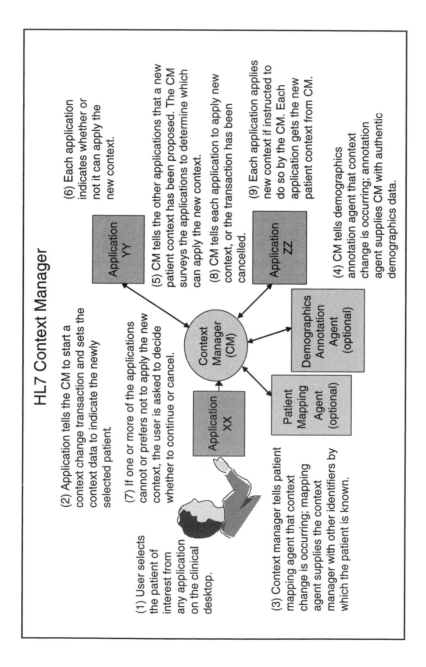

FIGURE 4-3 Overview of the HL7 Context Manager.
SOURCE: Seliger and Royer, 2001.

data currently held by the organization. Data are viewed in an integrated manner while the organization progressively builds a truly integrated, comprehensive clinical information system at the back end.

Patient Data Linkage

While not a data standard in the traditional sense, being able to link a patient's health care data from one departmental location or site to another unambiguously is important for maintaining the integrity of patient data and delivering safe care. The administrative simplification provisions of the Health Insurance Portability and Accountability Act (HIPAA) originally mandated the implementation of a unique health identifier for individuals. However, Congress withheld funding of the implementation pending adequate federal privacy protection. Now that the HIPAA privacy rules have been implemented nationwide, means to link patient data across organizations should be revisited.

In the meantime, pragmatic approaches to linking patient data have been emerging within the provider community. One approach used by many health care systems is the enterprise master patient index, which essentially creates a local unique patient identifier for persons cared for within a single health care system. Since most health care is local, and relationships among patients, physicians, and specific hospitals are ongoing, this approach has served as a viable interim solution; however, it is costly to maintain, does not address the issue of data coming from other systems of care, and requires the development of matching algorithims to solve such problems as patients with similar names. Because no algorithm is perfect, a small percentage of attempted matches will result in errors that can be recognized and reconciled only through human intervention.

Another approach under study, developed by the Patient Safety Institute (PSI) for its project to link health care providers statewide, is based on the Visa credit card network system which allows for connections among doctors' offices and hospitals (Carper, 2003). In PSI's network, PSI manages the automated system as a master patient index of only patient names and their identification numbers. Each hospital/clinic's method for identifying the patient data is mapped to this index, which is maintained by PSI. All medical data are retained by the health care organizations behind secure firewalls. Initially, authentication was accomplished through established hospital procedures. A three-key approach to authentication is in the process of being implemented: card and password for patient, digital certificate and password for physician, and permission key for the hospital or clinic. As of this writing, control features have not been implemented; access to medical information is "all or nothing." PSI is now in the process of implementing controls for two levels: general medical information and sensitive information (e.g., mental health, drug rehabilitation, HIV). Patients voluntarily opt into the program to allow their physicians access to past diagnoses, laboratory results, medications, allergies, and immunizations (Carper, 2003). Sensitive medical data (e.g., HIV status) are excluded from level-one access. PSI has also developed a set of guiding principles to safeguard access and limit exposure of patients' electronic medical data. These principles include avoiding use of a patient's social security number as their unique identifier, never releasing a patient's medical records to anyone without the patient's express authorization, physically separating a patient's clinical and demographic data, and using cutting-edge encryption technology and secure private networks (Carper, 2003).

The committee believes that the careful examination and development of innovative methods for patient data linkage should be undertaken against a background of changing technology, illness patterns, and consumer attitudes. In particular, changing demographics have resulted in the growth of chronic care conditions that involve multiple providers and data sources, making it more difficult to maintain and integrate relevant patient information. Consumers will be more involved in their self-care and disease management and will require the capability to utilize a personal health record and engage in electronic communication with their provider(s). Likewise, as they continue to become more savvy in accessing and understanding health information on the Internet, the demand for tools to incorporate this information into their care protocols and personal health records will likely increase. With HIPAA security rules in place, it is also possible to create patient data linkages in a manner that empowers patients to permit access to some of their data while restricting access to other, more sensitive data (e.g., mental health).

Terminologies

Standardized terminologies facilitate electronic data collection at the point of care; retrieval of relevant data, information, and knowledge (i.e., evidence); and data reuse for multiple purposes, such as automated surveillance, clinical decision support, and quality and cost monitoring. To promote patient safety and enable quality management, standardized terminologies that represent the focus (e.g., medical diagnosis, nursing diagnosis, patient problem) and interventions of the variety of clinicians involved in health care as well as data about the patient (e.g., age, gender, ethnicity, severity of illness, preferences, functional status) are necessary. Significant efforts during the last quarter-century have resulted in the development of standardized terminologies for the core phenomena of clinical practice: (1) diagnoses, symptoms, and observations (e.g., medical diagnoses, nursing diagnoses, problem list); (2) interventions, procedures, and treatments, including those focused on prevention and health promotion; and (3) health outcomes (e.g., disability, functional status, symptom status, quality of life) (Wang et al., 2002a). Although standardized measures for health outcomes have been developed, the incorporation of such measures into standardized terminologies has lagged behind that of measures for problems and interventions. Additionally, standardized terms for patient goals (i.e., expected outcomes) have been addressed only minimally and almost exclusively by the nursing community (Johnson et al., 2000). While no single current terminology has the breadth and depth needed for health care data, the National Library of Medicine (NLM) houses the world's largest database of standardized terminologies from a broad array of digital knowledge sources—the Unified Medical Language System (UMLS) (see Chapter 3). The terminology resources available through the UMLS are critical to initiatives to establish the NHII and to corresponding use of the EHR and patient safety systems.

Technical Criteria and Representation of Clinical Domains

Standardized terminologies vary along many dimensions; most important is the primary purpose of the terminology, as well as the extent to which it is concept oriented and possesses the semantic structures that enable computer (algorithmic) processing (Ingenerf, 1995; Rossi et al., 1998). To achieve the integrated approach to patient safety envisioned by the committee, the terminology must serve the purposes of decision support tools, the EHR, and knowledge resources (Chute et al., 1998). Terminology efforts for the EHR have focused on how to represent the history, findings, diagnoses, management, and outcomes of patients in a way that can preserve clinical detail and identify characteristics that enable improved risk adjustment, the development of common guidelines, aggregate outcome analyses, and shared decision support rules.

While a number of diverse terminologies are required for clinical care, patient safety, and other aspects of biomedicine, a central group of terminologies can serve as the backbone of clinical information systems. A number of technical criteria must be met for terminologies to function in a way that serves these purposes. The most basic criteria for a controlled medical vocabulary are identified by Cimino (1998); they include domain completeness, nonredundancy, synonymy, nonambiguity, multiple classification, consistency of views, and explicit relationships. In 1998, the ANSI Health Informatics Standards Board went a step further and created a detailed framework of informatics criteria for the development and evolution of terminologies with high functionality (Chute et al., 1998). The National Committee on Vital and Health Statistics (NCVHS) used these informatics criteria to evaluate and select a core set of well-integrated, nonredundant clinical terminologies that will serve as the national standard for medical terminology for the EHR (Sujansky, 2003) (Table 4-2).

Minimization of overlap in domain representation was another important criterion for selection of the NCVHS core terminology group. The CHI initiative is also evaluating the terminologies in this regard, as well as assessing their ability to meet the extensive data representation requirements for the common clinical domains that cut across the three dimensions of the NHII (i.e., provider health, personal health, and public health), points of overlap, and gaps in coverage. Issues related to data collection, sharing, and reuse are being addressed during the evaluations, as well as identification of the overlap and gaps in clinical representation. Table 4-3 provides an overview of the cross-cutting domains identified by CHI to date. The terminologies determined by CHI to best represent requirements of the clinical domain areas, after consultation with NCVHS, will be accepted for federal government–wide implementation. Additional areas within the clinical domains, including those relevant to patient safety, will be added as the process proceeds.

CHI is working rapidly and expects to make recommendations on terminologies to represent many, if not all, of the domain areas identified in Table 4-3 by late 2003. The first round of terminology evaluations includes laboratory results content, medications, demographics, immunizations, and interventions and procedures. Initially, CHI identified many of the domain areas that support the corresponding domains needed for patient safety reporting systems; however, the list is not comprehensive, and there will likely be a need to expand or extend the domains. For example, in the domain area for medications, CHI identifies clinical drugs, warnings, allergic reactions, and adverse drug events (ADEs) as primary areas for clinical representation. For patient safety, representation is also needed for subcategories, such as nutritional supplements and alternative medicines.

Expansion of the domain areas for comprehensive clinical and patient safety data is a subject for additional work. Appendix F provides a compre-

TABLE 4-2 Technical Criteria Used by the National Committee on Vital and Health Statistics for Evaluating and Selecting Terminologies

Required Technical Criteria

Concept orientation	Elements of the terminology are coded concepts, possibly with multiple synonymous text representations, and hierarchical or definitional relationships to other coded concepts. No redundant, ambiguous, or vague concepts are included (Sujansky, 2003).
Concept permanence	The meaning of each coded concept in a terminology remains forever unchanged. If the meaning of a concept needs to be changed or refined, a new coded concept is introduced. No retired codes are deleted or reused (Sujansky, 2003).
Nonambiguity	Concepts must have exactly one meaning. When a common term has two or more associated meanings, it must be separated into distinct concepts (Cimino, 1998).
Explicit version IDs	Each version of the terminology is designated by a unique identifier, such that parties exchanging data can readily determine whether they are using the same set of terms (Sujansky, 2003).

Desired Technical Criteria

Meaningless identifiers	Unique codes attached to concepts are not tied to hierarchal position or other contexts and do not carry any meaning (Chute et al., 1998).
Multihierarchies	Concepts are accessible through all reasonable hierarchical paths (i.e., multiple semantic patients) (Chute et al., 1998).
Nonredundancy	A mechanism must exist that can help prevent multiple terms for the same concept from being added to the terminology as unique concepts (Cimino, 1998).
Formal concept definitions	Concepts are defined by means of formal roles/attributes represented in description logic (Sujansky, 2003).
Infrastructure tools for terminology development	Software tools support and enforce a collaborative terminology development process (Sujansky, 2003).
Change sets	A complete change set is provided electronically as part of each update, including those concepts/terms that have been added, changed, and retired (Sujansky, 2003).
Mapping to other terminologies	Mappings to other terminologies should be algorithmic and derive from mapping tables or hierarchies within the classification or should be treated commonly (Chute et al., 1998).

TABLE 4-3 Clinical Domain Areas of the Consolidated Health Informatics Initiative

Priority 1 Task Groups Deployed	Priority 2 Forthcoming Task Groups
Demographics	History and physical, including:
Diagnosis/problem lists for:	History
Signs	Vital signs
Symptoms	Anatomy
Diseases	Exam findings
Social problems	Functional status
Interventions/procedures, including:	Immunizations
Laboratory orders	Population health, including:
Laboratory results contents	Nosocomial infections reporting
Encounters	Reportable infections reporting
Medications, including:	Other reportable conditions reporting
Clinical drugs	Hospital errors other than adverse drug
Warnings	reactions reporting
Allergic reactions	Emergency room trauma reporting
Adverse drug events	Other national health statistics
Text-based reports, including:	
Clinical document architecture	
Clinical document naming	

SOURCE: Office of Management and Budget, 2003.

hensive listing of the additional clinical domain areas needed to represent patient safety.

Evolution and Development of New Terms

In cases where domain coverage of a terminology is inadequate, the best sources of data for the development of new terms to represent clinical and patient safety information are the clinical measures within standardized datasets for a health condition derived from evidence-based guidelines, documentation of physical findings, and narrative text of patient safety reports. Once comprehensive datasets have been identified, it may be possible to develop extensions of existing terminologies for those areas that are insufficient in representing clinical or safety data. In other cases, it may be necessary to develop new terminologies. Each data element (e.g., measure, finding) should include definitions of patient safety terms for near misses,

Priority 3 Forthcoming Task Groups	Terminologies Used by Other Processes
Genes and proteins	Billing (HIPAA)
Multimedia, including but not limited to:	Chemicals (UMLS)
Image	Disability (International Classification of
Audio	Functioning, Disability and Health [ICF])
Waveforms	Scientific/fundamental (UMLS)
Nursing, including:	Units (UMLS)
Diagnoses	
Interventions	
Goals and outcomes	
Physiology	
Supplies, including	
Ontology for the ordering physician	
Medical devices	

adverse events, and medical errors for both commission and omission, as the basis for expanded clinical documentation in integrated systems. This approach takes into consideration the conceptual model for data integration discussed in Chapter 2.

For the 20 priority areas identified by the IOM in its 2003 report *Priority Areas for National Action,* efforts to extend and create complete terminologies for clinical and safety data should follow a process that:

- Supports evidence-based clinical guidelines.
- Clearly defines the condition in terms of clinical measurements and actions, and define safety in terms of what could go wrong with those measures or actions.
- Evaluates datasets to determine whether they truly represent data elements necessary to measure outcomes, including safety.

- Continues refining the taxonomy for safety by asking about the reasons for errors of omission and commission (e.g., why a foot exam was not given), in addition to using information extracted through natural language processing from the rich narrative in textual reports and data from surveillance and decision support systems.
- Determines precursors to potential adverse events (e.g., a fall) where possible.

The need for multiple levels of granularity and cross-organizational terminologies means that a dataset will need to be either initially represented by or mapped to a concept-oriented clinical reference terminology and further mapped to high-level taxonomies for comparative analysis and research. The committee encourages further work on developing standardized datasets with the capability to represent patient safety information in all clinical areas.

Selection of the Core Terminology Group

The NCVHS core terminology group comprises a core set of medical terminologies that together are sufficiently comprehensive, technically sound, mutually consistent, and readily available to deliver most of the envisioned functionality of a national standard medical terminology for the EHR (Sujansky, 2003). Having a common clinical reference terminology is expected to reduce the cost, increase the efficiency, and improve the quality of data exchange, clinical research, patient safety, sharing of computer guidelines, and public health monitoring. Terminologies to be included in the core group must have sufficient clinical granularity and serve multiple functions, including decision support, interoperability, aggregation and reporting, EHR data entry, order entry, indexing for data retrieval, and domain ontology. Supplemental terminologies should be mapped to the core terminologies to provide the functionalities associated with the use of data standards and information systems. Box 4-1 provides a brief overview of these terminologies.

On November 13, 2003, NCVHS officially recommended that the Department of Health and Human Services (DHHS) adopt five medical terminologies for use by federal health care services programs: SNOMED, Clinical Terms CT; Laboratory LOINC; RxNORM; the National Drug File Clinical Drug Reference Terminology (NDF RT); and the Food and Drug Administration's terminology sets for drug ingredient name, dosage form, and package form for drugs (National Committee on Vital and Health Statistics, 2003b). NCVHS continues to study additional terminologies that it may recommend for adoption at a later date. Also of note, NCVHS recently voted to recommend that HHS adopt the International Classification of Disease, 10th revision, or ICD-10, as the new coding system under the HIPAA rule, replacing the current ICD-9 system (National Committee on Vital and Health Statistics, 2003b).

SNOMED CT SNOMED CT is the most well-developed concept-oriented terminology to date. A concept-oriented reference terminology can be defined as one that has such characteristics as a grammar that defines the rules for automated generation and classification of new concepts, as well as the combining of atomic concepts to form molecular expressions (Spackman et al., 1997). SNOMED CT is based on a formal terminology model that provides nonambiguous definitions of health care concepts and contains the most granular concepts for representing clinical and patient safety information. For example, the atomic concepts of "diabetes mellitus," "self-management," and "education" could be combined to form "diabetes self-management and education," one of the priority areas identified by the IOM, as a precoordinated concept within a terminology or postcoordinated for a particular quality indicator report addressing errors of omission. SNOMED CT is designed to be the primary support for knowledge-based systems, the expression of clinical guidelines and datasets for the IOM priority conditions, and a key source for the development of new concepts for clinical and patient safety data. SNOMED CT's model was recently submitted to ANSI for approval as a standard. As part of the UMLS, it will serve as the core clinical reference terminology for the NHII (Department of Health and Human Services, 2003).

Laboratory LOINC Even with its comprehensiveness, SNOMED CT requires the support of additional terminologies to capture certain clinical data not currently available in the terminology with sufficient granularity or scope, namely laboratory, medication, and medical device data. LOINC has already been designated by CHI (in May 2003) as the terminology for representing laboratory test results and is a part of the NCVHS core terminology group (Consolidated Health Informatics Initiative, 2003). LOINC is the available terminology that most fully represents laboratory data in terms of naming for tests (e.g., chemistry, hematology) and clinical observations (e.g., blood pressure, respiratory rate). The LOINC terms are composed of up to eight dimensions derived from component (e.g., analyte), type of property

BOX 4-1
Overview of Core and Supplemental Terminologies

CORE TERMINOLOGIES

Systemized Nomenclature of Human and Veterinary Medicine, Clinical Terms (SNOMED CT)—developed by the College of American Pathologists, SNOMED CT is an inventory of medical terms and concepts for human and veterinary medicine arranged in a multihierarchical structure with multiple levels of granularity and relationships between concepts. Many nursing codes have been incorporated into the terminology. It is a comprehensive medical vocabulary and classification system with over 300,000 fully specified concepts and 450,000 supporting descriptions.

Logical Observation Identifiers, Names, and Codes (LOINC)—developed by the Regenstrief Institute, LOINC provides a set of universal names and numeric identifier codes for laboratory and clinical observations and measurements in a database structure without hierarchies whereby the records appear as line items. Currently, there are over 30,000 codes in the LOINC database.

RxNORM ("normalized" notations for clinical drugs)—developed in a joint project between the National Library of Medicine and the Veterans Health Administration to create a semantic normal form for a clinical drug, designed to represent the meaning of an expression typically seen in a physician's medication order. When released, RxNORM will represent the 81,165 clinical drugs in the Unified Medical Language System.

Universal Medical Device Nomenclature System (UMDNS)—developed by the Emergency Care Research Institute as a multihierarchical terminology for identifying, processing, filing, storing, retrieving, transferring, and communicating data about medical devices. UMDNS contains 17,221 terms.

SUPPLEMENTAL TERMINOLOGIES

Unique Ingredient Identifier (UNII)—developed by the Food and Drug Administration (FDA) as a method for coding molecular entities through their active and inactive ingredients.

Medical Dictionary for Drug Regulatory Affairs (MedDRA)—developed by the International Conference on Harmonization to harmonize international regulatory requirements for the drug development, marketing approval, and safety monitoring process. It provides a comprehensive vocabulary and coding system of 70,000 terms for safety-related events and adverse drug reactions.

Medicomp Systems Incorporated (MEDCIN)—a proprietary medical vocabulary designed as a controlled vocabulary of precorrelated clinical concepts from its nomenclature and associated knowledge base containing 175,000 clinical findings and diagnoses and 600,000 synonyms. It is considered a "user interface" terminology.

International Society for Blood Transfusion (ISBT)—developed by the American Blood Commission as a bar-code labeling specification for blood products. It was designed to capture additional and more complex information regarding the identification and content of blood and blood products on the label and to make that information universally accessible to the international blood banking community.

Diagnostic and Statistical Manual for Mental Disorders (DSM-IV)—developed by the American Psychiatric Association to provide a terminology and set of diagnosis codes for mental health conditions.

Pharmacy knowledge bases—developed by the vendor community, including FirstDatabank, Medi-Span, and Multum. These systems provide information about drug interactions, allergies, contraindications, drug–laboratory inferences, toxicology, and the like.

HIPAA Terminologies

International Classification of Diseases (ICD), Clinical Modifications (CM)—U.S. government expansion of the World Health Organization (WHO) coding system. ICD-9 CM provides approximately 15,500 terms and codes for diagnosis and inpatient services/procedures. The U.S. clinical modification of ICD-10 was published in late 2002. ICD-10 CM contains about 50,000 terms.

National Drug Codes (NDCs)—the standard code set developed by suppliers and maintained by the FDA to identify and regulate drugs and biologics marketed in the United States. The codes also are used for reimbursement of medicines. NDCs are employed for the approximately 10,000 drugs approved for use in the United States.

Current Procedural Terminology (CPT) and Health Care Financing Administration Common Procedure Coding System (HCPCS)—developed and maintained by the American Medical Association. CPT is the official code set for physician services in outpatient office practices. HCPCS provides codes for products, supplies, and services not in the CPT codes (e.g., ambulance service) and local codes established by insurers and agencies to fulfill claims processing needs. Together, CPT and HCPCS provide 7,300 terms.

Current Dental Terminology—developed by the American Dental Association to represent data related to dentistry.

Terminologies for Further Research

International Classification of Primary Care (ICPC)—developed by the World Organization of National Colleges and Academic Associations of General Practice/Family Doctors, ICPC allows simultaneous classification of the three elements related to an encounter in primary care: the process of care, the reason for the encounter, and the health problems diagnosed.

International Classification of Functioning, Disability and Health (ICF)—developed by WHO to provide a scientific basis for understanding information on health outcomes, determinants, and functional capacity that is complementary to the ICD.

(e.g., mass concentration), timing (e.g., 24-hour specimen), specimen (e.g., urine), and method (American National Standards Institute, 1997). LOINC also contains information for clinical observations that is not included in the core terminology group at this time, since it may be possible to represent many of the observations with SNOMED CT, and one of the criteria for selection is to minimize overlap in terminology representation. However, Clinical LOINC currently is and will continue to be used by a number of organizations.

For LOINC clinical measures, the code usually includes identification of the organ system. In addition, with Clinical LOINC, many measurements are distinguished for estimated, reported, and measured values (e.g., patient's report of his/her body weight versus a measured result or a physician's estimate) (American National Standards Institute, 1997). Varying degrees of precoordination for an observation are also provided for (e.g., cardiac output based on the Fick method versus based on the 2D method) (American National Standards Institute, 1997). Both Laboratory LOINC and those portions of Clinical LOINC that do not overlap with SNOMED CT are important terminologies for patient safety, as well as for the EHR.

Drug terminologies Drug terminologies are an important part of the core group. NCVHS has been evaluating which drug (and device) terminologies best represent these areas. The process for determining drug terminologies is more complex than that for identifying a comprehensive reference terminology and laboratory terminology. Representation of drug information involves both definitional and knowledge-based information (National Committee on Vital and Health Statistics, 2003a). Definitional information serves the purpose of interoperability by providing standardized terms to represent clinical drugs in clinical information systems. Knowledge-based information provides terminology for such phenomena as drug interactions, allergies, and contraindications, thus supporting greater functionality of clinical systems (National Committee on Vital and Health Statistics, 2003a). For purposes of standardizing data elements for patient medical records information, the core terminology group will be focused on definitional terms.

NLM has developed a normalized (i.e., standard) form for clinical drugs and their components—the RxNORM terminology. RxNORM assigns a standardized name for the active ingredient (i.e., generic), strength and physical form as given to the patient (e.g., 120 milligrams), and standard dosage form (e.g., tablet) (Brown et al., 2003). The semantic form provides the ability to link drug concepts from disparate vocabularies with naming variations developed by different pharmacy knowledge base vendors and drug manufacturers to match more closely the actual form a physician would order for a patient (Nelson et al., 2002). RxNORM was developed to be fully compatible with the FDA's system that provides identifiers/codes for active and inactive ingredients—the Unique Ingredient Identifier (UNII) project (Brown et al., 2003). Preliminary research on incorporating RxNORM into actual systems indicates that some refinements are needed (e.g., a few drugs need to be added) for greater precision and comprehensiveness; however, it will be possible to begin implementing it for use with clinical systems in the near term (National Committee on Vital and Health Statistics, 2003b).

In addition to RxNORM, other drug-related terminologies under consideration for inclusion in the core terminology group are the UNIIs and National Drug Codes (NDCs), both managed by the FDA, and the NDF RT being developed by the Veterans Health Administration. Following CHI's evaluation of the terminologies for representing the medication domain and presentation of findings in October 2003, NCVHS included these drug terminologies in its recommendation to DHHS.

Medical device terminologies A medical device terminology is also a must for the core terminology group. The two medical device terminologies being considered by NCVHS are the Global Medical Device Nomenclature (GMDN), developed by an international consortium to harmonize terms for regulatory purposes, and the Universal Medical Device Nomenclature System (UMDNS), developed and maintained by the Emergency Care Research Institute (ECRI). The terminology selected should be comprehensive in scope to cover the range of devices and their functions; capable of representing adverse events and malfunctions related to the devices; inclusive of emerging technologies used in investigative settings; sufficiently granular to capture essential data without losing critical information; and capable of being continuously maintained at a high level of technical quality, being mapped to other terms in use, and supporting high-quality translation to other languages for international use (Coates, 2003a).

Although the GMDN consortium initiated its activities using international standards and collaborated with six primary device terminology developers, the FDA found that the final resulting terminology did not meet the above criteria. The terminology that most closely meets these criteria is UMDNS. UMDNS provides a formal hierarchical system for representing complex medical device concepts, with content expressed in preferred terms and codes, entry terms, parent–child–sibling relationships, attributes, definitions, mappings, and linkages (Coates, 2003b). The process for maintaining the terminology is well developed at ECRI. In addition, ECRI functions as a collaborating center for the World Health Organization (WHO), an Agency for Healthcare Research and Quality (AHRQ) Evidence-Based Practice Center, a National Guideline Clearinghouse, and a National Quality Measures Clearinghouse, and it maintains an extensive patient safety reporting system (Coates, 2003b). These functions are important to the development of an integrated information infrastructure and the NHII, and the committee supports the inclusion of UMDNS in the NCVHS core terminology group. For international regulatory purposes, subsequent modifications and enhancements of the GMDN by the FDA may render it mappable to the terminologies in the core terminology group.

Mapping terminologies Mapping terminologies is a challenging task. The detailed terminologies of the core group and less granular classifications can be thought of as existing along a continuum of detail; for example, patient information can be expressed in a detailed nomenclature, such as SNOMED CT, funneling into a classification rubric, such as an ICD-9, Clinical Modification (CM) code (Chute, 2003). This is a limited one-way process in that once patient data have been expressed solely in the form of classifications, the original detail is lost and generally cannot be recovered. In many cases, this funneling process can be accomplished satisfactorily through a simple mapping or table that indicates which classification code subsumes a detailed description. However, such code-to-code mappings often fail since some terminologies incorporate complex criteria that can be reliably achieved only with rules for aggregating several patient details (Chute, 2003). Thus, such "aggregation logics" afford the automated and accurate mapping of detailed patient data into broader classifications, even for complex cases.

To satisfy the needs for the NHII and the EHR, computer-executable aggregation logic would stem from SNOMED CT and the other terminologies in the core group to the supplemental terminologies. It is also critical that the integration and mapping of the terminologies be based on the same information model as that of the data interchange standards—the HL7 RIM—to ensure optimum system functionality and interoperability (National Committee on Vital and Health Statistics, 2003a).

The committee believes that several supplemental terminologies are necessary to support the requirements for an integrated information infrastructure that supports multiple methods of collecting, analyzing, disseminating, and incorporating patient safety data with consideration for the differences among health care settings. As noted earlier, the terminologies must support system functionality and knowledge-based activities such as automated chart reviews and surveillance, voluntary reporting, natural language processing of narrative text, decision support tools (e.g., alerts and reminders), and the use of computer-readable evidence-based clinical guidelines. The supplemental terminologies outlined in Box 4-1 would be mapped through aggregation logic to the NCVHS core terminology group. These terminologies include HIPAA-designated code sets (i.e., ICD-9 CM, Current Procedural Terminology [CPT]-4, the Health Care Financing Administration Common Procedure Coding System [HCPCS], NDCs, Current Dental Terminology [CDT]), primary pharmacy knowledge bases (i.e., FirstDatabank National Drug Data File [NDDF]; plus MediSpan, Multum Lexicon), the Medical Dictionary for Drug Regulatory Affairs (MedDRA), UNII, International Society for Blood Transfusion [ISBT] 128, the Diagnostic and Statistical Manual for Mental Disorders [DSM-IV], and those nursing terminologies not already incorporated into SNOMED CT.

Terminologies for further investigation and research The NCVHS core terminology group and the supplemental terminologies support the basic functionalities of the conceptual model for integrated systems presented in Chapter 2. However, the committee has determined that two additional terminologies are also needed and warrant further investigation and research—the International Classification of Functioning, Disability and Health (ICF) to represent outcomes data, and the International Classification of Primary Care (ICPC) to represent the data needs of the office practice clinician.

Promising sources for standardized representation of functional status and outcome reporting include the WHO International Classification of Functioning and Disability (WHO ICF) and nursing terminologies such as the Nursing Outcomes Classification (Johnson et al., 2000). Functional status can be regarded as the demonstrated or anticipated capacity of an individual to perform or undertake actions or activities deemed essential for independent living and physiological sustenance (Ruggieri et al., forthcoming). Computer formats for clinical data describing the functional status of patients will be in increasing demand for measuring the impact of health care interventions and gauging quality of life (Ruggieri et al., forthcoming). These outcome measures can be used not only to capture the effect of an intervention on health status but also to control symptoms of a chronic condition, supplement specific clinical findings, or understand the patient's perception of care (Nerenz and Neil, 2001). Information on functioning as a supplement to diagnosis provides a broader, more meaningful picture of individual or population health over time that can be used for clinical decision making (World Health Organization, 2001), reporting and surveillance, and research and analysis.

The Mayo Clinic is undertaking a study to determine how well ICF can represent functional status data as they emerge traditionally within the health care setting (Ruggieri et al., forthcoming). Preliminary findings suggest that in their current state, ICF terms lack unambiguous clarity, fidelity, and hence usability across the ranges of clinical data and granularity required for the varied and extensive use cases that rely on the representation of functional status data (Ruggieri et al., forthcoming). However, ICF provides an important foundation from which clinical modifications and extensions can be developed to support robust functional status descriptions and representations in a broad spectrum of clinical domains and use cases (Ruggieri et al., forthcoming). Further study and development of outcome terminologies for patient safety applications, including nursing terminologies, are recommended.

ICPC was developed by the World Organization of National Colleges and Academic Associations of General Practice/Family Doctors (WONCA) to provide a system for classifying the broad range of symptoms, unease and difficulties, and conditions that make up those problems related to primary care that cannot be documented with the ICD codes (WONCA, 1998). More specifically, ICPC provides for simultaneous classification of the three elements of an encounter: the process of care, the reason for the encounter, and the health problem diagnosed (WONCA, 1998). Although ICPC is not widely used in the United States, it is the primary classification system used by much of the international community for electronic documentation of clinical practice in primary care or for reporting to national governments (Marshall, 2003). ICPC is used (in conjunction with ICD-9) extensively in the European Union and former U.K. countries, which have the most robust EHRs in the world. A study in Finland found repeatedly that ICPC permits coding of 95 percent or more of primary care visits (episodes of care), compared with 50 percent for ICD-9 (diagnosis) (Jamoulle, 2001). The ability to monitor episodes of care would support concurrent surveillance efforts by permitting a longitudinal look at patient symptoms, encounters (including diagnoses and treatments), and outcomes.

Because ICPC captures episodes of care, it has also been used to produce probability tables for presenting symptoms and diagnoses. This function could support the development of triggers in data monitoring or data mining systems and could be the basis for a much more robust decision support function. The ability of U.S. primary care practitioners to evaluate their practice and compare it with those of other physicians around the world relates directly to their ability to use the ICPC terminology in association with the NCVHS core terminology group.

With regard to patient safety, the University of Colorado Department of Family Medicine and numerous other organizations are involved in a collaborative project entitled Applied Strategies for Improving Patient Safety. This project, sponsored by AHRQ to analyze the causes and effects of adverse events in primary care and reduce the incidence of errors, is using ICPC as its classification system (Pace, 2003). Preliminary results are not available at this time.

A conceptual diagram of the core terminology group and associated mappings to supplemental terminologies is presented in Figure 4-4, which shows the possible relationships among the terminologies and the use of aggregation logic for mapping through various levels of granularity. This figure was developed as a modification of a presentation in August 2002 to

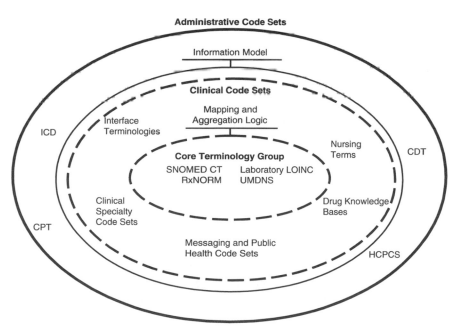

FIGURE 4-4 Conceptual diagram of the core terminology group and mappings to supplemental terminologies.
SOURCE: Adapted from Campbell, 2002.

NCVHS on clinical semantic interoperability by Dr. James R. Campbell of the University of Nebraska Medical Center (Campbell, 2002).

Knowledge Representation

Biomedical literature knowledge bases are powerful tools for clinical reference. These knowledge bases hold the vast body of medical research findings from both a historical perspective and the perspective of current best evidence-based practice. At present, most digital sources of evidence are operating as stand alone systems without the ability to link to clinical information systems. With the development and use of common data standards, this linkage for enhanced access to medical knowledge bases can occur.

Clinical Guideline Representation Model

An earlier IOM report defines practice guidelines as systematically developed statements to assist practitioners and patients in making decisions about health care for specific circumstances (Institute of Medicine, 1992). The National Guideline Clearinghouse alone contains nearly 1,000 publicly accessible guidelines (Maviglia et al., 2003). There are gaps and inconsistencies in the medical literature supporting one practice versus another, as well as biases based on the perspective of the authors, who may be specialists, general practitioners, payers, marketers, or public health officials (Maviglia et al., 2003). Few national guidelines can be implemented in clinical information systems because of the lack of a way to represent the knowledge in machine-executable formats.

Automating guidelines requires a computer-readable format that is unambiguous and makes use of stored patient data. A number of computational models and tools for extracting, organizing, presenting, and sharing clinical guidelines are currently in developmental use. Box 4-2 lists the most common of these.

Few guidelines have been successfully translated and incorporated into real clinical settings (Advandi et al., 1999) because the language of which most text-based guidelines are composed is ambiguous. Eligibility criteria and severity of disease or symptoms often are not explicitly defined, and when they are defined, they may not map to computable data within an EHR (Maviglia et al., 2003) or other decision support systems. Simpler decision support that has worked successfully has been in the form of "if–then" rules triggered by EHR data that result in alert/reminder messages (Maviglia

BOX 4-2
Guideline Representation Models and Tools

Arden Syntax, Columbia University
DILEMMA/PRESTIGE model, Europe
EON/DHARMA model, Stanford University
PROforma model, Imperial Cancer Research Center, United Kingdom
Siegfried system, Duke University
Guideline Interchange Format (GLIF) model, InterMed Collaboratory
Asbru model, Vienna University of Technology and Ben-Gurion University
GUIDE/PatMan model, University of Pavia
PRODIGY model, University of Newcastle, United Kingdom
GASTON framework, University of Maastricht
Torino model, University of Torino

SOURCE: Wang et al., 2002b.

et al., 2003). The multitude of guideline models are dissimilar—they capture different features of a guideline and were created for different purposes. For example, guidelines can be used to support clinical work flow, to foster background utilization review and monitoring, to drive consultations, or to capture the process flow in a clinical protocol. As a consequence, no single model enables all of the features of the various models to be fully encoded.

One potential approach to data sharing is a model known as Guideline Interchange Format (GLIF), developed by the InterMed Collaboratory (comprising Harvard, Stanford, and Columbia universities), that encodes the essential features of guidelines common to all models (i.e., a maximal subset of features, not a superset) (Greenes et al., 2001). The goal of GLIF is to be able to (1) encode different requirements of clinicians during decision making, (2) support automatic verification and validation of guidelines, (3) facilitate standard approaches to guideline dissemination and local adaptation, and (4) be used as a template for the integration of automated clinical guidelines with clinical information systems (Wang et al., 2002b).

Following a workshop hosted by InterMed in March 2000, the collaboratory decided to develop a standard model for representing guidelines with HL7. Rather than pursue agreement on one model, the group decided to focus on the building-block components that all guideline models must accommodate, such as a way to formulate queries and to express decision logic, a way to express the models' logical rules, a way to reference data (the data model), an approach to resolving terminology issues, and a way to represent the process flow/work flow of a guideline (Greenes, 2003). The common language for representing the components is GELLO (Guideline Expression Language, Object-Oriented), which was developed for GLIF. GELLO includes an object-oriented query language—that is, syntax for querying the EHR—thus specifying how one retrieves elements to be used in the logic expressions (Sordo et al., 2003). GELLO depends on the existence of an object-oriented data model (i.e., HL7 RIM). Additional work on GELLO is being undertaken by HL7 with the intent of making it an official standard. Sufficient resources should be made available for revisions to resolve specifications for GLIF and to complete GELLO.

Another aspect to consider with GLIF is recognition that guidelines most often are not executed in their entirety (Greenes, 2003). Instead, certain steps of a guideline may be implemented within different parts of a clinical information system (Greenes, 2003). For example, some steps may bear upon evaluation of clinical findings and may offer suggestions for diagnostic assessment or workup strategy; some may bear on the choice of particular medications or other procedures and may be implemented as order entry suggestions or templates; some may relate to the interpretation to be made and the action to be taken when an abnormal laboratory result is obtained and might be implemented as alerts; and some may trigger reminders or scheduling events (Sordo et al., 2003). Thus a guideline should be considered in terms of the application services or functions required by its various steps to be most effective (Sordo et al., 2003). These requirements will differ from one clinical information system to another based on functionality supported by the system (e.g., whether computerized physician order entry is present, or whether automatic alerts or time-driven scheduling reminders are supported), as well as institutional preferences about how to interface recommendations with actions (e.g., whether to offer them as suggestions or to trigger them as default actions that need to be overridden to be ignored, and what user interactions with the clinical information system will be affected by them) (Greenes, 2003). Thus work is proceeding on developing a taxonomy for application services that might be invoked by guidelines, as well as ways of marking up particular steps with the details of how the action is to be carried out in a specific clinical information system implementation (Greenes, 2003).

Representation of Medical Literature

The volume of medical information continues to grow exponentially, leaving some clinicians feeling that it has become unmanageable (Jerome et al., 2001). Yet the value of having the most recent medical literature for reference at the point of care is clear. Leveraging the efficiencies of information technology and expanding the services of medical libraries can facilitate this objective. Advances in communication technologies, application interface tools, and standardization in the representation of medical literature should allow such requests and retrievals to be completed through a fully automated system so that reliance on a librarian is not necessary, and information access is available to clinicians around the clock (Humphreys, 2003a). Since NLM holds the largest and most comprehensive database of medical literature, the development of application interface tools should initially be targeted to accessing the NLM databases. Automated data retrieval would require a direct connection to the various medical literature topics, rather than linkage through the NLM Web site as is now the case (Humphreys, 2003a). Such application interface tools would greatly enhance the usability of medical knowledge bases and capabilities for information seeking at the point of care (Humphreys, 2003a). The committee recommends further study into what characteristics of information and what design of the interface tools would be most useful to clinicians in this regard.

In addition, resources should continue to be provided to NLM to maintain its services in making medical literature available to consumers through its MEDLINEplus program. MEDLINEplus identifies information that is easy to read for the consumer and makes more than 150 interactive tutorials available in English, which include voice corresponding to the information printed on the screen (Humphreys, 2003b). The interactive tutorials are a popular feature in part because they are also suitable for those with low literacy (Humphreys, 2003b). In fact, those who select material for inclusion in MEDLINEplus actively seek low-literacy materials. NLM also encourages the institutes of the National Institutes of Health and producers of patient and consumer health materials to both convert their existing materials to electronic form and produce more of these materials.

The Cochrane Collaboration—an international effort for preparing, maintaining, and promoting the accessibility of systematic reviews of the effects of health care interventions—is another important source of medical knowledge. Its database was designed to produce up-to-date summaries of the results of reliable research and is now considered one of the world's best sources of medical evidence on treatments, diagnostic techniques, and preventive interventions (Cochrane Collaboration, 2003).

Other types of knowledge bases are highly important to patient safety and decision support tools. Disease registries are special databases that contain information about people diagnosed with a specific disease. Most registries are either hospital or population based and are used for a number of purposes, such as patient outcome tracking, support for self-care, epidemiological research, and public health surveillance (New York State Department of Health, 1999). They are also used for direct patient care, such as providing reminders for follow-up visits.

Knowledge bases, such as those for pharmacology and pharmacokinetics, hold a vast amount of medical knowledge critical to the accurate prescription drugs and surveillance of drug reactions. These knowledge bases provide information on drug–body interactions to support decisions about what drugs to prescribe; drug–drug comparisons; advice on administration (Duclos-Cartolano and Venot, 2003); information on contraindications, interactions, or therapeutic strategies related to the physiological conditions of a particular disease; and listings of drugs according to some of their properties (Duclos-Cartolano and Venot, 2003). Common data standards can facilitate interconnections with bar-code medication administration systems, computerized physician order entry systems, and other decision support tools for the clinician and can support the self-care of patients by providing access to drug interaction checking programs.

Clinician and patient access to vital information about medications contained in labeling (i.e., package inserts) is also important to patient safety. NLM is playing a key role in the standardization of the information on medication package inserts so the information can be made available in electronic format over the Internet. The DailyMed database, as its name suggests, is intended to provide updates of medication information to the public on a daily basis. Labels are also being restructured so they will be easier to understand and useful to both nonprofessionals and information systems (Brown et al., 2003). A major innovation will be the inclusion of labeling highlights that include recent label changes, indications, usage, dosage, administration, how supplied, contraindications, warnings/precautions, drug interactions, and use in special populations (Brown et al., 2003). Finally, NLM is working on the UNII project intended to code the molecular structure and other features of each new medication. With the pending market entry of about 1,500 new drugs in the next few years, the NLM Molfile database of molecular and manufacturing information on new drugs will augment pharmacy and pharmacogenetic databases by supplying more detailed information about medication functions and the prevention of adverse reactions.

Implementation of Data Standards

Implementing data standards is just as important as developing and selecting standards. In preparing to implement standards, several issues tend to arise that should be considered when establishing a mechanism for compliance; these issues include vendor readiness, organizational readiness, cost of compliance tools, unresolved issues related to terminologies and coding, identifiers for providers and patients, and interpretation of the implementation guides and standard specifications. Help in dealing with these issues is critical.

Most recently, in the implementation of HIPAA, the Workgroup on Electronic Data Interchange (WEDI) stepped forward to lead the Strategic National Implementation Process and provided guidance, assistance, and advice on the implementation of and compliance with HIPAA standards. The workgroup has developed a number of white papers that provide specific guidance on the technical aspects of implementing the associated code sets, messaging formats, security features, and privacy policies. It has also provided guidance on the testing and certification of clinical systems for compliance (i.e., conformity assessment) with the standards—testing organizational systems internally as well as testing systems externally with trading partners. The committee recommends that a similar entity be identified to assist with the implementation of clinical and patient safety data standards for the NHII. Such an entity might best be established with AHRQ as coordinator. The entity might assist organizations in increasing staff awareness and education; undertaking a gap analysis of current and desired standards; formulating a strategic plan, budget, and timeline to meet the CHI requirements; implementing the plan and certifying conformance; and providing an audit process for ongoing monitoring and enforcement. In contrast with HIPAA, however, self-certification should not be an option for compliance with clinical data standards.

In addition to the establishment of an oversight organization and a national implementation plan, a mechanism for assessing conformance with the data standards is needed. Conformity assessment, an integral part of the utilization of standards, is the comprehensive term for measures taken by manufacturers, their customers, regulatory authorities, and independent third parties to evaluate and determine whether products and processes conform to particular standards (National Research Council, 1995). The National Institute of Standards and Technology (NIST) could perhaps serve as the body supporting the implementation process as the developer of protocols for conformance tests, information assurance, and certification procedures to verify vendors' compliance with the standards.

Because the core terminology group for the EHR and other health-related applications will be housed for public availability within the UMLS, NLM will play a vital role in the coordination, mapping, and dissemination of the terminologies for national adoption. NLM will share responsibility for the maintenance and regular updating of the terminologies with the terminology developers. As the chief standards development organization for the EHR, HL7, in collaboration with government organizations (e.g., Centers for Medicare and Medicaid Services), will develop the specifications for the actual implementation of the terminologies.

As stated in Chapter 3, AHRQ can facilitate the standards adoption process by functioning as a coordinating body and provider of technical assistance for the efforts of CHI, NCVHS, NLM, FDA, and HL7 in the area of data standards and for the Quality Interagency Coordination Task Force, evidence-based practice centers, specialty societies, academic institutions, and professional organizations involved in the determination of best practices that become translated into electronic data systems. AHRQ should be fully funded to function in this capacity.

Assessing the costs related to the development, implementation, and dissemination of data standards will involve a coordinated set of evaluations by AHRQ and NLM. AHRQ would most likely have the responsibility for estimating the costs related to the establishment and operation of a WEDI-like entity for standards implementation and conformity assessment. NLM would have responsibility for estimating the costs related to the development and maintenance of the core terminology group and mappings to supplemental terminologies. Together, these organizations should engage in a comprehensive evaluation of the costs to provide the data standards needed for the NHII and patient safety systems.

REFERENCES

Advandi, A., S. Tu, M. O'Connor, R. Coleman, M. K. Goldstein, and M. Musen. 1999. *Integrating a Modern Knowledge-Based System Architecture with a Legacy VA Database: The ATHENA and EON Projects at Stanford.* Proceedings of the Annual American Medical Informatics Association Symposium. Philadelphia, PA: Hanley and Belfus.

American National Standards Institute. 2002. *ANSI Procedures for the Development and Coordination of American National Standards.* Online. Available: http://public. ansi.org/ansionline/Documents/Standards%20Activities/American%20National%20Standards/Procedures,%20Guides,%20and%20Forms/anspro2002r.doc [accessed June 1, 2003].

American National Standards Institute, Health Informatics Standards Board. 1997. *Inventory of Health Care Information Standards.* New York, NY: American National Standards Institute.

Association for the Advancement of Medical Instrumentation. 2001. *Human Factors Design Process for Medical Devices HE74.* Arlington, VA: Association for the Advancement of Medical Instrumentation.

Brown, S. H., R. Levin, M. J. Lincoln, R. M. Kolodner, and S. J. Nelson. 2003. *United States Government Progress Towards a Common Information Infrastructure for Medications.* Bethesda, MD: National Library of Medicine.

Campbell, J. R. 2002. *Presentation and Testimony on Converging the Clinical Care Model.* National Committee on Vital and Health Statistics, Subcommittee on Standards and Security.

Carper, T. 2003. *Health Information on Demand.* Online. Available: http://www.ndol.org/print.cfm?contentid=251495 [accessed April 15, 2003].

Chute, C. 2003. *Terminology Mappings and Aggregation Logic.* Personal communication to Institute of Medicine's Committee on Data Standards for Patient Safety.

Chute, C. G., S. P. Cohn, and J. R. Campbell. 1998. A framework for comprehensive health terminology systems in the United States. *J Am Med Inform Assoc* 5 (6):503–510.

Cimino, J. J. 1998. Desiderata for controlled medical vocabularies in the twenty-first century. *Methods Inf Med* 37 (4–5):394–403.

Coates, V. H. 2003a. *Medical Device Terminologies.* Personal communication to Institute of Medicine's Committee on Data Standards for Patient Safety.

———. 2003b. *ECRI's Universal Medical Device Nomenclature System.* Presentation to the NCVHS Subcommittee on Standards and Security.

Cochrane Collaboration. 2003. *Cochrane Collaboration Brochure.* Online. Available: http://www.cochrane.org/software/docs/newbroch.pdf [accessed July 14, 2003].

Consolidated Health Informatics Initiative. 2003. *Standards Adoption Strategy and Portfolio.* Presentation to the NCVHS Subcommittee on Standards and Security.

Department of Health and Human Services. 2003. *HHS Launches New Efforts to Promote Paperless Health Care System.* Online. Available: http://www.hhs.gov/news/press/2003pres/20030701.html [accessed July 7, 2003].

Dolin, R. H., L. Alschuler, C. Beebe, P. V. Biron, S. L. Boyer, D. Essin, E. Kimber, T. Lincoln, and J. E. Mattison. 2001. The HL7 Clinical Document Architecture. *J Am Med Inform Assoc* 8 (6):552–569.

Duclos-Cartolano, C., and A. Venot. 2003. Building and evaluation of a structured representation of pharmacokinetics information presented in SPCs: From existing conceptual views of pharmacokinetics associated with natural language processing to object-oriented design. *J Am Med Inform Assoc* 10(3):271–280.

Greenes, R. A., M. Peleg, A. T. S. Boxwala, V. Patel, and E. H. Shortliffe. 2001. Sharable computer-based clinical practice guidelines: Rationale, obstacles, approaches, and prospects. *Medinfo* 10 (Pt 1):201–205.

Greenes, R. A. 2003. *Electronic Representation of Clinical Guidelines (Attachments: 1).* Personal communication to Institute of Medicine's Committee on Data Standards for Patient Safety.

Hammond, W. E. 2002. *Overview of Health Care Data Standards.* Commissioned paper for IOM Committee on Data Standards for Patient Safety.

Health Level Seven. 2001 (March). *HL7 V3 Standard: Backbone, Draft 1.0, Version 3.0,* K. Blyler, ed.

Humphreys, B. June 2, 2003a. *Medical Knowledgebases.* Personal communication to Institute of Medicine's Committee on Data Standards for Patient Safety.

———. June 20, 2003b. *Medical Knowledgebases.* Personal communication to Institute of Medicine's Committee on Data Standards for Patient Safety.

Ingenerf, J. 1995. Taxonomic vocabularies in medicine: The intention of usage determines different established structures. *MedInfo 95* 136–139. R. A. Greenes, H. E. Peterson, and D. J. Protti, eds. Vancouver, British Columbia: Health Care Computing and Communications, Canada, Inc.

Institute of Medicine. 1992. *Guidelines for Clinical Practice: From Development to Use.* Washington, DC: National Academy Press.

———. 2003. *Priority Areas for National Action: Transforming Health Care Quality.* Washington, DC: The National Academies Press.

Jamoulle, M. 2001. *ICPC Use in the European Community.* Durban, South Africa: WONCA International Classification Committee at the 16th WONCA World Congress of Family Doctors.

Jerome, R. N., N. B. Giuse, K. W. Gish, N. A. Sathe, and M. S. Dietrich. 2001. Information needs of clinical teams: Analysis of questions received by the clinical information consult service. *Bulletin of the Medical Library Association* Apr 2001 177–185.

Johnson, M., M. Maas, and S. Moorehead, eds. 2000. *Nursing Outcomes Classification.* St. Louis, MO: Mosby.

Marshall, I. 2003. ICPC around the world. *WONCA News: An International Forum for Family Doctors* 29 (4):14–18.

Maviglia, S. M., R. D. Zielstorff, M. Paterno, J. M. Teich, D. W. Bates, and G. J. Kuperman. 2003. Automating complex guidelines for chronic disease: Lessons learned. *J Am Med Inform Assoc* 10:154–165.

National Committee on Vital and Health Statistics. August 19-20, 2003a. *Proceedings: Subcommittee on Standards and Security.* Personal notes of Institute of Medicine Staff to Committee on Data Standards for Patient Safety taken during proceedings.

———. 2003b. *Letter to Tommy G. Thompson, Secretary of the Department of Health and Human Services, Recommendations on Uniform Data Standards for Patient Medical Record Information.* Online. Available: http://www.ncvhs.hhs.gov/031105lt3.pdf [accessed December 5, 2003].

National Research Council. 1995. *Standards, Conformity Assessment, and Trade: Into the 21st Century.* Washington, DC: National Academy Press.

Nelson, S. J., S. H. Brown, M. S. Erlbaum, N. Olson, T. Powell, B. Carlsen, J. Carter, M. S. Tuttle, and W. T. Hole. 2002. *A Semantic Normal Form for Clinical Drugs in the UMLS: Early Experiences with the VANDF.* Proceedings of the Annual American Medical Informatics Association Symposium. Philadelphia, PA: Hanley and Belfus, 557–561.

Nerenz, D. R., and N. Neil. 2001. *Performance Measures for Health Care Systems.* Commissioned paper for the Center for Health Management Research.

New York State Department of Health. 1999. *Chronic Disease Teaching Tools—Disease Registries.* Online. Available: http://www.health.state.ny.us/nysdoh/chronic/diseaser.htm [accessed August 2003].

Office of Management and Budget. 2003. *Consolidated Health Informatics.* Online. Available: http://www.whitehouse.gov/omb/egov/gtob/health_informatics.htm [accessed April 21, 2003].

Pace, W. 2003. *Applied Strategies for Improving Patient Safety: Making the Health Care System Safer.* Denver, CO: Agency for Healthcare Research and Quality.

Rossi, M., F. Consorti, and E. Galeazzi. 1998. Standards to support development of terminological systems for healthcare telematics. *Methods Inf Med* 37 (4–5):551–563.

Ruggieri, A. P., S. V. Pakhomov, and C. G. Chute. Forthcoming. *A Corpus Driven Approach Applying the Frame Semantic Method for Modeling Functional Status Terminology.* Proceedings of the Annual American Medical Informatics Association Symposium. Philadelphia, PA: Hanley and Belfus.

Russler, D. C. 2002. Chapter 5: Patient safety and the HL7 reference information model. In: Russell Lewis, ed. *The Impact of Information Technology on Patient Safety.* Chicago, IL: Healthcare Information and Management Systems Society. Pp. 67–79.

Seliger, R. 2003. *HL7 Context Manager.* Personal communication to Institute of Medicine's Committee on Data Standards for Patient Safety.

Seliger, R., and B. Royer. 2001. *HL7: Standards for E-Health. CCOW Context Management Standard.* Online. Available: http://www.hl7.org/special/Committees/ccow_sigvi.htm [accessed September 5, 2003].

Sordo, M., O. Ogunyemi, A. A. Boxwala, and R. A. Greenes. 2003. *Software Specifications for GELLO: An Object-Oriented Query and Expression Language for Clinical Decision Support.* Boston, MA: Brigham and Women's Hospital and Harvard Medical School.

Spackman, K. A., K. E. Campbell, and R. A. Cote. 1997. SNOMED RT: A reference terminology for health care. *Proc AMIA Annu Fall Symp* 640–644.

Sujansky, W. 2003. *Summary and Analysis of Terminology Questionnaires Submitted by Developers of Candidate Terminologies for PMRI Standards: A Draft Report to the National Committee on Vital and Health Statistics Subcommittee on Standards and Security.* National Committee on Vital and Health Statistics Meeting 5.

van Bemmel, J. H., and M. A. Musen. 1997. *Handbook of Medical Informatics.* Heidelberg, Germany: Springer-Verlag.

Van Hentenryck, K. 2001. *HL7: The Art of Playing Together.* Online. Available: www.medicalcomputingtoday.com [accessed September 25, 2001].

Wang, A. Y., J. H. Sable, and K. A. Spackman. 2002a. The SNOMED clinical terms development process: Refinement and analysis of content. *Proc AMIA Symp* 845–849.

Wang, D., M. Peleg, S. W. Tu, A. A. Boxwala, R. A. Greenes, V. L. Patel, and E. H. Shortliffe. 2002b. Representation of primitives, process models and patient data in computer-interpretable clinical practice guidelines: A literature review of guideline representation models. *Int J Med Inf* 68:59–70.

Washington Publishing Company. 1998. *Overview of Healthcare EDI Transactions: A Business Primer.* Online. Available: http://www.wpc-edi.com/Default_40.asp [accessed February 2002].

World Health Organization. 2001. ICF Introduction: International Classification of Functioning, Disability and Health. Geneva: World Health Organization.

WONCA—World Organization of National Colleges, Academies and Academic Associations of General Practitioners and Family Physicians. 1998. International Classification of Primary Care-2. Oxford, UK: Oxford University Press.

Part II

Establishing Comprehensive Patient Safety Programs

This part of the report begins by providing an overview of the components of a patient safety program (Chapter 5). It then reviews in more detail adverse event analysis (Chapter 6) and near-miss analysis (Chapter 7).

ESTABLISHMENT OF COMPREHENSIVE PATIENT SAFETY PROGRAMS

Traditionally, adverse event reporting systems have focused on past events, logging serious events and facilitating root-cause analysis and the formulation of system improvements. While submitting and analyzing patient safety–related reports of past events is extremely important, insufficient attention has been paid to improving patient safety by preventing adverse events from occurring in the first place. Patient safety considerations are integral to each clinical decision and surveillance. Thus, the committee believes patient safety cannot be considered separately from the delivery of quality care. Chapter 5 outlines the components of a comprehensive patient safety program implemented within a culture of safety. To facilitate the implementation of such a program, a strong patient safety research agenda is needed.

> **Recommendation 5. All health care settings should establish comprehensive patient safety programs operated by trained personnel within a culture of safety. These programs should encompass (1) case find-**

ing—identifying system failures, (2) analysis—understanding the factors that contribute to system failures, and (3) system redesign—making improvements in care processes to prevent errors in the future. Patient safety programs should invite the participation of patients and their families and be responsive to their inquiries.

Recommendation 6. The federal government should pursue a robust applied research agenda on patient safety, focused on enhancing knowledge, developing tools, and disseminating results to maximize the impact of patient safety systems. AHRQ should play a lead role in coordinating this research agenda among federal agencies (e.g., the National Library of Medicine) and the private sector. The research agenda should include the following:

- Knowledge generation
  - High-risk patients—Identify patients at risk for medication errors, nosocomial infections, falls, and other high-risk events.
  - Near-miss incidents—Test the causal continuum assumption (that near misses and adverse events are causally related), develop and test a recovery taxonomy, and extend the current individual human error/recovery models to team-based errors and recoveries.
  - Hazard analysis—Assess the validity and efficiency of integrating retrospective techniques (e.g., incident analysis) with prospective techniques.
  - High-yield activities—Study the cost/benefit of various approaches to patient safety, including analysis of reporting systems for near misses and adverse events.
  - Patient roles—Study the role of patients in the prevention, early detection, and mitigation of harm due to errors.
- Tool development
  - Early detection capabilities—Develop and evaluate various methods for employing data-driven triggers to detect adverse drug events, nosocomial infections, and other high-risk events (e.g., patient falls, decubitus ulcers, complications of blood product transfusions).
  - Prevention capabilities—Develop and evaluate point-of-care decision support to prevent errors of omission or commission.
  - Data mining techniques—Identify and develop data mining techniques to enhance learning from regional and national patient safety databases. Apply natural language processing techniques to facilitate the extraction of patient safety–related concepts from text documents and incident reports.

   • **Dissemination—Deploy knowledge and tools to clinicians and patients.**

ADVERSE EVENT ANALYSIS

The Institute of Medicine's (IOM) report *To Err Is Human: Building a Safer Health System* report (Institute of Medicine, 2000) boosted existing patient safety initiatives and stimulated new ones. Today in the United States, there are many types of patient safety reporting systems in operation or under development at the federal, state, and private-sector levels. Overseas, Australia (Australian Council for Safety and Quality in Health Care, 2001; Runciman and Moller, 2001) and the United Kingdom (National Patient Safety Agency, 2001) are implementing nationwide patient safety reporting systems.

The federal government operates patient safety reporting systems as part of its role of performing regulatory oversight of the health care industry and as part of its caregiver role through the Veterans Health Administration and the Department of Defense. Many states operate reporting systems as part of their regulatory oversight role of health care providers. In addition, many health care institutions operate patient safety systems for internal quality improvement purposes, and a few private-sector organizations operate such systems on a national basis. Appendix C provides summaries of a sampling of major U.S. patient safety reporting systems.

The aim of adverse event analysis is to identify ways to improve the delivery of health care through the analysis of adverse events. Accomplishing this objective involves defining the adverse events to investigate, establishing methods for the detection of such events, and identifying the data needed for analysis purposes. The functional requirements of adverse event analysis systems and the implications for data standards are examined in Chapter 6.

NEAR-MISS ANALYSIS

Current patient safety reporting systems are nearly always focused on adverse events and usually neglect near-misses (sometimes called "close calls"). Of the patient safety reporting systems currently operational in the United States, only a small proportion collect and analyze information on near misses (see Appendix C). None of the reporting systems used for federal regulatory oversight include near misses as reportable events. Of the 21 states mandating patient safety reporting systems, only Pennsylvania and

Kansas collect near-miss information (Rosenthal, 2003). Private-sector reporting systems are much more likely to collect information on near misses.

The committee believes that near-miss reporting and analysis systems should be fostered. Near misses are often precursors of adverse events, and analysis of their root causes can provide important insights into how to prevent adverse events from happening. In addition, near misses involve some planned or unplanned recovery procedures. These responses to system breakdowns are a key element of learning from near misses. Identifying what recovery procedures work in practice helps in developing better care delivery systems. The functional requirements of near-miss analysis systems and the implications for data standards are examined in Chapter 7.

REFERENCES

Australian Council for Safety and Quality in Health Care. 2001. *Safety in Numbers: A Technical Options Paper for a National Approach to the Use of Data for Safer Health Care (Work in Progress)*. Online. Available: http://sq.netspeed.com.au/articles/Publications/numbers.pdf [accessed March 4, 2002].

Institute of Medicine. 2000. *To Err Is Human: Building a Safer Health System*. Washington, DC: National Academy Press.

National Patient Safety Agency, Department of Health, United Kingdom. 2001. *Doing Less Harm (Version 1.0a)*. Online. Available: http://www.npsa.org.uk/admin/publications/docs/draft.pdf [accessed April 16, 2002].

Rosenthal, J. 2003. *State Reporting Systems Collecting Information on Near Misses*. Personal communication to Institute of Medicine's Committee on Data Standards for Patient Safety.

Runciman, W. B., and J. Moller. 2001. *Iatrogenic Injury in Australia*. Adelaide, Australia: Australian Patient Safety Foundation, Inc.

5

Comprehensive Patient Safety Programs in Health Care Settings

CHAPTER SUMMARY

Based on the premise that patient safety is an integral part of the delivery of quality care, health care settings should establish comprehensive patient safety programs. The committee sets forth in this chapter a complete program for improving patient safety within a culture of safety. This program needs to be pilot tested, with the results discussed widely and supported by a research program.

The key elements of a culture of safety include (1) a shared belief that although health care is a high-risk undertaking, delivery processes can be designed to prevent failures and harm to participants; (2) an organizational commitment to detecting and analyzing patient injuries and near misses; and (3) an environment that balances the need for reporting of events and the need to take disciplinary action. Improving patient safety requires a multiphased process beginning with the detection of injuries and near misses and ending with a mechanism for ensuring that improvements in patient safety are maintained. A model for the introduction of safer care is presented. The application of these ideas is illustrated through two case studies—one relating to adverse drug events and the other to postoperative deep wound and organ space infections.

A key aspect of a patient safety program is the involvement of patients and their families in the process. Finally, to foster the development and implementation of comprehensive patient safety programs, a research agenda for knowledge generation, tool development, and dissemination is needed.

A CULTURE OF SAFETY

Improvements in patient safety are best achieved when health care delivery organizations adopt a culture of safety. A culture of safety can be defined as an integrated pattern of individual and organizational behavior, based upon shared beliefs and values, that continuously seeks to minimize patient harm that may result from the processes of care delivery (Kizer, 1999).

A measurement strategy based on a culture of safety is sometimes called a just (i.e., fair) system. Such a strategy implements two complementary ideas. First, it describes a system within which health professionals can report injuries and near misses safe from blame, humiliation, and retaliation (O'Leary, 2003). Second, such open and complete reporting is key in creating an environment that reliably avoids injuries and near misses—that is, a care delivery system that is safe for patients.

A culture of safety encompasses the following elements (adapted from Kizer, 1999): shared beliefs and values about the health care delivery system; recruitment and training with patient safety in mind; organizational commitment to detecting and analyzing patient injuries and near misses; open communication regarding patient injury results, both within and outside the organization; and the establishment of a just culture. Aspects of organizational leadership relating to the implementation of information technology systems were addressed in Chapter 2.

Systemic improvements in the way health care is delivered should not be made at the expense of a weakening of the sense of professional responsibility. Health care professionals still need to be adequately prepared both mentally and physically to carry out their responsibilities. They also need to be aware of the environment in which they practice and seek to eliminate distractions that can be avoided. In addition, they need to be vigilant in identifying hazardous situations and able to respond to these situations when they occur.

Shared Beliefs and Values

A culture of safety requires a shared recognition among all members of a health care delivery organization, reinforced regularly and rigorously by professional and organizational leaders, that health care is a highly complex, error-prone, and thus high-risk undertaking. Failures are inevitable when dealing with humans and complex systems, regardless of how hard the humans involved try to avoid errors. However, hazards and errors can be anticipated, and processes can be designed both to avoid failures and to prevent patient harm when a failure occurs.

Recruitment and Training with Patient Safety in Mind

A culture of safety requires organizational understanding that knowledge and skills are an essential foundation for safe practices. Also required is a recognition that such competence is ephemeral and must be actively maintained. At present, health professions education does not address many subjects critical to a safe care delivery environment.

Organizational Commitment to Detecting Patient Injuries and Near Misses

As part of a culture of safety, organizations need to commit to detecting as many patient injuries and near misses as possible through the following means:

- Active surveillance based on case finding through real-time, interventional, prospective data-based clinical trigger systems, as well as retrospective chart review driven by code-based trigger systems.
- Routine self-assessments to identify error-prone or high-risk processes, systems, or settings that could jeopardize patient safety (see Box 5-1).
- Standardized, widely understood, and easily accessible mechanisms for voluntary reporting, with an independent team completing all the paperwork. These mechanisms could include a simple computerized reporting system allowing front-line care professionals to mark possible injuries for independent review; telephone and e-mail tip lines enabling front-line professionals, patients, and family members to report potential adverse events or near misses; and a system for asking front-line health professionals, as they leave work, whether they experienced any unsafe conditions or observed any injuries or near misses during their just-completed workday.

BOX 5-1
Examples of High-Risk Areas That Deserve
Special Attention

- Many and varied interactions with diagnostic and/or treatment technology; many different types of equipment being utilized
- Multiple individuals involved in the care of individual patients and many hand-offs of care
- High acuity of patient illness or injury
- Ambient atmosphere prone to distractions or interruptions
- Need for rapid care management decisions; care givers being time pressured
- High-volume and/or unpredictable patient flow
- Use of diagnostic or therapeutic interventions having a narrow margin of safety, including high-risk drugs
- Communication barriers with patients and/or co-workers
- Instructional setting for care delivery, with inexperienced caregivers

These procedures could be augmented by internal safety experts and organizational leaders conducting regular "walk-around" reviews to identify potential weaknesses in patient safety.

- Appropriate protections and rewards for individuals who report injuries and near misses. The most potent reward for front-line health professionals may be seeing their reports lead to real changes in systems that result in a safer care environment.

Organizational Commitment to Analyzing Patient Injuries and Near Misses

In parallel with a commitment to detecting as many patient injuries and near misses as possible, there should be an organizational commitment to developing a management structure for tracking and rigorously analyzing injury-related events. There should also be a commitment to monitoring proven solutions from outside the organization that may address sources of injury the organization has yet to encounter. In addition, there should be a commitment to identifying and prioritizing possible actions to reduce injury rates; verifying actions taken, their effectiveness, and whether there were untoward secondary effects; and ensuring leadership involvement in and coordination of all these activities.

Open Communication

Another key element of a culture of safety is an organizational commitment to open communication. This commitment begins with leadership setting clear expectations regarding patient safety through publicized organizational goals. It also includes open sharing of patient injury results, both within and outside the organization (i.e., with front-line professionals, boards of directors or trustees, patients and patient representatives, and health care overseers) as part of a transparent care delivery system.

A Just Culture

A "just" culture is a key element of a safe culture (Reason and Hobbs, 2003). If data to support a learning environment are to be collected, employees must be willing to report adverse events and near misses without threat of retribution. On the other hand, a totally blame-free environment, sometimes referred to as a "bungler's charter," is not acceptable. A just culture seeks to balance the need to learn from mistakes and the need to take disciplinary action (Marx, 2001). Processes for differentiating between blameless and blameworthy acts have been proposed (Reason and Hobbs, 2003).

On the basis of experience from other industries and with some important exceptions given later, the committee believes protection from disciplinary action should be afforded to front-line workers when they report injuries, errors, and near misses even if they were personally involved. This belief derives from proven performance in other endeavors, such as airline transportation, nuclear power, safe manufacturing environments, and high-reliability military operations (e.g., aircraft carrier operations). Without such protections, injury reporting rates drop drastically, and with them the ability to prevent future injuries. Such protections reflect an acknowledgment that errors are nearly never intentional, nor are they caused by simple human failures alone. Health care delivery organizations should be held accountable for designing and implementing safe processes, which in turn make it possible for front-line health professionals to deliver safe care.

Three important exceptions apply, however. Protection is not granted for criminal behavior (e.g., a physician treating a patient while inebriated), for active malfeasance (e.g., a nurse who purposely violates safety policies or short-circuits built-in protections), or cases in which an injury is not reported in a timely manner (usually within 1 to 2 days).

A MODEL FOR INTRODUCING SAFER CARE

The ultimate aim of standardized patient safety data is safer care. While not all change produces improvement, safer care requires change. Data standards and data collection have no utility unless they lead to change that produces safer care. The process for positive change has the following elements (see Figure 5-1):

- Injury and near-miss detection
- Epidemiological analyses
- Generation of hypotheses for change—develop a list of system fixes that could potentially improve safety results
- Prioritization of improvement opportunities
- Rapid-cycle testing
- Deployment and implementation
- Holding the gains

Each of these elements is discussed in turn below.

Injury and Near-Miss Detection

Detection of injuries and near misses contributes to safety improvement at four key points by:

- Providing information for epidemiological analyses.
- Using relative failure rates to help formulate research priorities.
- Demonstrating what changes work in practice.
- Checking to see whether the expected improvements are sustained over time.

Traditional reporting systems can grossly underdetect injuries, significantly impeding the ability to improve. A balanced detection system necessarily relies on case finding through surveillance, working together with voluntary incident reporting systems. Injury surveillance uses data-based clinical trigger systems that lead to prospective expert review, as well as retrospective review of patient records identified by International Classification of Diseases (ICD)-9, Clinical Modification (CM) discharge codes, and External Causes of Injury Codes (E-Codes) (Xu et al., 2003). Until research efforts (discussed later in this chapter) make more such tools available, data-

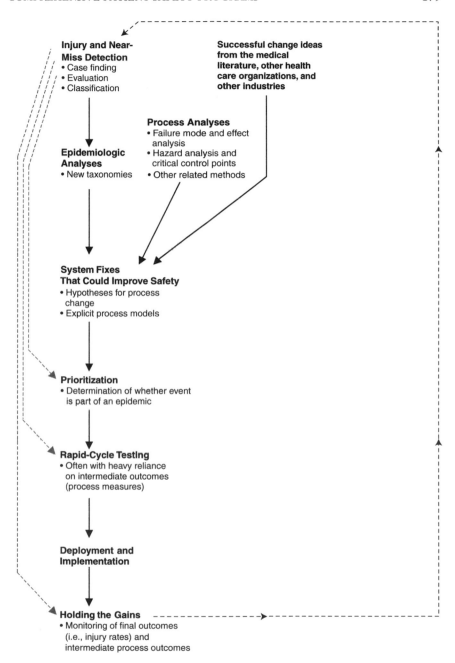

FIGURE 5-1 Use of standardized patient safety information to improve care.

based clinical trigger systems would initially focus on adverse drug events (ADEs) and hospital-acquired infections, then move on to other common causes of injuries. This injury detection and tracking effort should start with hospitals and then be introduced into other care delivery settings, such as nursing homes, surgical centers, and outpatient offices.

In the future, adverse event detection should become much more a part of the routine fabric of care. Systems for adverse event detection and prevention should be embedded within the broader proactive hazard analysis framework—an approach to identifying and minimizing or eliminating hazards.

Epidemiologic Analyses, Hypotheses for Change Generation, and Prioritization

Effective, standardized injury detection and reporting plays a key role in patient safety by providing the information with which patient safety officers and other researchers can conduct epidemiologic analyses of injury data. Improvement teams often must try several different ways of organizing and analyzing injury data before finding an approach that leads to successful change and improvement. Good patient safety data systems need to be capable of supporting new, innovative classification approaches, or taxonomies, as health professionals seek system solutions that can prevent future failures.

Other proven sources of change hypotheses include failure mode and effect analysis (FMEA) and hazard analysis and critical control points (HACCP) (McDonough, 2002) (see also Appendix D), as well as process changes that have been demonstrated to work in other settings within and outside health care delivery. Failure mode and effect analysis and hazard analysis and critical control points are used to analyze process work flow, with the aim of identifying likely failure points, rather than relying upon epidemiologic analysis of actual injuries and near misses. They thus offer the possibility of preventing failures even before the first patient has been injured.

Human beings cannot think about a problem—for example, how to deliver patient care or collect and analyze data—without an underlying mental model (Smith, 1998). When measuring, managing, and improving care delivery processes, it is highly useful to make underlying models visible by writing them down. Written models help produce consensus and enable critical examination, leading to improvement of the underlying mental models themselves (James, 2003). Just as important, a written model helps identify key measurement factors and grounds those measurements within the care delivery context. Successful process change often relies as much on data about the performance of process steps—intermediate outcomes—as on final near-miss and injury rates.

A cause-and-effect diagram such as that shown in Figure 5-2 is one relatively unstructured way of making a mental model explicit (Sholtes et al., 2003). Other, more highly organized methods for displaying models include conceptual flow diagrams (a form of flow charting, leading to traditional decision flow charts) and outcome chains.

All sources of injury are not created equal. A Pareto chart (see Table 5-1) ranks causes or possible solutions from most to least frequent, with the aim of targeting improvement activities to those areas that will achieve the most benefit for patients (Sholtes et al., 2003).

Other factors beyond injury rates may be important for setting improvement priorities. For example, existing leadership, available measurement systems, the local culture of health professionals, readiness for change at the front-line level, and sound theory identifying likely process improvements can all greatly affect the likelihood of success within a particular area. However, actual failure rates always play an essential part in the choice of points of attack for safety improvement—the second key role for an effective, standardized patient safety data system. The same principle applies at a larger scale: some sources of injury, such as ADEs, hospital-acquired infections, and decubitus ulcers—are orders of magnitude more common than some other, more sensational, sources of injury, such as wrong-side surgery.

Rapid-Cycle Testing

Having helped choose an aim for safety improvement and generate a list of potential changes that might lead to that goal, effective, standardized patient injury detection and reporting plays a third critical role: it allows an improvement team to determine whether a change is an improvement (Langley et al., 1996). As noted earlier, an improvement team often must try a series of change ideas before finding a combination that results in demonstrated better performance. Often, some elements of the final, successful change strategy are unique to the particular local environment within which the improvement effort occurred. Local circumstances, such as available data systems, clinical culture, the nature of patient populations being served, and organizational readiness for change, can make a large difference in what works. Local injury and near-miss tracking can therefore play an important role as a team discovers what works in its particular circumstances.

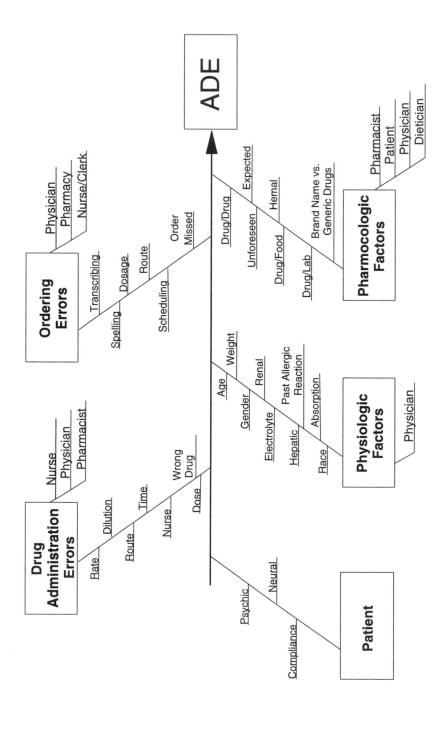

FIGURE 5-2 A cause-and-effect diagram of potentially preventable causes of adverse drug events.

TABLE 5-1 Frequency of Adverse Drug Events by Cause

Class	Percent	Description	Preventable
Allergic reaction with no prior history	28.0	Allergic or idiosyncratic reactions in patients with no prior history of allergy	Unclear
Renal dysfunction	23.0	Failure to adjust dosage in the face of declining renal function, among drugs excreted through the kidneys	Yes
Patient age	14.2	Failure to adjust dosage for patient age	Yes
Patient weight	5.7	Failure to adjust dosage for patient body mass	Yes
Dosage error	5.0	Simple error in dosage ordered (excluding other sources on this list)	Yes
Hematologic factors	4.6	Failure to appropriately adjust for other known hematological factors	Yes
Patient compliance	3.8	Failure of patient to comply with medical instructions	Unclear
Drug administration rate	2.7	Error on rate of administration of medication	Yes
Liver dysfunction	2.3	Failure to appropriately adjust for reduced liver function, for hepatically excreted drugs	Yes
Known allergies	1.5	Failure to recognize and respond to known allergies	Yes
Electrolyte imbalances	1.5	Failure to appropriately adjust dosage for known electrolyte imbalances	Yes
Dosage schedule error	1.5	Error on medication order regarding dosing schedule	Unclear

NOTE: The first cause accounted for 28 percent of all events recorded; the second an additional 23 percent. Among almost 40 causes originally hypothesized in the cause-and-effect diagram, the first 6 shown here accounted for 80 percent of all ADEs detected.

Deployment and Implementation

"Pilot and deploy" is an approach to implementing improvements that has been successful in a number of care delivery organizations. The idea is simple: choose an important systemwide safety problem; then determine methods for achieving demonstrated performance within a small group using rapid-cycle improvement tools. A small group often avoids larger organizational change issues and thus can discover effective process steps more rapidly. Once the necessary process steps are known, they can be implemented in other parts of the organization. Demonstrated success in the pilot group makes the discovered changes concrete and often provides a potent incentive to other teams. Pilot team members frequently become natural advocates and consultants, with high credibility at the peer-to-peer level.

Deployment and implementation methods, when used as part of an improvement strategy, differ from traditional clinical research in two ways. First, improvement often focuses more on clinical work flow and operational process than on patients' clinical response to treatment. It aims to make the process do the right thing, the right way, the first time, every time (James, 1989) to achieve demonstrated excellent performance. Often, this means carefully designing care delivery systems so that health professionals find it easy to do it right (James, 2001). It involves building best care into standard work processes, with publication of new biomedical science as a secondary goal. Second, even though the pilot project may have identified key process factors that play important roles in implementation in other settings, most delivery settings, as noted above, include unique local factors. Therefore, successful deployment requires the ability to try change ideas locally and determine whether they do in fact produce better results in the particular setting. In other words, effective, standardized detection and reporting of injuries and near misses is a key part of deployment. Under a pilot and deploy strategy, ideas tried during the deployment phase have the advantage of having shown success in at least one previous setting. When such ideas are implemented with local testing in other settings, the rate of successful change accelerates.

Holding the Gains

The aim of improvement is to establish a new baseline, but achieving this aim often requires new work processes, support systems, and professional habits. These requirements feed back to the need for new case finding methods, evaluation procedures, and classification systems. An effective, standardized injury detection and reporting system therefore plays a fourth key role: once successful change has been implemented, it helps the care delivery team maintain the gains (Juran, 1989). Otherwise, processes and performance can drift back to their old baselines as attention shifts.

TWO CASE STUDIES

The application of the above ideas is illustrated through two case studies. One concerns ADEs and the other postoperative deep wound and organ space infections. Throughout these case studies, the key elements of the model for introducing safer care detailed in the preceding section are high-lighted in bold print.

CASE STUDY 1
Detecting and Preventing Adverse Drug Events

In 1988, researchers working within a 520-bed, tertiary teaching hospital's departments of clinical epidemiology, pharmacy, and medical informatics (the improvement team) questioned whether the hospital's existing nurse incidence reporting system adequately detected ADEs. They compared three different ADE detection systems in a parallel trial: (1) traditional nurse incidence reporting; (2) enhanced reporting; and (3) prospective expert case review, driven by a data-based clinical trigger system. Enhanced reporting allowed nurses to simply flag a patient through the computerized charting system, avoiding the time and effort of filling out an incident report. A representative from the improvement team reviewed the patient's chart, determined whether an ADE had occurred, and completed the documentation. The clinical trigger system involved a series of treatment markers for ADEs, such as the use of antidote drugs (e.g., naloxone to counteract an opiate), abnormal values on specific laboratory tests (e.g., a twofold increase in blood creatinine), or other clinical indicators (e.g., reports of rash or itching in nursing notes). A positive clinical trigger led to prospective review by a clinical pharmacist within 24 hours, using explicit criteria. A clinical pharmacist from the improvement team also used explicit criteria to review all cases detected by traditional nurse incidence reporting to confirm whether an actual ADE had occurred. During the review, all ADEs were staged as mild, moderate, or severe, and their causes and patient outcomes were documented.

Over 18 months (May 1, 1989, through October 31, 1990), covering 36,653 hospitalizations, standard nurse incidence reporting, enhanced reporting, and prospective expert review driven by data-based clinical triggers found, respectively, 9, 92, and 731 confirmed ADEs (Classen et al., 1991). While enhanced reporting increased ADE detection rates by an order of magnitude, prospective expert review driven by data-based clinical triggers increased detection 80-fold.

Three members of the improvement team, expert in ADEs, reviewed more than 200 charts to identify ADE causes. Early analyses that classified ADEs by hospital location (e.g., emergency department versus operating room versus nursing unit) and by drug type (i.e., narcotics versus antibiotics) were not as useful as those that classified failures by process mechanism (**epidemiological analyses** and **hypotheses for change generation**). The team organized its findings as a cause-and-effect diagram (see Figure 5-2), then tallied actual ADEs to generate a Pareto chart of prioritized causes

(Evans et al., 1994). Table 5-2 lists the most common sources of detected ADEs.

On the basis of its ADE causal analysis, the improvement team began to devise, test, and implement changes to drug ordering, delivery, and review systems within the hospital (**rapid-cycle testing**) (Classen et al., 1992; Evans et al., 1994). Figure 5-3 shows ADE rates at the hospital as the detection system was enhanced (1988–1990) and then as system fixes were implemented to prevent or reduce the consequences of ADEs (1993–1999). Several changes produced better performance. Under the data-based clinical trigger system, rapid case review by a pharmacist led to more rapid recognition of an event with immediate clinical reaction, averting some ADEs in earlier, less severe stages. The hospital's electronic pharmacy system was programmed to recommend safer alternatives when a physician ordered highly allergenic medications. The electronic pharmacy system was also programmed to calculate ideal medication doses for each dose delivered, based on patient age, gender, and body mass; estimates of kidney function; estimates of liver function; and other blood chemistry values. It was demonstrated that similar results can be obtained without an electronic medication decision support system by having a pharmacist join physicians and nurses as they conduct patient rounds each day or by having pharmacists conduct their own independent patient rounds (Leape et al., 1999).

The same ADE prevention system was later deployed to sister hospitals in the region (**deployment and implementation**). The hospital system continued to monitor ADE rates to ensure that its investment in safer patient care did not deteriorate as organizational attention was shifted to other major sources of injury (**holding the gains**).

In March 2000, a visiting clinical researcher analyzed almost 10 years of data on ADEs detected by the hospital's data-based clinical trigger system (Henz, 2000). As Table 5-2 shows, among more than 70 clinical triggers in active use during the trial, 14 accounted for more than 95 percent of all ADEs detected. A number of groups have used the resulting list of high-yield clinical triggers to build manual and automated ADE detection systems, with the aim of delivering safer care. More recent internal investigation has suggested that the data-based clinical triggers could be improved even further through examination of interactions among triggers on the list (Kim, 2003).

Other researchers have investigated enhanced case finding based on ICD-9 CM discharge abstract codes and E-Codes, followed by retrospective chart review using explicit criteria to detect ADEs. Initial results suggest that such methods can roughly double the total number of ADEs detected relative to those found by the data-based clinical trigger system (Xu et al., 2003). Such activities represent the start of a second major improvement cycle, which if successful, could lead to a further decline in the single largest source of care-related injuries Americans face when hospitalized.

TABLE 5-2 Major Causes of Adverse Drug Events

ADE Alert	Location	True Positive Rate (%)	% of All ADEs Detected	Cumulative % Detected
1. Use of naloxone	Pharmacy	21.9	28.3	28.3
2. Use of benadryl	Pharmacy	21.0	20.8	49.1
3. Use of inapsine	Pharmacy	39.2	20.4	69.5
4. Use of lomotil	Pharmacy	26.8	7.5	77.0
5. Nurse reports of rash/itching	Nurse reporting	17.9	5.1	82.1
6. Use of loperamide	Pharmacy	22.3	3.4	85.5
7. Test for c.difficile toxin	Clinical laboratory	24.3	3.1	88.6
8. Digoxin level > 2	Clinical laboratory	2.3	2.2	90.8
9. Abrupt med. stop/reduction	Pharmacy	48.0	1.0	91.8
10. Use of vitamin K	Pharmacy	4.8	0.9	92.7
11. Doubling of blood creatinine	Clinical laboratory	0.4	0.8	93.5
12. Use of kaopectate	Pharmacy	21.8	0.7	94.2
13. Use of paregoric	Pharmacy	9.8	0.7	95.0
14. Use of flumazenil	Pharmacy	77.3	0.7	95.7

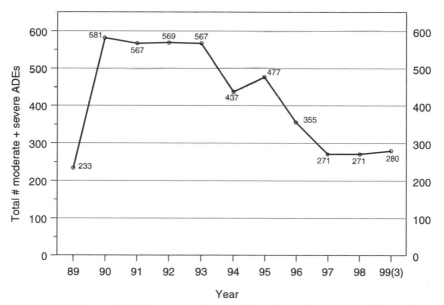

FIGURE 5-3 Detected ADE rates at a large teaching hospital, as a more effective detection system was put in place (1988–1990) and as a series of medication ordering, delivery, and follow-up systems were implemented (1994–1999). Comparing 1990–1993 (pre-intervention period) with 1997–1999 (postintervention period), the detected ADE rate fell from 571 to 274 ADEs per year on average—a 52 percent decline.

CASE STUDY 2
Postoperative Deep Wound and Organ Space Infections

The second most common source of significant inpatient injuries is postoperative deep wound infection (Gawande et al., 1999; Leape et al., 1991). The same hospital-based improvement team as that in case study 1 recognized that infection detection within its hospital, based upon recommendations developed and widely distributed by the Centers for Disease Control and Prevention (CDC), represented a data-based clinical trigger system. The team enhanced the hospital's ability to detect postoperative deep wound infections by implementing careful patient follow-up after hospital discharge through calls to attending physicians' offices and, occasionally, directly to patients (**injury and near-miss detection**). The improvement team also created a working model for infection prevention (**hypotheses for change generation**), then used expert opinion to focus its model on the timing of delivery of prophylactic antibiotics for clean or clean-contaminated surgery cases (**prioritization**). For most case types, postoperative infection rates were significantly lower if the antibiotics were started within 2 hours before the initial surgical incision was made, which produced high antibiotic levels in the patient's blood and tissue at the time the surgery started (Classen et al., 1992).

Having established a strong link between a key intermediate outcome (timing of antibiotic prophylaxis) and the primary outcome of interest (postoperative deep wound and organ space infection rates), the improvement team was able to use a process factor (whether the antibiotic prophylaxis was started within the ideal 2-hour time window) to drive change. Failure to deliver antibiotic prophylaxis within the ideal time window is usually a near miss; only in a minority of cases does the process failure produce an outcome failure. However, use of a process step as a primary performance measure greatly increased the sample size (compared with infection rates) and enhanced the improvement team's ability to tell when a change had resulted in improvement.

The improvement team then devised (**hypotheses for change generation**) and tested (**rapid-cycle testing**) a series of process change hypotheses to bring the hospital closer to the established clinical ideal. Table 5-3 shows on-time antibiotic prophylaxis rates and associated postoperative deep wound and organ space infection rates over time as the hospital's process improved. The process change that finally worked best in this hospital's care delivery environment involved fully preparing the intravenous prophylactic antibiotic, then having the anesthesiologist start the medicine immediately after initial induction of surgical anesthesia.

TABLE 5-3 Postoperative Deep Wound and Organ Space Infection Rates, as Process Changes Were Implemented to Improve Timing of Delivery of Antibiotic Prophylaxis

Prophylaxis and Infection Rates	1985	1986	1991
Rate (%) prophylactic antibiotics started during optimal 2-hour time window	40	58	96
Deep wound and organ space infection rate (%)	1.8	0.9	0.4

NOTE: No efforts were undertaken to change the patients who received prophylaxis or the choice of antibiotic used.
SOURCE: Larsen et al., 1989.

The care delivery group of which the improvement team was a part deployed its proven process steps to all other sister hospitals within its system (**deployment and implementation**). Other groups achieved similar success in the timing of antibiotic prophylaxis and subsequent infection rates through changes that involved other members of the operating room staff. Figure 5-4 shows rates of deep wound and organ space infections for the system as a whole as the pilot was deployed.

Since initial deployment, the improvement team has shifted its attention to other aspects of the infection prevention process. Current efforts are focused on applying published national guidelines to ensure that all the right patients, and only the right patients, receive antibiotic prophylaxis; that all patients receive the recommended antibiotics; and that antibiotic prophylaxis is discontinued at the appropriate time. Other infectious disease specialists, surgeons, and infection control nurses have examined the conceptual model used by the team and suggested improvements. For example, recent research indicates that process changes addressing blood sugar control, tissue oxygen tension, and tissue temperature could make further contributions to lowering infection rates. The injury and near-miss detection system continues to play a vital role in helping to maintain the gains already achieved (**holding the gains**) and in driving and supporting further improvement in the future.

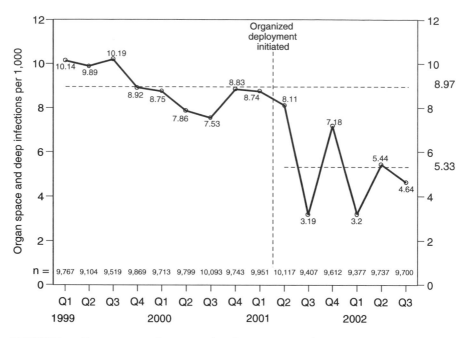

FIGURE 5-4 Postoperative deep wound and organ space infections per 1,000 clean and clean-contaminated elective surgical cases, as process changes to improve timing of antibiotic prophylaxis were deployed across a hospital system.

Engaging Patients and Their Families More in Patient Safety

Patients generally assume a basic level of quality in health care—though recent media reports on adverse events have raised questions and concerns among the public. Assuring safety and quality in health care requires an integrated effort that includes a new role for patients. With regard to adverse events and near misses, patients are possibly the last point at which event detection and prevention can occur.

Qualitative research conducted through focus groups has contributed to an understanding of the patient's role in assuring safe and high-quality care. Focus groups conducted by Voluntary Hospitals of America, Inc., revealed that for the most part, consumers perceived quality in terms of service issues (Voluntary Hospitals of America, 2000). However, it was also found that specific information about clinical quality and reports (i.e., evidence-based guidelines and system design approaches to reduce medical error) generated participant interest and changed attitudes about the ability to differentiate hospitals on the basis of quality. These findings led to a recommendation that initial education efforts target information about the role of hospitals in monitoring and controlling quality and the definition and dissemination of information on clinical quality that can be used by consumers in monitoring their care.

Other focus groups conducted by the Centers for Medicare and Medicaid Services revealed that patient safety messages receiving the highest rankings tended to be those that indicated *specific* ways for patients to inform their health professionals and themselves about what the health professionals were doing. Messages that stressed keeping one's doctor informed and informing oneself were better received than those seen as embarrassing or rude (e.g., asking health providers whether they had washed their hands). The conclusion of this research was that consumer messages on reducing medical errors work best if they:

- Advocate a collaborative doctor–patient relationship.
- Specify action to be taken.
- Clearly indicate how that action can be taken.

A number of organizations have sponsored educational activities to assist patients and their families in becoming more involved in their care. The National Patient Safety Foundation (www.npsf.org) has produced a number of publications that emphasize what patients can do to make health care safer. The Agency for Healthcare Research and Quality (AHRQ) also has developed patient materials setting forth ways to help prevent medical errors. One document in particular is designed for low-literacy patients and is presented in a comic strip format (Agency for Healthcare Research and Quality, 2001). The Institute for Safe Medication Practice sponsors a series of newsletters designed to help patients protect themselves from medication errors (www.ismp.org). Several state-based patient safety coalitions have developed and disseminated patient education materials. Finally, in March 2002 the Joint Commission on Accreditation of Healthcare Organizations launched the SPEAK UP campaign to help patients get involved in their care (Joint Commission on Accreditation of Healthcare Organizations, 2002).

Similar activities have taken place in Australia. Following consumer pressure in the late 1980s, legislation was passed in 1992 to ensure that consumer information on medicines would be available for new and existing drugs by 2004. In addition, the Medicine Information Persons project began in the early 1990s. This project trains older people as volunteer peer educators and aims to reduce the inappropriate use of medications among older people (Pharmaceutical Health and Rational Use of Medicines Committee, 2001).

Evaluating the Approach

To achieve an acceptable standard of patient safety, the committee recommends that all health care settings establish comprehensive patient safety programs operated by trained personnel within a culture of safety and involving adverse event and near-miss detection and analysis. The program put forward in this chapter is innovative and needs to be pilot tested to determine which levels of investment will bring the best returns. The results of these rigorous evaluations should then be widely circulated and discussed by all the key stakeholders.

APPLIED RESEARCH AGENDA

To foster the implementation of comprehensive patient safety systems, a robust applied research agenda for knowledge generation, tool development, and dissemination is needed. As noted earlier, near-miss analysis in health care is a much less mature discipline than adverse event analysis. As a consequence, fundamental research is needed on a number of topics related to near misses to improve analysis of these events and thereby enhance patient safety. Research is also needed in a number of areas to improve analysis of adverse events.

Knowledge Generation

High-Risk Patients

A greater focus is needed in adverse event systems on enhancing knowledge about risks and about how to identify patients at risk for medication errors, nosocomial infections, falls, and other high-frequency adverse events. Such knowledge is necessary to implement better prevention strategies.

Testing a Fundamental Assumption of Near-Miss Analysis

Near-miss analysis is predicated on the "causal continuum" assumption—that the causal factors of consequential accidents (adverse events) are similar to those of nonconsequential incidents (near misses) (Wright, 2002). This vital assumption, according to which the causes of near misses can be used predictively in preventing actual adverse events, needs to be examined for every major medical domain to optimize the cost/benefit ratio for investments in patient safety. Equally important is the strong motivation provided to potential near-miss reporters if they are aware that their contributions to achieving better insight into small, relatively trivial events indeed help in foreseeing and preventing real harm to patients.

Developing and Testing a Suitable Recovery Taxonomy

Prevention of failure factors has been the traditional approach to improving safety and will continue to play a vital role. However, when insight into recovery factors derived from near-miss analysis rounds out our understanding of what jeopardizes patient safety, a potentially powerful alternative means of improving patient safety becomes available: strengthening the (in)formal barriers and defenses between (partially unavoidable) errors/failures and their adverse consequences. Ideally, the active components of the recovery factors can be linked to the static components of the organizational structure that are positively associated with reliability and safety.

Integrating Individual Human Error/Recovery Models with Team-Based Error/Recovery Models

In most cases, health care is delivered by teams, not isolated individuals. However, the current models of individual human error and recovery have not yet been integrated with those of group and team processes as necessary to achieve the better understanding required to improve the safety performance of health care teams. In particular, there are advantages to developing specific crisis management algorithms in response to certain constellations of clinical signs or signals from monitors of vital signs. In addition, simulators have been demonstrated to have a role in training teams to respond to common crises (Jha et al., 2001).

Integration of Retrospective and Prospective Techniques

Retrospective risk analysis techniques (such as incident analysis) and prospective ones (such as hazard analysis and critical control points and failure mode and effect analysis) should be integrated for mutual validation and increased efficiency. Both techniques aim at insight into weaknesses (and strengths) at the system level: retrospective approaches, such as analysis of reported incidents, achieve such insight on the basis of actual deviations in an operational system, while prospective/predictive approaches, such as hazard analysis and critical control points and failure mode and effect analysis attempt to predict such deviations in the design/operational phases. Combining the two approaches may make it possible to validate predictions, feed failure scenarios with real data, and check reporting systems for biases.

Cost/Benefit Analysis of Patient Safety Programs

The qualitative changes resulting from the introduction of patient safety programs, including adverse event and near-miss analysis, must be documented. Comparing various introduction strategies across different types of health care organizations may make it possible to achieve continuing improvements in best practices. In the longer term, it would be desirable to quantify the benefits of patient safety programs—the reduction of adverse events in terms of frequency and/or severity—and the resources used to achieve this reduction. It would also be desirable to quantify the reduction of negative consequences in other areas, such as equipment failure, environmental releases, and logistic and operational costs, as they would be expected to stem from the same underlying organizational characteristics.

Patient Roles

Applied research is needed on how patients and their families can help with the prevention, early detection, and mitigation of harm due to errors. Health care organizations should implement policies and procedures designed to assist patients and their families in understanding their role in assuring the safety of patients while in a health care institution. Specific strategies should be designed to meet the needs of vulnerable populations, such as those with limited English, low literacy, and cognitive impairment, as well as others whose ability to understand and take action on health care information may be compromised. In particular, patient safety systems should be designed to elicit and receive information on adverse events and near misses from patients, their families, and their designees. Mechanisms should be in place to provide feedback to patients on the disposition of this information.

Evaluating the Impact of New Technologies for Detecting Near Misses

Technologies such as smart pumps, intensive care unit monitoring systems, and computerized physician order entry can be used to identify near misses. There is a need to investigate these systems and how the near misses they identify can be used to improve patient safety.

Tool Development

Early Detection

Automated triggers already allow for the detection of some types of adverse events, such as nosocomial infections (Evans et al., 1986) and ADEs (Classen et al., 1991; Jha et al., 1998), and it appears likely that this general approach could be extended to other types of adverse events (Bates et al., 2003). The approach works through detection of a signal, such as a high serum drug level, use of an antidote, or a laboratory abnormality in the context of use of a specific medication. A program called an event monitor is integrated with the clinical database to detect the presence of such a signal. Once a signal has been identified, it can be sent to the appropriate person or written to a file for later action. Currently, such detection approaches have high false-positive rates (Bates et al., 2003; Jha et al., 1998). Further research is needed to reduce false-positive rates for ADEs and nosocomial infections and to develop and validate computerized clinical trigger detection systems for other high-frequency sources of injury, such as decubitus ulcers, patient falls, complications of blood product transfusions, and complications of central and peripheral venous lines.

Prevention Capabilities

Tools such as computerized physician order entry incorporate capabilities to prevent adverse events, for example, by checking to see whether drug interactions with negative side effects could occur. Further research is needed to convert the growing knowledge base on patient safety risks into existing and new point-of-care decision support tools.

Verifying Adverse Events

Verification of adverse events can be problematic, and issues regarding the reliability of such assessments have been raised (Sanazaro and Mills, 1991; Thomas et al., 2002). For some types of adverse events, such as ADEs, scales having high interrater reliability, such as the Naranjo algorithm, have been developed (Naranjo et al., 1981). Overall, reliability in identifying adverse events can be expected to be higher with the use of triggers than with chart review because the evaluation relates to a discrete event. Nonetheless, greater standardization in the verification of adverse events is important—for example, using highly structured definitions of events, as is the case for nosocomial infections, or tools similar to the Naranjo algorithm.

Developing Data Mining Techniques for Large Patient Safety Databases

The size of patient safety databases at the state and regional levels will quickly become far too great for any individual to oversee their contents. Data mining will therefore be necessary to uncover patterns, test hypotheses, and even recognize whether individual new reports have been seen before.

Natural Language Processing

Much clinical information is contained in clinical notes and incident reports. Natural language processing can be used to analyze such data. Research is needed to develop natural language processing tools for patient safety applications.

Dissemination

Knowledge Dissemination

New methods are needed for promoting and speeding up the dissemination of knowledge and tools related to patient safety to aid and support health care administrators, care providers, and patients.

Audit Procedures

Existing knowledge and tools regarding patient safety need to be incorporated into audit criteria used to determine whether a health care organization is detecting most adverse events that occur. The term "audit" can describe a series of activities ranging from unstructured self-assessments (National Quality Forum) to comprehensive reviews of structure, process, and outcomes (Joint Commission on Accreditation of Healthcare Organizations). For patient safety data standards, audit means independent review of injury case finding, evaluation, and classification using explicit criteria for the structure and function of the data systems and for the review process itself. The aim of a data system audit should be to provide assurance that the numbers reported are reasonably complete, accurate, and reproducible and thus useful for shared analysis and comparison. By design, such an audit does not address how a health care organization responds to the injury data obtained or produce judgments about safety performance. In other industries, such audit assurance is an essential element of transparency and a potent antidote to misrepresentation, cheating, and corruption. Research is needed to develop fully functional quality-of-care audit criteria and to determine how such systems might be administered.

REFERENCES

Agency for Healthcare Research and Quality. 2001. *Ways You Can Help Your Family Prevent Medical Errors.* Online. Available: http://www.ahcpr.gov/consumer/5tipseng/5tips.pdf [accessed July 30, 2003].

Bates, D. W., R. S. Evans, H. Murff, P. D. Stetson, L. Pizziferri, and G. Hripcsak. 2003. Detecting adverse events using information technology. *J Am Med Inform Assoc* 10 (2):115–128.

Classen, D. C., S. L. Pestotnik, R. S. Evans, and J. P. Burke. 1991. Computerized surveillance of adverse drug events in hospital patients. *JAMA* 266 (20):2847–2851.

Classen, D. C., R. S. Evans, S. L. Pestotnik, S. D. Horn, R. L. Menlove, and J. P. Burke. 1992. The timing of prophylactic administration of antibiotics and the risk of surgical-wound infection. *N Engl J Med* 326 (5):337–339.

Evans, R. S., R. A. Larsen, J. P. Burke, R. M. Gardner, F. A. Meier, J. A. Jacobson, M. T. Conti, J. T. Jacobson, and R. K. Hulse. 1986. Computer surveillance of hospital-acquired infections and antibiotic use. *JAMA* 256 (8):1007–1011.

Evans, R. S., S. L. Pestotnik, D. C. Classen, S. D. Horne, S. B. Bass, and J. P. Burke. 1994. Preventing adverse drug events in hospitalized patients. *Ann Pharmacother* 28 (4):523–527.

Gawande, A. A., E. J. Thomas, M. J. Zinner, and T. A. Brennan. 1999. The incidence and nature of surgical adverse events in Colorado and Utah in 1992. *Surgery* 126 (1):66–75.

Henz, S. 2000. *Improved ADR Detection Without Using a Computer-Assisted Alert System.* Salt Lake City, UT: Institute of Healthcare Delivery Research.

James, B. C. 1989. *Quality Management for Health Care Delivery.* Chicago, IL: Hospital Research and Education Trust (American Hospital Association).

————. 2001. Making it easy to do it right. *NEJM* 345 (13):991–992.

————. 2003. Information system concepts for quality measurement. *Med Care* 41 (1):supplement I-71–I-79.

Jha, A. K., G. J. Kuperman, J. M. Teich, L. Leape, B. Shea, E. Rittenberg, E. Burdick, D. L. Seger, M. Vander Vliet, and D. W. Bates. 1998. Identifying adverse drug events: Development of a computer-based monitor and comparison with chart review and stimulated voluntary report. *J Am Med Inform Assoc* 5 (3):305–314.

Jha, A. K., B. W. Duncan, and D. W. Bates. 2001. Chapter 45: Simulator-based training and patient safety. In: *Making Health Care Safer: A Critical Analysis of Patient Safety Practices: Evidence Report/Technology Assessment No. 43*. Rockville, MD: Agency for Health Care Research and Quality.

Joint Commission on Accreditation of Healthcare Organizations. 2002. *SPEAK UP: National Campaign Urges Patients to Join Safety Efforts*. Online. Available: http://www.jcaho.org/news+room/press+kits/speak+up+national+campaign+urges+patients+to+join+safety+efforts+.htm [accessed August 5, 2003].

Juran, J. M. 1989. *Juran on Leadership for Quality*. New York, NY: Free Press.

Kim, Y. 2003. *Interaction Among Data-Based Clinical Triggers*. Personal communication to Institute of Medicine's Committee on Data Standards for Patient Safety.

Kizer, K. W. 1999. Large system change and a culture of safety. In: *Enhancing Patient Safety and Reducing Errors in Health Care*. Chicago, IL: National Patient Safety Foundation.

Langley, G. J., K. M. Nolan, C. L. Norman, L. P. Provost, and T. W. Nolan. 1996. *The Improvement Guide: A Practical Approach to Enhancing Organizational Performance*. San Francisco, CA: Jossey-Bass.

Larsen, R. A., R. S. Evans, J. P. Burke, S. L. Pestotnick, R. M. Gardner, and D. C. Classen. 1989. Improved perioperative antibiotic use and reduced surgical wound infections through the use of computer decision analysis. *Infect Control Hosp Epidemiol* 10 (7):316–320.

Leape, L. L., T. A. Brennan, N. M. Laird, A. G. Lawthers, A. R. Localio, B. A. Barnes, H. L. Newhouse, P. C. Weiler, and H. Hiatt. 1991. Incidence of adverse events and negligence in hospitalized patients: Results of the Harvard Medical Practice Study II. *N Engl J Med* 324:377–384.

Leape, L. L., D. J. Cullen, M. D. Clapp, E. Burdick, H. J. Demonaco, J. I. Erickson, and D. W. Bates. 1999. Pharmacist participation on physician rounds and adverse drug events in intensive care unit. *JAMA* 282 (3):267–270.

Marx, D. 2001. *Patient Safety and the "Just Culture": A Primer for Health Care Executives*. Funded by a grant from the National Heart, Lung, and Blood Institute, National Institutes of Health (Grant RO1 HL53772, Harold S. Kaplan, M.D., Principal Investigator). New York, NY: Trustees of Columbia University.

McDonough, J. E. 2002. *Proactive Hazard Analysis and Health Care Policy*. New York, NY: MilBank Memorial Fund/ECRI.

Naranjo, C. A., U. Busto, E. M. Sellers, P. Sandor, I. Ruiz, E. A. Roberts, E. Janecek, C. Domecq, and D. J. Greenblatt. 1981. A method for estimating the probability of adverse drug reactions. *Clin Pharmacol Ther* 30 (2):239–245.

O'Leary, D. S. 2003. *Perspectives and Insights*. Council on Teaching Hospitals, Spring Meeting. Phoenix, AZ: Joint Commission on Accreditation of Healthcare Organizations.

Pharmaceutical Health and Rational Use of Medicines Committee, Australian Pharmaceutical Advisory Council. 2001. *Quality Use of Medicines: A Decade of Research, Development and Service Activity 1991–2001.* Canberra: Commonwealth Department of Health and Aged Care.

Reason, J., and A. Hobbs. 2003. *Managing Maintenance Error: A Practical Guide.* Burlington, VT: Ashgate.

Sanazaro, P. J., and D. H. Mills. 1991. A Critique of the Use of Generic Screening in Quality Assessment. *JAMA* 265 (15):1977–1981.

Sholtes, P. R., B. L. Joiner, and B. J. Streibel. 2003. *Team Handbook, Third Edition.* Madison, WI: Oriel.

Smith, E. R. 1998. Mental representation and memory. In: D. T. Gilbert, S. T. Fiske, and G. Lindzey, eds. *The Handbook of Social Psychology.* Boston, MA: McGraw-Hill. Pp. 391–445.

Thomas, E. J., S. R. Lipsitz, D. M. Studdert, and T. A. Brennan. 2002. The reliability of medical record review for estimating adverse event rates. *Ann Intern Med* 136 (11):812–816.

Voluntary Hospitals of America. 2000. *Consumer Demand for Clinical Quality: The Giant Awakes: VHA's 2000 Research Series—Volume 3.* Irving, TX: Voluntary Hospitals of America, Inc.

Wright, L. B. 2002. *The Analysis of UK Railway Accidents and Incidents: A Comparison of Their Causal Patterns.* Glasgow: University of Strathclyde.

Xu, W., P. Hougland, S. Pickard, C. Masheter, G. Petratos, and S. D. Williams. 2003. *Detecting Adverse Drug Events Using ICD-9-CM Codes.* Arlington, VA: AHRQ Second Annual Patient Safety Research Conference.

6

Adverse Event Analysis

CHAPTER SUMMARY

Iatrogenic injury often arises from the poor design and fragmentary nature of the health care delivery system. The detection and analysis of adverse events, both individually and in the aggregate, can reveal organizational, systemic, and environmental problems. This chapter examines the functional requirements for the two fundamental components of adverse event systems—methods for detecting adverse events and methods for analyzing such events—and the implications for data standards.

The primary method of adverse event detection is voluntary reporting, and as result, most adverse events in health care today are not detected. Even if larger numbers of adverse events were detected, the information would be of limited value because of differing definitions of adverse events and varying data collection and analysis methods.

There are many ways to detect adverse events—through reporting systems, document review, automated surveillance of clinical data, and monitoring of patient progress. These approaches are ultimately complementary and require a broad range of data elements covering demographic information, signs and symptoms, medications, test results, diagnoses, therapies, and outcomes. While all the available methods are complementary and each has its strengths and weak-

nesses, automated surveillance is likely to become the most important source of adverse event data. More research is needed to improve the effectiveness of these detection systems and to broaden the types of adverse events that can be detected through automated triggers. Ultimately, an integrated approach, using patient safety data standards, will evolve, with electronic health record systems providing decision support at the point of care, preventing adverse events to the extent possible and facilitating the collection of reporting data when adverse events do occur.

Use of adverse event systems is also aimed at identifying improved health care processes through the analysis of adverse event data. This process involves selecting and defining the adverse events to survey, defining the analysis population, collecting surveillance data, analyzing surveillance findings (identifying causal factors), and using the findings to develop interventions. The process requires standard definitions of adverse events, minimum datasets for describing the events, standard definitions of dataset variables, and standard approaches for collecting and integrating the data.

INTRODUCTION

An adverse event is defined as an event that results in unintended harm to the patient by an act of commission or omission rather than by the underlying disease or condition of the patient. The understanding that adverse events are common and often result from the poor design of health care delivery systems (Institute of Medicine, 2000) has led to the development of institutional adverse event systems. These systems are used to collect data on adverse events that make it possible to learn from such events and identify trends that may reveal organizational, systemic, and environmental problems.

Despite these developments, most adverse events are undetected. The reason is that most health care organizations rely on voluntary reporting for the detection of adverse events (Bates et al., 2003; Cullen et al., 1995), and spontaneous reporting has been demonstrated to be a minimally effective way of detecting such events (Classen et al., 1991; Cullen et al., 1995; Jha et al., 1998).

Even if larger numbers of adverse events were detected, the value of the information would be limited because existing adverse event systems use widely differing definitions, characterizations, and classification approaches.

In this emerging field of study, many different definitions of adverse events are used, and a common terminology has yet to emerge. One of the more difficult problems in discussing patient safety is imprecise taxonomy, since the choice of terms has implications for how the problems related to patient safety are addressed. This imprecision makes comparison of different studies and reporting systems difficult. With few exceptions, existing studies each report data for different populations, and they frequently differ in the way they define, count, and track adverse events. Major variations in nomenclature with no fixed and accepted consensus hamper further research and application.

Adverse event systems have two fundamental components—methods for detecting adverse events and methods for analyzing such events. The remainder of this chapter explores in turn the requirements for each of these components and the implications for data standards. The final section presents a future vision for the use of adverse event systems.

DETECTION OF ADVERSE EVENTS: MULTIPLE APPROACHES REQUIRING A BROAD SET OF DATA ELEMENTS

Sources of Adverse Event Data

There are many sources of adverse event data. These include the following:

- Voluntary and mandatory reporting from internal hospital systems, state and federal systems, and patients themselves and their relatives.
- Document review, including patient charts, medical–legal documents, death certificates, coroners' reports, complaint data, and media reports.
- Automated surveillance of patient treatment data, including clinical patient records, hospital discharge summaries, and Medicare claims data that may be a response to a patient injury.
- Monitoring of the progress of patients to anticipate conditions that could lead to adverse events or to identify adverse events and implement corrective actions.

Reporting and chart review approaches identify adverse events that have already occurred. The focus is on the analysis of a subset of adverse events to determine root causes and identify improvements in care processes, ultimately improving patient safety.

Automated surveillance of data and monitoring of patient progress, referred to as concurrent surveillance methods, are prospective in that they start with a clinical care process and seek to identify critical points in that process at which failures are likely to occur (e.g., when medication is prescribed). These approaches aim to prevent adverse events from happening in the first place or to quickly identify an adverse event once it has happened. For example, a concurrent surveillance system might monitor pharmacy orders for the use of antidote medications, then quickly send a trained professional to review any such case detected. The reviewer determines whether an injury or near miss has occurred and then investigates and classifies the event. More important, because such a review occurs in real time, a clinician can often intervene to prevent or ameliorate resulting harm. While prospective surveillance systems can be created and operated effectively using solely manual methods, automated methods offer more cost-effective and elegant solutions when automated clinical data systems are available. The committee believes increased attention should be devoted to concurrent surveillance methods since many common causes of adverse events are already known (Agency for Healthcare Research and Quality, 2001).

Comparison of the Various Approaches for Adverse Event Detection

Broad-based studies of the relative effectiveness of the detection methods outlined above have not yet been carried out. However, a number of epidemiological studies have examined the relative strengths and weaknesses of voluntary reporting, retrospective chart review, and automated surveillance for detection of adverse drug events (ADEs).

Using inpatient data, Classen et al. (1991) established that automated surveillance could effectively detect ADEs at a much higher rate than voluntary reporting. Cullen et al. (1995), again using inpatient data, demonstrated that voluntary reporting uncovered only a small fraction of the ADEs identified by a nurse investigator reviewing charts daily.

Jha et al. (1998) compared automated surveillance with chart review and voluntary reporting using inpatient data. They found that automated surveillance and chart review each identified many more ADEs than did voluntary reporting. They also found that automated surveillance and chart review identified different types of events. Automated surveillance was more effective at identifying events associated with changes in laboratory results, such as renal failure. Chart review was more effective at identifying events manifested primarily through symptoms, such as changes in mental state.

In addition to ADEs, automated surveillance approaches have proven to be effective in identifying nosocomial infections and falls (Bates et al., 2003), although these approaches are not used routinely. Evans et al. (1986) demonstrated that computerized surveillance is at least as effective as traditional surveillance methods used by infection control practitioners for identifying hospital-acquired infections. Natural language processing was used to search radiology reports for indications that a patient fall after the second day of hospitalization was a reason for the radiological examination (Bates et al., 2003).

Although there has been considerable success in using automated surveillance techniques for detecting certain types of adverse events, there will continue to be many problems that will make automated detection without manual over-read challenging. For example, in searching anesthesia records for problems arising from the management of diabetes in the peri-operative period, large amounts of redundant information might be picked up as a result of patients having iatrogenic diabetes in the peri-operative period.

In conclusion, for ADEs, and probably for other types of adverse events as well, the three approaches to event detection reviewed—automated surveillance, chart review, and voluntary reporting—complement each other, with voluntary reporting being most effective at identifying potential adverse events or near misses (see Chapter 7). It is also likely that these three methods complement patient monitoring systems. Any patient safety data standards developed must be supportive of all the above detection methods.

Data Requirements for Adverse Event Detection

Voluntary and Mandatory Reporting

To encourage people to report, voluntary reporting tends not to be prescriptive about what types of events are to be reported or what information should be supplied. Generally, just a short description of what happened is required. The recipient of the report is then tasked with creating a report for analysis purposes.

Mandatory reporting systems usually specify in some detail the types of adverse events that must be reported and analyzed. For example, in New York State all hospitals (inpatient and outpatient) and freestanding clinics must report a wide range of adverse events to the New York Patient Occurrence Reporting and Tracking System (see Appendix C).

Chart Review

Chart review to identify possible adverse events involves reading physician and nurse progress notes and carefully examining the chart if certain indicators are present. For ADEs, these indicators might include an unexpected need for blood transfusion, the transfer of the patient to an intensive care unit, falls, explicit comments in the chart about a drug reaction, abnormal laboratory values, unexpected hypotension, and recent changes in mental state (Cullen et al., 1995). More recently, chart review has begun to use the rules incorporated in automated surveillance techniques. The Institute for Healthcare Improvement and Premier, Inc., have modified the automated surveillance methodology (Classen et al., 1991) created at LDS Hospital, Salt Lake City, to develop an ADE trigger that does not require computerized technology. The tool has about 20 triggers, outlined in Box 6-1,

---

BOX 6-1
Triggers for Chart Review to Detect Adverse Drug Events

- Receiving diphenhydramine
- Receiving vitamin K
- Receiving Flumazenil
- Receiving Droperidol or Ondanestron Promethazine or Hydoxyzine or Trimethobenzamide or Prochlorperazine or Metoclopramine
- Receiving naloxone
- Receiving Diphenoxylate or Loperamide or Kaopectate of Pepto-Bismol
- Receiving sodium polystyrene
- Partial thromboplastin time >100 seconds
- International normalized ratio >6
- White blood count <3,000
- Serum glucose <50
- Rising serum creatine
- Clostridium difficile positive stool
- Digoxin level >2
- Lidocaine level >2
- Gentamicin or Tobramycin levels: peak >10, trough <2
- Vancomycin level >26
- Theophylline level >20
- Oversedation, lethargy, fall, hypotension
- Rash
- Abrupt cessation of medication
- Transfer to a higher level of care

SOURCE: Rozich et al., 2003.

relating to medications, laboratory results, and signs and symptoms. Using this tool, it takes a reviewer about 20 minutes to review an average inpatient chart. This low-tech tool has produced consistent, reliable, and relevant data, although the cost of its use is not low (Rozich et al., 2003); indeed, relative to computer screening, the cost per event is very high.

Automated Surveillance of Clinical Data

An epidemiological study at Brigham and Women's Hospital using primary care data collected in 1995–1996 exemplifies some of the different approaches to automated surveillance. This study demonstrated the feasibility of identifying ADEs using automated surveillance of outpatient electronic medical records (Honigman et al., 2001). The study used four different approaches for identifying ADEs:

- International Classification of Diseases (ICD)-9 codes—Each patient record is scanned for ICD-9 codes that are often associated with the presence of possible ADEs.
- New allergies—An ADE may be present when a patient has a known allergy or a medication is listed as a new allergy. This approach requires knowing the patient's medications, including dose, interval, and quantity.
- Computer detection rules—These are Boolean combinations of medical events, for example, new medication orders or laboratory results outside certain limits that suggest an ADE might be present. One such rule is "If patient is receiving phytonadione (vitamin K) AND on Coumadin, then an ADE may be present." A list of such rules is given in Box 6-2.
- Data mining—Free-text searching of the electronic medical record is used to identify for each medication taken an indication of its known adverse reactions. For the drug type "diuretic," fatigue is a potential adverse reaction and "drowsiness," "drowsy," and "lassitude" are some of the synonyms used instead of the word "fatigue." Box 6-3 lists some potential adverse reactions (plus synonyms) for the diuretic drug group.

Monitoring of the Progress of Patients

The progress of patients can be monitored as they pass through the care process both to anticipate and protect against circumstances that could lead to adverse events and to implement corrective actions based on analysis of patient injuries discovered in the past. Monitoring systems are particularly important when addressing potential injuries of omission. One example of

BOX 6-2
Rules for Detecting Possible Adverse Drug Events Using Automated Surveillance

Receiving new diphenhydramine AND no diphenhydramine within last 7 days AND patient not on paclitaxel AND no blood transfusion in last 1 day AND no diphenhydramine at bedtime
Receiving oral vancomycin
Blood alkaline phosphatase >350 units/liter (L)
Receiving phytonadione (vitamin K) AND on Coumadin
Receiving ranitidine AND platelet count has fallen to less than 50 percent of previous value or below 100,000
Serum carbamazepine >12.0 micrograms/milliliter (µg/mL)
Serum digoxin >1.7 nanograms (ng)/mL
Serum bilirubin >10 milligrams/deciliter
Serum cyclosporine >500 µg/L
Serum potassium >6.5 millimoles/L
Blood eosinophils >6 percent
Receiving kaopectate
Receiving loperamide
Serum n-acetyl procainamide >20 µg/mL
Serum phenytoin results >20 µg/mL
Serum phenobarbital results >45 µg/mL
Receiving prednisone AND diphenhydramine
Serum procainamide >10 µg/mL
Serum aspartate amino transferase >150 U/L AND no prior result >150 U/L
Serum theophylline >20 µg/mL
Serum valproate >120 µg/mL
Serum quinidine >5 µg/mL
Serum alanine aminotransferase >150 U/L AND no result >150 U/L in last 7 days

SOURCE: Honigman et al., 2001.

this approach is monitoring the progress of individual patients and groups of patients with the same condition as they pass through the care process using measures for assessing the quality of care given, such as those of the Diabetes Quality Improvement Project (DQIP). Another example is monitoring all patients at a particular point in the care continuum, such as through use of a validation system for medical prescribing based on computerized physician order entry. This section examines the general data requirements of these two examples.

BOX 6-3
Sample of Triggers for Outpatient Adverse Drug Events

In the case of an outpatient taking a diuretic, the following adverse reactions (and their synonyms) would serve as triggers for detection of a potential ADE:

- Dizziness (also syncope, lightheaded, vertigo, "wooziness")
- Fainting (also blackout, loss of consciousness, syncope or near syncope, vagal reaction, vasometer collapse, vasovagal reaction, "swooning")
- Fall(s)
- Fatigue (also drowsiness, drowsy, lassitude, lethargic, lethargy, listless, listlessness, malaise, tired)
- Hypokolemia (also low potassium, muscle cramps, potassium decreased, potassium deficiency)
- Hyponatremia (also low serum sodium)
- Hypotension (also arterial blood pressure decreased, low blood pressure, postural hypotension)
- Renal failure (also kidney shutdown, chronic renal insufficiency)
- Weakness (also decreased muscle strength, lack of strength)

SOURCE: Bates, 2002.

DQIP has developed a core set of evidence-based measures[1] for assessing the quality of adult diabetes care. These measures are used to monitor the progress of individual patients and groups of patients with diabetes as they pass through the care process.

The measures include those used for external accountability and internal quality improvement. The core set for accountability encompasses measures in seven areas of outpatient care: hemoglobin A1C (HbA1C) management, lipid management, urine protein testing, eye examination, foot examination, blood pressure management, and smoking cessation. The set for quality improvement includes measures in these seven areas and in two additional areas—influenza immunization and aspirin use.

---

[1] These performance measures were initially developed by the Centers for Medicare and Medicaid Services, the Foundation for Accountability, the American Diabetes Association, and the National Committee for Quality Assurance. In 2002, DQIP merged with a performance collaboration of the American Medical Association, the Joint Commission on Accreditation of Healthcare Organizations, and the National Committee for Quality Assurance to form the National Diabetes Quality Improvement Alliance.

Making the determination that a particular patient is a diabetic and applying the DQIP measures requires a number of data elements:

• Presence of the following data elements: insulin medication, oral hypoglycemic medication, date of ambulatory encounter, diagnosis of ambulatory encounter, medication prescribed at ambulatory encounter, date of inpatient encounter, diagnosis at inpatient encounter, date of emergency room (ER) encounter, and diagnosis at ER encounter (see Table 6-1).
• The two annual accountability measures for hemoglobin management—percent of patients receiving one or more HbA1C tests and percent of patients with most recent HbA1C level >9.0 percent—require the data elements HbA1C test, date of HbA1C test, and HbA1C level (see Table 6-2).

Computerized physician order entry systems accept physician orders (e.g., for medications and for laboratory/diagnostic tests) electronically in lieu of the physician's handwritten orders on a prescription pad or an order sheet. Order entry systems offer the potential to reduce medication errors through a number of validation procedures. One procedure is to determine the extent of therapeutic duplication between the newly prescribed medica-

TABLE 6-1 Data Requirements for the Definition of an Adult Diabetes Patient

Definition	Data Requirements
Those who were dispensed insulin and/or oral hypoglycemics/antihypoglycemics OR Those who had *two* face-to-face encounters in an ambulatory setting or non-acute inpatient setting or *one* face-to-face encounter in an inpatient or emergency room setting with a diagnosis of diabetes	• Insulin medication • Oral hypoglycemic medication • Date of ambulatory encounter • Diagnosis of ambulatory encounter • Medication prescribed at ambulatory encounter • Date of inpatient encounter • Diagnosis at inpatient encounter • Date of ER encounter • Patient age

NOTE: Patients with gestational diabetes excluded.
SOURCE: American Medical Association, Joint Commission on Accreditation of Healthcare Organizations, National Committee for Quality Assurance, 2001.

TABLE 6-2 Data Requirements for Diabetes Quality Improvement Project Measures

Performance Measure	Quality Improvement Measures (per year)
HbA1C management	Per patient: • Number of HbA1C tests received • Trend of HbA1C values Across all patients: • Percent of patients receiving one or more HbA1C test(s) • Distribution of number of tests done (0, 1, 2, 3, or more) • Distribution of most recent HbA1C value by range
Lipid management	Per patient: • Trend of values of each test Across all patients: • Percent of patients receiving at least one lipid profile (or all component tests) • Distributions of most recent test values for total cholesterol, high-density lipoprotein (HDL) cholesterol, low-density lipoprotein (LDL) cholesterol, and triglycerides by range
Urine protein testing	Per patient: • Any test for microalbuminuria received • If no urinalysis or urinalysis with negative or trace urine protein, a microalbumin test received Across all patients: • Percent of patients receiving any test for microalbuminuria • Percent of patients with no urinalysis or urinalysis with negative or trace urine protein who received a test for microalbumin
Eye examination	Per patient: • Dilated retinal eye exam performed by an ophthalmologist or optometrist • Funduscopic photo with interpretation by an ophthalmologist or optometrist Across all patients: • Percent of patients receiving a dilated retinal eye exam by an ophthalmologist or optometrist • Percent of patients receiving funduscopic photo with interpretation by an ophthalmologist or optometrist

Public Reporting Measures (per year)	Data Requirements
• Percent of patients receiving one or more HbA1C test(s) • Percent of patients with most recent HbA1C level >9.0%	• Glycohemoglobin test • Date of glycohemoglobin test • HbA1C level
• Percent of patients receiving at least one low-density lipoprotein cholesterol (LDL-C) test • Percent of patients with most recent LDL-C level <130 milligrams/deciliter	• Lipid profile test • Date of lipid profile test • Result of lipid profile test (total cholesterol, HDL cholesterol, LDL cholesterol, and triglycerides)
• Percent of patients with at least one test for microalbumin during the measurement year or who had had evidence of medical attention for existing nephropathy (diagnosis of nephropathy or documentation of microalbuminuria or albuminuria)	• Microalbumin test • Date of microalbumin test • Result of microalbumin test • Urinalysis test • Urinalysis test date • Urinalysis test result (amount of protein found—negative, trace, positive—for all test components • Evidence of nephropathy—an allowable diagnosis code/description or an eligible treatment code/description • Insulin medication • HbA1C level
• Percent of patients who received a dilated eye exam or evaluation of retinal photographs by an ophthalmologist or optometrist during the reporting year, or during the prior year, if patient is at low risk of retinopathy (i.e., patient not taking insulin, and HbA1C <8%, and no evidence of retinopathy in prior year)	• Eye exam • Date of eye exam • Types of eye exams performed (dilated examination of the retina or funduscopic photographs) • Specialty of clinician performing eye exam (ophthalmology, optometry, or other) • Retinopathy • Insulin medication • HbA1C level

Continued

TABLE 6-2 Continued

Performance Measure	Quality Improvement Measures (per year)
Foot examination (exclusions: patients with bilateral foot amputation)	Per patient: • At least one complete foot exam received (visual inspection, sensory exam with monofilament, and pulse exam) Across all patients: • Percent of eligible patients receiving at least one complete foot exam (visual inspection, sensory exam with monofilament, and pulse exam)
Influenza immunization (exclusions: patients allergic to eggs)	Per patient: • Immunization status Across all patients: • Percent of patients who received an influenza immunization during the recommended calendar period • Percent of eligible patients who received an influenza immunization or refused immunization during the calendar period
Blood pressure measurement	Per patient: • Most recent systolic and diastolic blood pressure reading Across all patients: • Distribution of most recent blood pressure values by range
Aspirin use (exclusions: patients under 40 years old, aspirin contraindication/ allergy)	Per patient: • Patient receiving aspirin therapy (dose $\geq$ 75 mg) Across all patients: • Percent of patients receiving aspirin therapy (dose $\geq$ 75 mg)
Smoking cessation	Per patient: • Patient assessed for smoking status • Patient identified as a smoker was recommended or offered counseling or pharmacologic therapy Across all patients: • Percent of patients who are smokers • Percent of patients assessed for smoking status • Percent of smokers who were recommended or offered an intervention for smoking cessation (i.e., counseling or pharmacologic therapy)

SOURCE: National Diabetes Quality Improvement Alliance (2003).

Public Reporting Measures (per year)	Data Requirements
• Percent of eligible patients receiving at least one foot exam, defined in any manner	• Foot exam • Date of foot exam • Type of foot exam (including visual inspection, sensory exam with monofilament, and pulse exam)
None	• Influenza immunization • Date influenza immunization given • Influenza immunization refused • Date influenza immunization refused • Allergy to eggs
• Percent of patients with most recent blood pressure <140/90 millimeters/hemoglobin	• Blood pressure measurement • Date of blood pressure measurement • Most recent blood pressure level
None	• Patient age • Aspirin therapy • Aspirin dose • Aspirin contraindications/allergies
• Percent of patients whose smoking status was ascertained and documented annually	• Smoking status • Date smoking status documented • Counseling offered or recommended • Pharmacologic therapy offered or recommended

TABLE 6-3 Computerized Physician Order Entry Validation Modules for
Medication Prescribing

Validation Module	Generic Data Requirements
Therapeutic duplication	Medications, medication ingredients
Single and cumulative dose limits	Medications, dose levels
Allergies and cross-allergies	Allergies, drug allergies
Contraindicated route of administration	Medications, route of administration
Drug–drug and drug–food interactions	Medications
Contraindication/dose limits based on patient diagnosis	Medications, diagnoses
Contraindication/dose limits based on patient age and weight	Medications, medication dose levels, patient age, weight
Contraindication/dose limits based on laboratory studies	Medications, medication dose levels, laboratory results
Contraindication/dose limits based on radiology studies	Medications, contrast media used in radiology

SOURCE: Kilbridge et al., 2001.

tion and the patient's existing medications. To do this requires data on all
the patient's medications and the ingredients of each.

A list of validation modules that could be incorporated in a computerized physician order entry system is given in Table 6-3, together with the
generic data requirements. A full set of validation modules requires a wide
range of data elements: medications (including ingredients, dose levels, and
administration routes), allergies (including drug allergies), diagnoses, patient age, weight, laboratory results, and contrast media used in radiology.

Implications for Data Standards

The various approaches to adverse event detection discussed above demonstrate that it is not possible to simply identify a small set of clinical data
elements specifically for adverse event detection, especially when addressing
potential injuries due to errors of omission as well as injuries due to errors of
commission. On the contrary, a broad range of data elements encompassing
demographic information, signs and symptoms, medications, test results,
diagnoses, therapies, and outcomes are required to: (1) detect adverse events
through voluntary and mandatory reporting, chart review, and automated
surveillance; (2) implement performance measures (e.g., DQIP measures);

and (3) use decision support tools (e.g., computerized physician order entry). Thus, comprehensive clinical and patient safety data are necessary for adverse event detection and monitoring.

ANALYSIS OF ADVERSE EVENT SYSTEMS

Functional Requirements

Understanding an Adverse Event

> An outside physician calls hospital administration after one of her patients develops a near-fatal adverse reaction thought to be secondary to a drug–drug reaction to a medication prescribed in an emergency department 2 days previously. The patient safety team is assembled and after some careful detective work determines that the cause of the problem was that house staff rotating into the hospital from outside institutions were trained inadequately in use of the hospital electronic health record.

Determining which of many interwoven processes should be implicated in a typical case of error is a critical step in eliminating sources of risk in the health care system. Making this determination involves asking four main questions.[2] First, *what* is the event we are trying to eliminate? In this case we are trying to prevent patients from receiving an inappropriate drug. Second, *which* roles or processes must occur for this event to happen? Here, steps include recognizing a patient's need for a medication, prescribing, filling the prescription, delivering it to the patient, and so on. Next, *when* did the event occur, and were there co-occurring events that could be related? Here, the fact that this reaction occurred in close proximity to the initiation of a new medication is helpful. Finally, *where* did the event or associated processes take place? In this case, characteristics of emergency departments, outpatient pharmacies, and homes are important.

In the parlance of public health professionals, adverse event surveillance should characterize a latent[3] problem within a complex system, placing the event in context rather than characterizing it as primarily the failing of a single upstream process, such as a hospital, patient, or provider. The

---

[2] A similar approach is adopted for the analysis of a near miss; see the next chapter.

[3] James Reason distinguishes two types of errors—active and latent (Reason, 1990). Active errors are associated with the performance of front-line operators, such as doctors and nurses. Latent errors result from underlying system failures.

focus should be more on enhancing knowledge about risks and how to prevent them rather than on blaming, shaming, and punishing individuals. This process of understanding is the lynchpin of an effective safety culture, and its importance points to the main deficiencies in existing standards for representing potential or actual adverse medical events. One hallmark of effective analysis of adverse events is that it leads to system changes that inherently make it easier for those working in a health care delivery environment to do the job right, as opposed to a constant emphasis on more education or closer oversight—both second-hand markers for blame. Since much of health care is organized around the convenience of clinicians, however, it is important to note that interventions that alter the sequence of work flow are more challenging to implement.

Addressing Errors of Omission

Efforts such as those of ORC Macro[4] and DQIP extend the breadth of the nomenclature needed for adverse event systems by including errors of omission. In the latter cases, in addition to characterizing errors and near-miss events by specifying what, which, when, and where, there is a need for additional elements or classification.

For example, an error of commission, such as the ICD-9, Clinical Modification (CM) measure of *foreign body left in during a procedure*, may be adequately characterized by knowing the probable cause for leaving the foreign body in (why), the conditions under which it occurred (when and where), and the people present for the procedure (who). On the other hand, analysis of an error of omission (e.g., DQIP measure for HbA1C count), could benefit from more data about the patient. The DQIP measures indicate the specific patient data required to confirm a diagnosis of diabetes (prescription or dispensing of insulin and/or oral hypoglycemics/antihyperglycemics during the reporting year, exclusion of women with gestational diabetes). To assess errors of omission, the dataset to compare HbA1C test rates should be expanded to include data about how the diagnosis was established, in addition to data for risk stratification or covariate analysis.

---

[4]ORC Macro is a research, management consulting, and information technology firm based in Calverton, Maryland.

Implications for Data Standards

The above examples and requirements of adverse event analysis point to the need to enhance existing data standards to support adverse event reporting. The most usable of standards will include clear and unambiguous event definitions, minimum datasets that characterize the population and setting, explicit data collection processes, and methods for integrating data across systems and settings.

Definitions of Terms

An examination of the literature on patient safety raises many questions. Paramount among these is the problem of definitions of terms, with differing definitions of errors, adverse events, and near misses being used from one publication to another. Often, the addition of a single word creates ambiguity across the entire spectrum of reporting. For example, are potential adverse events synonymous with near misses? Do nonpreventable adverse events stem from errors? Will medication errors include actions taken by a family member who, for example, might administer insulin injections in an area with poor absorption of the medication?

As with data collected for clinical trials, strict definitions of terms, including processes by which the data may be obtained, are critical to acquiring information on adverse events in a reproducible fashion. For example, each type of adverse event must be precisely defined, including examples and events that are outside the definition. Unfortunately, few standard terminologies include such definitions. DQIP represents a model for both the use of terms and the standardization of data collection. Each measure encompasses inclusion and exclusion definitions, confounding patient demographic or other data, the rationale for the importance of the measure, and a process by which the measure should be obtained. In contrast, many clinical terminologies contain terms that do not have precise definitions or conditions of use. For example, the ICD code for diabetes without ketoacidosis could refer to a patient with either Type II diabetes or well-controlled Type I diabetes. Moreover, it is not clear for many terms whether they are used to describe a point in time or a chronic condition. The ICD code for diabetes with ketoacidosis, for instance, should be applied only to a single encounter because the ketoacidosis will resolve, while the underlying diabetes will remain. In the case of a patient with Alzheimer's disease, however, the presence of any encounter with that diagnosis passes forward to all subsequent encounters.

Term definitions should also include a precise description of the groups of patients who are included and excluded. As noted above, for example, DQIP excludes patients with diagnoses such as gestational diabetes, a condition that generally resolves once the pregnancy is over.

Precise definitions facilitate the prospective collection of data on similar events and an understanding of how the rate of these events is altered by interventions. They also allow large numbers of near misses and minor incidents to be analyzed (see Chapter 7). From a practical standpoint, health care workers need assistance when collecting data using such detailed definitions. For example, the appropriate definitions might appear on a computer screen when the data are being collected.

Minimum Datasets

To specify definitions and potential uses of terms to be included in an adverse event system, it is necessary to have minimum data requirements for the system. These minimum requirements should be stated and defined explicitly.

Regardless of how an adverse event is detected, the process for reporting and analyzing is essentially the same. Data are collected on each adverse event. Using these data, a subset of adverse events (as well as near misses; see Chapter 7) is analyzed to determine their root causes and recovery procedures. Improvements in the delivery of care are then devised and implemented. Aggregate analyses of adverse events for which the more detailed analyses were not carried out may also lead to improvements in the delivery of care.

Once an adverse event has been validated, the committee believes a report of the event should be a combination of narrative and coded elements. Coding is essential if large numbers of events are to be analyzed efficiently. However, any given coding system reflects a particular understanding of the key features of adverse events. Additional research can lead to new perspectives on what constitutes such features, and the availability of a narrative enables the adverse event to be recoded based on this new understanding.

At a minimum, the narrative text should give a brief description of what happened and the reporter's view of why it happened. Using the narrative and further information from the medical record, and possibly from the reporter, an adverse event record should be coded along the following dimensions (at a minimum):

- The discovery
  - Who discovered/reported the event—role, not names
  - How it was discovered
- The event itself
  - What happened—the type of adverse event
  - Where in the care process the event was discovered and/or occurred
  - When it occurred
  - Who was involved—functions, not names
  - Why—the most dominant cause based on a preliminary analysis
  - Likelihood of recurrence of similar adverse events
  - Severity of the event
  - Preventability of the event
- Ancillary information
  - Product information (blood, devices, drugs) if involved in the adverse event
  - Patient information, including age, gender, ethnicity, diagnoses, procedures, and comorbid conditions
- Detailed analysis

On the basis of the above information, a decision should be made as to whether a formal root-cause analysis should be carried out (a similar decision is required to investigate a near miss; see Chapter 7). Using automated surveillance together with other detection methods will lead to the detection of a much greater number of adverse events that might warrant such an analysis than would otherwise be possible. All such events cannot feasibly be investigated. Thus if root-cause analyses are not focused on a critical subset, then (1) useless analyses will be carried out because there is no time to do them properly, and (2) effort will be devoted to performing root-cause analyses at the expense of testing and implementing real system changes that can reduce injury rates. The decision to carry out a root-cause analysis will normally depend on the following factors:

- The likelihood of recurrence of similar adverse events—the assessment is facilitated by access to a database of adverse events. If a similar case has recently been investigated, full root-cause analysis will have only marginal utility.
- The severity of the adverse event—can be assessed by direct observation.

  – Whether the adverse event potentially represents a previously un-
    known problem—a judgment call drawing on the collective exper-
    tise of the patient safety team. Access to a database of adverse
    events also helps here.
  – The resources available to carry out such analyses—another judg-
    ment call for the patient safety team.
  – The potential for correction—depends on the expertise of the pa-
    tient safety team.

A number of risk assessment indices have been developed to help in making
the decision as to whether a root-cause analysis should be carried out. Chapter 9 provides further discussion on risk assessment as well as on methods
for classifying root cause data.

  • Results

Once a root-cause analysis has been completed, its results, including the
following, should be fully documented and acted upon:

  – Failed (and successful) defenses and recoveries for the patient
  – Outcome for the patient
  – Lessons learned and ways to improve patient safety

Here there is an important difference between adverse events and near
misses. Adverse events require the formal instigation of defenses (for example, a medication is discontinued, a prescription for diphenhydramine is
written), whereas near misses involve built-in defenses (for example, automatic compensation through stand-by equipment; see Chapter 7).

An examination of public health surveillance systems reveals the importance of refining these datasets, while health services research reminds us
that collecting less structured data early in the process will reduce respondent burden and potentially remove inherent biases in the types of data
collected. Therefore, it may be important to define an outcome of interest
precisely and then allow knowledge gained from the reporting process (both
accountability and learning) to inform system developers about data whose
collection in the aggregate will be useful. As knowledge about these outcomes and known or suspected causes accrues, the inclusion of elements in
a minimum dataset will evolve.

Explicit Data Collection Processes

Whenever possible, but especially if data are to be compared across institutions, standards for data in an adverse event system should describe how the data elements should be collected. Descriptions of patient populations that should be included or excluded and specification of whether a patient may be included multiple times during the same encounter will help clarify the group to be investigated. Data sources—including reports from health care providers' hospital discharge summaries, emergency department notes, computer triggers, electronic clinic notes, and administrative incident reports—should be described.

Uniformity of systems and applications for collecting the data (such as surveys, interviews, or claims data) will ensure that the data are comparable across time and location. As noted for the DQIP initial measure set, articulating the collection process and environment exposes cultural or other barriers to data collection (or sharing), facilitates auditing, and improves the data's external validity.

Integrating Data Across Systems and Settings

Clearly, one goal of adverse event systems is to allow aggregate reporting of events for purposes of both assessing known problems before and after interventions and detecting new problems. Attention to other requirements will allow appropriate comparisons of events. Standards such as Health Level Seven (HL7) (discussed in Chapter 4) and specifications such as extensible markup language (XML) may help improve data sharing but only if the contents of these shared items are based on the same terminology—for both items and responses. Ensuring that responses are easily combined is often beyond the realm of data standards but must be considered if large datasets will be generated. For example, different systems may allow a male to be represented as "Male," "1," "0," or "M." Integrating these terms will be a challenge.

FUTURE VISION

Increasing Importance of Automated Triggers

Looking to the future, it is likely that spontaneous reporting will be important indefinitely, especially for near misses; however, use of automated triggers is likely to grow as more computerized information becomes available and automated detection becomes increasingly feasible (Bates et al., 2003). The result will be the detection of a much higher proportion of adverse events than are found today. Events may be detected through sending signals to quality personnel who can evaluate them, yet increasingly, electronic records will prompt providers to assess in real time whether signals represent an adverse event. For example, when one medication is discontinued and a prescription for diphenhydramine is written, the clinician should be asked whether the patient is allergic to the first medication. Note that it will be important to determine how much data point-of-care providers can handle, since warnings and messages may be ignored if they are too numerous, especially if their relevance is not immediately apparent. Therefore, although automated triggers have enormous potential and have been shown to be highly valuable, the committee recognizes that in the end they will be suitable for certain types of problems but not others.

Definitions of Core Constructs

As noted above, a fundamental and nettlesome issue has been defining the key concepts relating to patient safety—adverse events and near misses. The failure to use standard definitions for these core concepts has made comparisons among institutions challenging at best. Broad adoption of the patient data safety standards recommended by this committee (and, where necessary, further refinement of the individual constructs) would represent a major step forward in enabling meaningful aggregation and comparison of rates of such incidents from different settings.

Detection of Adverse Events Using Claims Data

Another approach to detecting adverse events involves using claims data (Iezzoni et al., 1994). While this approach has been fairly effective for surgical patients, it has not worked well for medical patients. However, a recent tool developed by the Agency for Healthcare Research and Quality has demonstrated excellent specificity, although its sensitivity is still quite low (Zhan and Miller, 2003).

Improving the coding sets for patient safety–related conditions and events used in claims data (i.e., ICD-9) and employing incentives more broadly could represent an extremely attractive approach, especially if combined with the collection of clinical data (Classen, 2003). For example, codes to distinguish between preexisting conditions prior to a hospital admission and those predating the performance of a procedure would assist in automatically detecting complications of medical management. In addition, diagnoses that arise from complications due to a procedure (e.g., surgical procedure, medication order, absent safety procedure) should be associated with the procedure on claims submissions as a condition of participation.

Integrated Approach to Detecting and Preventing Adverse Events

If patient safety systems were integrated with electronic health record (EHR) systems, the EHR could prompt the provider to enter certain information when it appeared that an adverse event might have occurred. In the longer term, adverse event systems need to be embedded within the broader proactive hazard analysis framework—an approach to identifying and minimizing/eliminating hazards. Use of hazard analysis techniques would bring us closer to the ultimate goal of eliminating latent system defects and increasing the chances of preventing medical errors and adverse events. Such techniques have proven useful in manufacturing (failure modes and effects analysis) and the food sector (hazard analysis and critical control points) (McDonough, 2002; also see Appendix D). Proactive hazard analysis involves the following cycle:

- Analyzing the care process to identify for each step of the process known failure points and high-risk events.
- Identifying the reports/data needed to monitor the key clinical performance variables and patient outcomes and to collect information on failures and near failures (adverse events and near misses).
- Redesigning the care process to improve patient safety following analysis of the data collected and root-cause analyses of the more serious adverse events and near misses.
- Analyzing the redesigned process to identify known failure points and high-risk events for each step, paying particular attention to the hazards that may have been introduced at points where the redesigned portions of the care process intersect with the original portions.
- Identifying for the redesigned care process the reports/data needed to monitor the key clinical performance variables and patient outcomes and to collect information on failures and near failures (adverse events and near misses), then returning to process redesign, and so on.

Detailed investigations will doubtless remain the province of patient safety officers, but detection of adverse events could be made much more efficient if front-line providers became more involved in the detection and reporting of events and the dissemination of preventive measures. Such involvement cannot, of course, be allowed to substantially delay providers in delivering care, but it nonetheless could have a major impact. Early trials of this sort of approach (Bates et al., 1998) have already demonstrated that it can be efficacious, though it has rarely been used to date.

REFERENCES

Agency for Healthcare Research and Quality. 2001. *Making Health Care Safer: A Critical Analysis of Patient Safety Practices.* Washington, DC: Agency for Healthcare Research and Quality.

American Medical Association, Joint Commission on Accreditation of Healthcare Organizations, National Committee for Quality Assurance. 2001. *Coordinated Performance Measurement for the Management of Adult Diabetes.* Online. Available: http://diabetes-mellitus.org/diabetes.pdf [accessed January 27, 2004].

Bates, D. W. 2002. *Diuretics: Adverse Reactions and Their Synonyms.* Personal communication to Institute of Medicine's Committee on Data Standards for Patient Safety.

Bates, D. W., R. S. Evans, H. Murff, P. D. Stetson, L. Pizziferri, and G. Hripcsak. 2003. Detecting adverse events using information technology. *J Am Med Inform Assoc* 10 (2):115–128.

Bates, D. W., M. A. Makary, J. M. Teich, L. Pedraza, N. M. Ma'luf, H. Burstin, and T. A. Brennan. 1998. Asking residents about adverse events in a computer dialogue: How accurate are they? *Jt Comm J Qual Improv* 24 (4):197–202.

Classen, D. C. 2003. Medication safety: Moving from illusion to reality. *JAMA* 289:1154–1156.

Classen, D. C., S. L. Pestotnik, R. S. Evans, and J. P. Burke. 1991. Computerized surveillance of adverse drug events in hospital patients. *JAMA* 266 (20):2847–2851.

Cullen, D. J., D. W. Bates, S. D. Small, J. B. Cooper, A. R. Nemeskal, and L. L. Leape. 1995. The incident reporting system does not detect adverse drug events: A problem for quality improvement. *Jt Comm J Qual Improv* 21 (10):541–548.

Evans, R. S., R. A. Larsen, J. P. Burke, R. M. Gardner, F. A. Meier, J. A. Jacobson, M. T. Conti, J. T. Jacobson, and R. K. Hulse. 1986. Computer surveillance of hospital-acquired infections and antibiotic use. *JAMA* 256 (8):1007–1011.

Honigman, B., P. Light, R. M. Pulling, and D. W. Bates. 2001. A computerized method for identifying incidents associated with adverse drug events in outpatients. *Int J Med Inf* 61 (1):21–32.

Iezzoni, L. I., J. Daley, T. Heeren, S. M. Foley, E. S. Fisher, C. Duncan, J. S. Hughes, and G. A. Coffman. 1994. Identifying complications of care using administrative data. *Med Care* 32 (7):700–715.

Institute of Medicine. 2000. *To Err Is Human: Building a Safer Health System.* Washington, DC: The National Academies Press.

Jha, A. K., G. J. Kuperman, J. M. Teich, L. Leape, B. Shea, E. Rittenberg, E. Burdick, D. L. Seger, M. Vander Vliet, and D. W. Bates. 1998. Identifying adverse drug events:

Development of a computer-based monitor and comparison with chart review and stimulated voluntary report. *J Am Med Inform Assoc* 5 (3):305–314.

Kilbridge, P., E. Welebob, and D. Classen. 2001. *Overview of the Leapfrog Group Evaluation Tool for Computerized Physician Order Entry.* Washington, DC: The Business Roundtable.

McDonough, J. E. 2002. *Proactive Hazard Analysis and Health Care Policy.* New York, NY: MilBank Memorial Fund/ECRI.

National Diabetes Quality Improvement Alliance. 2003. *Performance Measurement Set for Adult Diabetes.* Online. Available: http://www.nationaldiabetesalliance.org [accessed Jan 27, 2004].

Reason, J. 1990. *Human Error.* Cambridge, UK: Cambridge University Press.

Rozich, J. D., C. R. Haraden, and R. K. Resar. 2003. Adverse drug trigger tool: A practical methodology for measuring medication-related harm. *Qual Saf Health Care* 12:194–200.

Zhan, C., and R. M. Miller. 2003. Excess length of stay, charges, and mortality attributable to medical injuries during hospitalization. *JAMA* 290 (14):1868–1874.

7

Near-Miss Analysis

Trivial events in nontrivial systems should not go unremarked (Perrow, 1984).

CHAPTER SUMMARY

Although near-miss events are much more common than adverse events—as much as 7–100 times more frequent—reporting systems for such events are much less common. As the airline industry has realized, analysis of near-miss data provides an opportunity to design systems that can prevent adverse events. Near-miss data for the health care domain should be analyzed more extensively than is currently the case. The data provide two types of information relevant to patient safety—on weaknesses in the health care system and, equally important, on recovery processes. The latter data are an underutilized source of valuable patient safety information. This chapter examines the functional requirements of near-miss systems and the implications for data standards.

With some exceptions, near-miss data (and adverse event data) should be examined in the aggregate to determine priorities for health care improvement. The analysis of aggregate event data requires the use of standardized taxonomies to describe the root causes of failure, recovery processes, and situational contexts uniformly. Since near misses and adverse events are thought to be part of the same causal con-

tinuum, there should be identical taxonomies for failure root causes and context variables for both types of events.

The development of near-miss systems works best when the systems are initially established and designed for the benefit of those delivering care, for example, a hospital department. Data from this level can be aggregated for higher-level purposes—reports for hospital-wide systems and domain-specific nationwide systems. However, uses of the data require that the same data standards be applicable across all domains and at all levels of aggregation. Near-miss systems should be an integral part of clinical care and quality management information systems. To foster data reuse across all health care applications, the same data standards should be used for all applications.

In safety management literature, a near miss is defined in various ways. According to one definition, a near miss is an occurrence with potentially important safety-related effects which, in the end, was prevented from developing into actual consequences (Van der Schaaf, 1992). Near misses are also synonymous with "potential adverse events" (Bates et al., 1995b) and "close calls" (Department of Veterans Affairs, 2002). In this report, a near miss is defined as an act of commission or omission that could have harmed the patient but did not cause harm as a result of chance, prevention, or mitigation. In most cases, definitions of a near miss imply a model such as the incident causation model (see Figure 7-1), consisting of the following components or phases (Van der Schaaf, 1992):

• Initial failures—some instigating failure process (triggered by a human error, a technical or organizational failure, or a combination of the two).
• Dangerous situation—a state of temporarily increased risk resulting from an initial failure but still without actual consequences.
• Inadequate defenses—a failure of the official barriers (such as double-check procedures, automatic compensation by standby equipment, or problem-solving teams) built into the system to deal with this risk.
• Recovery—a second informal set of (mainly human-based) barriers by which a developing risky situation is detected, understood, and corrected in time, thus limiting the sequence of events to a near-miss outcome instead of letting it develop further into an adverse event or worse.

According to the incident causation model, near misses are the immediate precursors to later possible adverse events. Examining near misses provides two types of information relevant for patient safety: (1) that on weak-

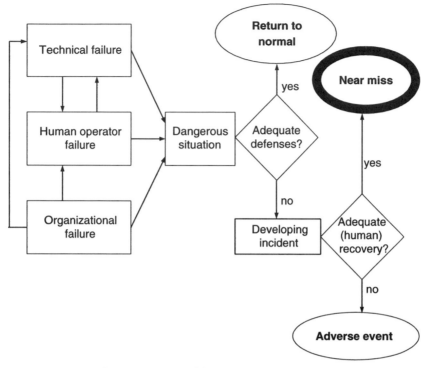

FIGURE 7-1 Incident causation model.
SOURCE: Van der Schaaf, 1992.

nesses in the health care system (errors and failures, as well as inadequate system defenses) and (2) that on the strengths of the health care system (unplanned, informal recovery actions) which compensate for those weaknesses on a daily basis, often making the essential difference between harm and no harm to a patient. Informal recovery actions are similar to the characteristic strengths of a highly reliable organization or a culture of safety, as identified by Roberts (2002).

Health care is an example of a low-reliability system, where frquently all that stands between an adverse event and quality health care is the health care provider. Health care professionals are continually detecting, arresting, and deflecting potential adverse events, sometimes even subconsciously. Data on recovery processes represent valuable patient safety information, a fact that often goes unrecognized.

The remainder of this chapter makes the case for the importance of near-miss reporting and analysis. The next two sections outline, respectively, the fundamental aspects and functional requirements of near-miss systems. Implementation and operational considerations are then reviewed. Next, a general framework is presented for processing near-miss reports and briefly address gaps between ideal and current systems. The final section describes the implications of the preceding discussion for data standards.

THE IMPORTANCE OF NEAR-MISS REPORTING AND ANALYSIS

The committee believes near-miss data should be analyzed more extensively than they currently are. Such analysis provides opportunities for learning about both weaknesses in the health care delivery system and ways in which the system is able to recover from dangerous or risky situations.

Three Goals for Near-Miss Systems

In an overview of near-miss systems in the industrial and transportation domains, Van der Schaaf et al. (1991) distinguish three different goals[1] of near-miss reporting and analysis:

• *Modeling*—to gain a *qualitative insight* into how (small) failures or errors develop into near misses and sometimes into adverse events. Eventually this insight should make it possible to identify the set of factors leading to the initial failures, as well as those enabling/promoting timely and successful recovery. As compared with adverse events, the added advantage of the recovery component should enable a more balanced view of how patient safety can be improved, focused not only on preventative measures to address the failure factors identified but also on means of building in or strengthening the recovery factors that come into play once errors have occurred.

• *Trending*—to gain a *quantitative insight* into the relative distribution of failure and recovery factors by building a database of underlying root causes of a large number of near misses. This database allows trending of the relative frequency of the various factors over time and thus provides a way to prioritize the most prominent factors as possible targets for error-reduction or recovery promotion interventions. Near misses, being 7–100 times more

---

[1]The first two goals, modeling and trending, are also applicable to adverse event systems (see Chapter 6).

frequent than adverse events (Bates et al., 1995a; Bird and Loftus, 1976; Heinrich, 1931; Skiba, 1985), allow for a much faster buildup of such databases, even at the lowest levels of a national reporting system (e.g., a single hospital department, a primary care provider's practice). Although *To Err Is Human* (Institute of Medicine, 2000) estimates the numbers of adverse events and associated fatalities to be very large nationwide, they are still infrequent at the lowest levels of the health care system and thus offer little insight into fundamental, frequently recurring underlying system factors on which to base the most efficacious safety improvements.

• *Mindfulness* (Kaplan, 2002)/*alertness*—to maintain a certain level of alertness to danger, especially when the rates of actual injuries are already low within an organization. For those employed in work environments with a mature safety culture, it eventually becomes difficult to maintain a minimum level of risk awareness in the absence of clearly visible adverse events. A weekly or monthly reminder in the form of a near miss in that same work situation may serve to reinforce awareness of specific safety risks that continue to exist, as well as demonstrate informal recovery defenses in action. It may be necessary to publicize the details of such near misses to ensure that all front-line workers are alerted to the continuing risks.

The Causal Continuum Assumption

Since the 1930s (Heinrich, 1931), most safety experts have assumed (based on anecdotal evidence) or claimed that the causal factors of consequential accidents are similar to those of nonconsequential incidents or near misses. Yet this so-called causal continuum assumption has not yet been firmly established as a scientific fact in health care. To date, this relationship has been documented only in recent transportation safety research (Wright, 2002). The pattern of failure factors for near misses in the railway sector was, by and large, not statistically different from that for train accidents involving injuries and damages. The claim in the health care domain that addressing the causes of near misses will also aid in preventing actual adverse events and fatalities will have to based on more than anecdotal evidence if that claim is to be widely accepted and therefore worth acting upon.

Currently available databases could be used to test the causal continuum assumption in health care. In fact, in one study that evaluated this assumption in health care, the characteristics of near misses were found to be somewhat different from those of errors that resulted in harm (Bates et al., 1995a). In particular, for medication errors, near misses involving a modest overdose were more likely to result in harm than errors involving massive overdoses since the former actions were more likely to be carried out. However, the underlying causes of near misses and adverse events (a lack of medication knowledge) were similar.

The Dual Pathway

One aspect of near-miss versus adverse event reporting that is relatively unknown but highly valued in practice is that near-miss reporting provides a dual pathway to improved system performance:

• The direct, *analytical* pathway, which near-miss and adverse event systems have in common, is based on collecting incident data; analyzing root causes; and acting upon the most important causes, thereby gradually improving the system and achieving better (safety) performance.

• In addition, near-miss systems appear to offer a second, indirect, *cultural* pathway to better performance: when reporters increasingly learn to trust the near-miss system as a means for communicating about and gradually improving patient safety, each voluntary decision on their part to report another near miss (instead of keeping it to themselves) helps change their attitude and ultimately their behavior as well, again leading to better performance. This slower, less visible, but fundamental and long-lasting cultural pathway is even regarded by some health care managers as more valuable in the long term than the straightforward analytical path (Joustra, 2003).

The Role of the Patient

As stated above, the dependence of near-miss systems on (voluntary) reporting by health care staff affects staff attitudes much more profoundly than is the case with systems not dependent on such personal commitment. However, playing an active role in detecting risks to patient safety is not necessarily limited to staff; patients themselves may be put in a position to contribute, for example, by being encouraged to ask questions about their care. In some cases, patients may help monitor their daily medications or medical treatment procedures, provided this information is supplied to them in an accessible format.

In this sense, patients (and by extension their family and friends) may be viewed as an extra, highly motivated line of defense. At the same time, involving patients in monitoring their own care clearly must be approached with caution and must be additional to, not a substitute for, the monitoring provided by systems and individual caregivers. Where patients provide an additional layer of monitoring, there could be a tendency in rushed circumstances to place total reliance on this mechanism. Moreover, many patients may be unable to contribute anything toward monitoring their own care because they lack the required information or have impaired cognitive or sensory skills.

In general, however, patients (and their family and friends) are a vastly underutilized resource for identifying things that go wrong in health care. Where possible, they should be encouraged to report incidents, especially those in which they averted potentially harmful consequences (e.g., by refusing to accept pills that differed in appearance or meals that did not conform to their dietary requirements).

FUNDAMENTAL ASPECTS OF NEAR-MISS SYSTEMS

To fulfill the goals outlined above, near-miss systems should be integrated into complete systems capable of capturing, analyzing, and disseminating information about patient safety. They should be able to support management decisions on how and where to invest in safety-oriented system improvements. They should describe the failure and recovery mechanisms behind the reported incidents; analyze the root causes of failures; and recommend specific actions, based on the root causes most prominent in the database, within a prioritization strategy. A complete system also entails covering the entire range of consequences, from very minor, easily corrected near misses to catastrophic adverse events and fatalities.

Learning from Databases, Not Just from Single Incidents

One of the consequences of the traditional focus on incidents in which patients were actually harmed in the belief that such incidents can yield more fundamental lessons is a lack of data at lower levels of the health care system. Rarely (if ever) do errors or failures end up causing severe damage to a patient in any single hospital department or primary care practice. Inevitably, such occasions receive a great deal of media attention. The result is often massive investments designed to prevent such (possibly very rare) mishaps from recurring, at least in part because of the attention they attract and the desire of hospital managers to be seen as acting swiftly. Because of the salience of the outcome, the analysis is subject to hindsight bias.

An incident-by-incident learning mode is reactive, based on specific characteristics of single events, and in most organizations consumes a major portion, if not the entirety, of the budget available for improving the system.

An alternative proactive learning approach (Reason, 1990), at least with regard to adverse events and fatalities, is to collect data on large numbers of events; analyze the root causes; build a database of these causes; and then act upon the underlying patterns of causes, which are much more likely than single events to point to systemic or latent (Reason, 1990) problems. Indeed, some systemic or latent causes that can be uncovered through aggregate databases can be identified not at all, or not as efficiently, by analysis of single incidents. Given that the majority of adverse events occur infrequently, large incident databases may be necessary to provide sufficient examples for purposes of analyzing rare events such as gas embolism or anaphylaxis.

Need for Root-Cause Taxonomies

If one wants to rise above the level of single events and their causes and base interventions on the most frequent and important root causes found in large databases, a root-cause taxonomy is needed. The causal factors fed into these databases should be made comparable at a general, abstract level so that they are quantifiable. Various aspects of the event will require different (sub)taxonomies:

- *Failure root causes* require a generic, fixed taxonomy, which should be identical over all medical/health care domains so that the system can be optimized overall, rather than within each domain This taxonomy should also acknowledge that patients themselves sometimes contribute to near misses and adverse events.
- *Recovery root causes* require a similar taxonomy. This taxonomy is likely to overlap somewhat with the categories of the failure taxonomy but will differ in some respects because of the more complex recovery phases of detection, diagnosis, and correction, each with their specific enablers (Van der Schaaf and Kanse, 2000).
- *Context variables*, although not causal, provide additional useful background information, such as the who, what, when, where, and consequences of an event. Context variables may well be largely domain specific, allowing analysis tailored to a specific reporting system. There is considerable overlap in the context variables collected for near-miss and adverse event analysis.
- *Free text* encompasses the reporters' narratives on which the event analysis was originally based. These narratives should be stored with the analysis results, with consideration of requirements for deidentification, to allow for later, off-line analysis, especially by external researchers.

FUNCTIONAL REQUIREMENTS OF NEAR-MISS SYSTEMS

General Functional Specifications

Van der Schaaf (1992) outlines four essential characteristics of near-miss systems:

- *Integration with other systems*—Not only should a near-miss system contribute to and benefit from adverse event reporting systems, it should also be integrated, wherever possible, with other approaches used to measure, understand, and improve the performance of health care systems, such as audits of employee safety conducted by the National Institute for Occupational Safety and Health, total quality programs, environmental protection programs, maintenance optimization efforts, and logistics cost reduction programs.

- *Comprehensive coverage* (in a qualitative sense) of possible inputs and outputs—The system should be able to handle not only safety-related near misses but also events with actual adverse consequences and with a range of different types of consequences (i.e., quality-, environment-, reliability-, and cost-related). It should cover not only negative deviations from normal system performance (errors, failures, faults) but also positive deviations (successful recoveries). Finally, it should focus not only on human errors or technical failures as factors contributing to a near miss but also on underlying latent organizational/managerial causes.

- *Model-based analysis*—To the extent possible, a system model of health care work situations, including a suitable description of individual behaviors in a complex technical and organizational environment, should be the basis for the design of the information processing portion of the near-miss system. Effective handling of the data encompasses (1) the required input data elements (taken from free-text near-miss reports), (2) methods for analyzing a report to identify root causes, and (3) methods for interpreting the resulting database to generate suggestions to management for specific countermeasures.

- *Organizational learning as the system's only focus*, that is, the development of progressively better insight into system functioning—As discussed in Chapter 6, except for clear instances of willful criminal acts (which are unlikely to be managed through such channels), the output of a near-miss system should never lead to assigning blame to or punishing individual employees or even be used to evaluate them. Rather, the emphasis should be on learning how to continuously improve patient safety by building feedback loops into the near-miss system. At the individual level, organizational learning can be improved by staff education and learning.

Types and Levels

In designing a near-miss system, two important dimensions are the medical domain it will cover and the level (from local hospital department or primary care practice, to hospital, to nationwide) at which it will function. An example is shown in Table 7-1. The four cells in this table can be divided into three levels of complexity of a near-miss system:

- The *basic* level of the local, one-domain system (I)
- The *intermediate* level of the hospital-wide or the domain-specific nationwide system (II and III)
- The *upper* level of the nationwide system covering all domains (IV)

Ideally, the design of a near-miss system should progress from the lowest to the highest level of complexity. Doing so will ensure a continuous flow of voluntary reports, which can be expected to be produced mainly by the cell I systems; to be passed on to the aggregate intermediate-level systems; and finally to reach the highest, comprehensive level of cell IV. Continued willingness to provide such input will depend greatly on its direct effects on those reporting, that is, insight into their work situation with regard to patient safety, specifically for their single-domain department. Considering the need for root-cause taxonomies cited earlier, this approach to designing a near-miss system means that:

- To the extent possible, all of these types and levels should have identical causal taxonomies (for both failure and recovery factors) and identical free-text structures (for the original input narratives).

TABLE 7-1 Examples of Two Dimensions of a Near-Miss System

Level	One Domain	Many/All Domains
One location	I: a single hospital department	II: a single hospital-wide system
Nationwide	III: a domain-specific national system	IV: a nationwide system of multiple domains

• Some basic context variables (i.e., those for type of patient, type of consequences) should also be fixed across levels and domains, while other specific context variables will vary with domain (i.e., type of treatment, medication, diagnosis) and/or level (i.e., codes for (sub)departments, protocols) to ensure enough specificity to provide useful and therefore motivational feedback.

As long as standard terminologies and taxonomies are used, data can be reported and acted upon at different levels of granularity. Coarser classification is necessary with the smaller collections available at the local level, but much finer granularity is possible when analyzing data from a large number of institutions. The strength of large-scale collections is that rare events can be well characterized.

IMPLEMENTATION AND OPERATIONAL CONSIDERATIONS

An overview of systems for the collection of human performance data in industry (Lucas, 1987) identifies five practical aspects that contribute significantly to such a system's success or failure and must be addressed when defining data standards:

• *The nature of the information collected*—It is obvious from arguments presented earlier in this chapter that descriptive reports are not sufficient; a causal analysis should be possible as well. A free-text description of an event will always be provided, sometimes guided by a standard set of questions (e.g., what the reporter was doing at the time, whether he/she was alone or with colleagues, what happened next, how the reporter reacted, whether there was a full recovery, what improvements the reporter would suggest).
• *The use of information in the database*—There should be regular and appropriate feedback to personnel at all levels. It should be easy to generate summary statistics and clear examples from the database and to identify specific error reduction and recovery promotion strategies that can be proposed to management.
• *The level of help provided for collecting and analyzing the data*—Analyst aids should be provided in the form of interview questions, flow charts, software, and the like.
• *The nature of the organization of the reporting scheme*—A local reporting system maintains close ties with reporters of events, but a central system may be more efficient in certain situations, for example, if there is widespread trust in the operation of the near-miss system. Probably for all

near-miss programs, voluntary reporting is to be preferred over mandatory. Only in the case of certain well-defined, near-catastrophic events should there be a legal obligation to report.

• *Whether the scheme is acceptable to all personnel*—All of the above considerations should lead to a feeling of shared ownership. Whether the data are best gathered by a well-known colleague (most commonly in a local system) or by an unknown outsider (usually in a more central system) again depends on the specific situation. Everyone involved should at least be familiarized with the purpose and background of the reporting scheme.

Problems of Data Collection

The following specific problems involved in data collection (Lucas, 1987) must be addressed to achieve a successful near-miss system:

• *Action oriented*—a tendency to focus on what rather than why.

• *Event focused*—analyzing individual incidents rather than looking for general patterns of causes in a large database. The result is anecdotal reporting systems.

• *Consequence driven*—making the amount of attention and the resources devoted to investigation directly proportional to the severity of the outcome.

• *Technical myopia*—a bias toward hardware rather than human failures.

• *Variable quality*—both within and between reporting systems, leading to incomparable investigation methods and results.

Key Issues: Willingness to Report, Trust, and Acceptance

Although the above discussion stems from experiences in (high-tech) industries and date from 1987, by and large they still hold today and for health care as well. Here we focus on those aspects most relevant to the key issues in near-miss systems for health care—willingness to report, trust, and acceptance:

• Input optimal in terms of both quantity and quality may be facilitated by providing multiple channels for reporting, including forms, computer linkup, and telephone; at multiple locations, including the nurses' station, the doctors' meeting room, from the patient's bedside, and from home; by multiple groups, not just medical staff but also lab technicians, administrative employees, patients themselves, and their relatives/visitors; and at all times during the day/shift.

• The reporting threshold (i.e., the difficulty and effort involved in making a near-miss report) should be minimal. A simple form should be used with just a few questions (who is reporting, how he/she can be reached for further information, what happened, why the reporter thinks it happened this way, how bad the outcome could have been if recovery had not occurred), taking not more than a few minutes to complete.

• The opportunity, importance, and procedures of contributing to patient safety by voluntary reporting should be well known to all target groups. To this end, substantial investments must be made in publicizing, explaining, and discussing these issues before the formal launching of the near-miss system (i.e., opening of the reporting channels).

• Especially important is clear, continued, visible support by top management. Managers should be open and consistent in their communication about the importance, use, and accessibility of the data and their commitment to actually using the recommendations from the database analysis to choose, justify, and implement focused actions aimed at improving local performance on patient safety.

• Optimum investments in system change depend not only on the scientific aspects of the root-cause analysis method and other tools employed but also on the more practical aspects of their usability and clarity and the training and support provided to the staff designated to carry out these analyses. Variability among individual analysts in identifying and then assigning classification codes to root causes should be checked at regular intervals using interrater reliability trials (Wright, 2002).

• All of the above preparations and aspects should culminate in an optimal stream of frequent, meaningful, convincing, and therefore motivating feedback to all levels of staff and patients. Within 24 hours of a report being made, an acknowledgment of its receipt should be sent to the reporter, thanking him/her for the contribution and stating when (within days) a request for further information required for a complete analysis might be expected. If prioritization requires a full root-cause analysis, the descriptive portion of the analysis (not the classifications themselves) should be fed back to the reporter for validation. After prioritization and analysis at the database level (i.e., every 2 or 3 months), the resulting insights and suggestions for focused action should be fed back, combined with the justified choice by management of where and how to concentrate resources for improvement. These visible changes in the system will serve as a major motivator, as will evaluation of their effects in a later phase.

Keeping It Manageable

Instituting and running a near-miss system should not burden an organization unduly. As noted in Chapter 6, automated surveillance systems, augmented by other detection methods, will increase the number of detected adverse events that might warrant further analysis. Since near misses occur much more frequently than adverse events (Bates et al., 1995b), an organization could become overwhelmed by the number of near misses that might warrant further analysis. Once a near-miss system has been functioning for a while, it is crucial to establish selection criteria that can identify a manageable number of reported events with enough learning potential to warrant full root-cause analyses.

In addition to the criteria mentioned in Chapter 6, likely candidates would include the novelty or surprise factor—new elements not seen before, even considered impossible. Another criterion could be potential fatal consequences or the realization that this event must have been latent in the organization for a long time, passing through many barriers that should have caught it earlier. Also, when an event is one that should have been prevented by a recent focused intervention, one would like to know why it still occurred.

Finally, an organization may have selected a certain type of medical event (such as wrong-side surgery or switching of patients' identities) as a topic of special concern for a limited period; in that case, it might prefer to select all such reports for full analysis until the end of the project.

Integration with Adverse Event Systems

Near misses are regarded as being on the same continuum as adverse events in terms of failure factors but differing in terms of the additional information they provide on recovery factors and in their significantly higher frequency of occurrence. Because the assumption of the causal continuum implies that the causes of near misses do not differ from those of adverse events, this leads to the claim that near misses are truly precursors to later potential adverse events and therefore valuable to report. The primary focus for improving patient safety is on identifying and eliminating the system faults that can lead to adverse events. This objective can be approached by analyzing both adverse events and near misses to identify the system faults involved.

A direct causal comparison between near misses and adverse events requires shared taxonomies for sets of events in terms of both root causes and context variables. After enough adverse events or other serious medical mishaps have been reported and analyzed to build a statistically sound database for a health care organization, the amount of overlap between the causes of near misses and adverse events should be examined. Doing so will not only clarify the relationship between these two sets of events but also demonstrate clearly and convincingly to all potential reporters the importance of near-miss systems. In some cases, adverse event descriptions also encompass recovery actions that were obviously too late, too weak, or of the wrong type to have been successful. In these cases, such failed opportunities at recovery, or at least damage limitation, can be classified using the taxonomy for near-miss recovery factors and compared with successful recoveries to understand the predictors of success.

GENERAL FRAMEWORK FOR PROCESSING NEAR-MISS REPORTS

Summarizing the main points for designing, implementing, and operating a near-miss system, Table 7-2 uses a seven-module framework to describe what is required in each step of the processing of near-miss reports (Van der Schaaf et al., 1991):

1. *Detection*—This module contains the registration mechanism, aiming at easy entry of complete (or at least nonbiased), valid reporting[2] of all near-miss situations detectable by employees, patients, and others.

2. *Selection*—A mature near-miss system will probably generate many duplications of earlier reports, increasing the workload of the safety staff coping with sizable piles of reports. To maximize the learning process using limited resources, a selection procedure is necessary to filter out the most interesting reports for further analysis in the subsequent modules.

3. *Description*—Any report selected for further processing should lead to a *detailed, complete, neutral* description of the course of events and situations resulting in the reported near miss, with appropriate deidentification. These causal elements should be shown in their logical order (what caused

---

[2]Computerized detection using a signal approach has not been as effective for detecting near misses as for detecting adverse events (Jha et al., 1998). Increasingly, however, new technologies such as computerized order entry (Bates et al., 1998) and "smart" intravenous pumps that record exactly what an operator tried to do (Bates and Gawande, 2003) will become useful as sources of data on large numbers of near misses.

TABLE 7-2 Seven-Module Framework for Processing

Module	Function	Role of Patient Safety Data Standards
1. Detection	Recognition and reporting	Reporting mechanisms (e.g., input form)
2. Selection	According to local and national criteria	Prioritization criteria
3. Description	All relevant technical, organizational, and human elements	Event investigation (e.g., by causal-tree building)
4. Classification	Using a suitable sociotechnical model of system failure	Taxonomies for root causes
5. Computation	Compiling a database; performing periodic statistical analysis to uncover dominant causal factors	Data exploration and problem diagnosis
6. Interpretation and Implementation	Translation of database analysis into corrective and preventative interventions	Linking of diagnosis to countermeasures
7. Evaluation	Measuring the effectiveness of interventions in subsequent periodic analyses	Learning-cycle mechanism

SOURCE: Van der Schaaf et al., 1991.

what) as well as their chronological sequence (e.g., using causal-tree techniques).

4. *Classification*—As the most fundamental of causal elements, root causes should each be classified according to a suitable taxonomy. In this way, the fact that every incident usually has multiple causes is fully recognized, and each analyzed near miss thus adds a set of root causes to the database. Severity should also be assessed.

5. *Computation*—In exceptional cases only (e.g., on first discovering a technical design fault or a new side effect of a drug), immediate action is required. Generally, however, the database is allowed to build up gradually over a certain period, after which a periodic statistical analysis of the entire or the most recent part of the database is performed, with the aim of identifying patterns of root causes instead of unique, nonrecurring symptoms.

6. *Interpretation and implementation*—Once the most dominant causes have been identified, a mechanism should be in place that suggests types of

interventions that may influence these causes by preventing them in the case of failure factors or promoting them in the case of recovery factors. Management can then select one or more focus areas on the basis of these model-based options for intervention and other dimensions, such as time to effect, cost, and regulator requirements. The associated interventions can then be implemented.

7. *Evaluation*—Once the selected interventions have had some time to take effect, they should be monitored for their effectiveness in bringing about the expected change. Subsequent periodic database analyses should be used for this purpose by checking for decreased (for failure factors) or increased (for recovery factors) presence in the near-miss reports generated after implementation. Such system feedback is essential for establishing a learning cycle.

GAPS BETWEEN IDEAL AND CURRENT SYSTEMS

A comparison of the requirements for designing and implementing near-miss systems (as summarized in the seven-module framework presented in Table 7-2) and the actual operational experience with the few existing near-miss systems reveals a number of gaps between ideal and current systems. Given that near-miss reporting and analysis is a new and evolving area, pilot testing of the principles set forth in this chapter is essential. In addition, a solid research program should be undertaken to quantify the benefits and costs of near-miss reporting and analysis. Chapter 5 details the committee's proposals for a research program.

IMPLICATIONS FOR DATA STANDARDS

The following subsections summarize the implications of the above discussion for the development of standards for data related to patient safety (excluding the research outlined in Chapter 5).

Definitions and Models

Clear, workable definitions and models should be formulated for all system and data elements necessary for collecting, analyzing, and learning from near-miss events, as well as for sharing these data and analysis results within and among all levels and domains of the health care system. Care should be taken to ensure maximum overlap between such near-miss standards and those for adverse events. Where possible, tested definitions and models from both within and outside the medical field should be preferred.

The various possible goals of near-miss systems should be reflected in these definitions and models, as well as potential roles of patients and their relatives.

Taxonomies

Classification systems for root causes (both failure and recovery) and context variables are essential for aggregating and comparing near-miss data. Failure taxonomies should allow a balanced, unbiased analysis of the human, technical, and organizational causes involved in an event. Recovery taxonomies will need further development but should at least distinguish among the detection, diagnosis, and correction phases of the recovery process. Contextual variables should be shared where possible among all domains and levels and remain specific as necessary to furnish enough detail within a certain domain or level to provide useful feedback and lessons for local improvement.

Design and Operation of System Components

Following the seven-module framework outlined above, system design and operation standards should address the following issues:

- *Detection*—Reporting should be as easy and quick as possible, through multiple channels, for medical staff, patients, and others present. The low threshold means that in this first module a report cannot be anonymous, as additional information may be required from the reporter. The report should, however, be strictly confidential at this phase.
- *Selection*—Predictably large numbers of incoming reports should be evaluated for their learning potential to determine whether root-cause analysis will be worthwhile; criteria for selection are essential to prevent the near-miss system from being flooded and should be specific for the local and national levels.
- *Description*—A concise description of all relevant elements, from root causes to the reported event, in their chronological and logical (i.e., cause–effect) order demands tree-like techniques. For near-miss data, these techniques should allow/be adapted for describing recovery elements as well as failure elements. After any additional information needed to complete and validate the event description has been furnished, the reporter's name is no longer needed and should be deleted, along with other possible identifiers.

• *Classification*—Identified failure and recovery factors and context variables require a set of transferable, learnable (and therefore relatively simple) taxonomies based on accepted safety management models and local/domain needs.

• *Computation*—At higher levels especially, near-miss database structures should allow for large numbers of coded events, easy queries, data mining, and state-of-the-art statistical analysis. At lower local levels, ease of use and preprogrammed recurring analyses for feedback to the reporting community are essential as well.

• *Interpretation and implementation*—Targeted (dominant) root causes should be linked to suggestions for methods of addressing them. The matrix should be based on accepted safety management models. Management should be supplied with this advice in a form that supports optimal decision making on the allocation of resources to patient safety improvement actions and then monitored with regard to whether these improvement programs have been implemented.

• *Evaluation*—It is essential that the effects of implemented programs be monitored. Monitoring not only allows for the establishment of a learning cycle (whether the right action was taken on that problem) but also provides highly motivating feedback to all (potential) reporters, who can then see for themselves how their contributions to the database help increase patient safety.

REFERENCES

Bates, D. W., and A. A. Gawande. 2003. Improving safety with information technology. *N Engl J Med* 348 (25):2526–2534.

Bates, D. W., D. L. Boyle, M. B. Vander Vliet, J. Schneider, and L. Leape. 1995a. Relationship between medication errors and adverse drug events. *J Gen Intern Med* 10 (4):199–205.

Bates, D. W., D. J. Cullen, N. Laird, L. A. Petersen, S. D. Small, D. Servi, G. Laffel, B. J. Sweitzer, B. F. Shea, R. Hallisey, M. Vander Vliet, R. Nemeskal, and L. L. Leape. 1995b. Incidence of adverse drug events and potential adverse drug events: Implications for prevention. *JAMA* 274 (1):29–34.

Bates, D. W., L. L. Leape, D. J. Cullen, N. Laird, L. A. Petersen, J. M. Teich, E. Burdick, M. Hickey, S. Kleefield, B. Shea, M. Vander Vliet, and D. L. Seger. 1998. Effect of computerized physician order entry and a team intervention on prevention of serious medication errors. *JAMA* 280 (15):1311–1316.

Bird, F. E., and R. G. Loftus. 1976. *Loss Control Management.* Loganville, GA: Institute Press.

Department of Veterans Affairs. 2002. *Veterans Health Administration (VHA) National Patient Safety Improvement Handbook.* Washington, DC: U.S. Department of Veterans Affairs.

Heinrich, H. W. 1931. *Industrial Accident Prevention.* New York, NY: McGraw-Hill.

Institute of Medicine. 2000. *To Err Is Human: Building a Safer Health System.* Washington, DC: National Academy Press.

Jha, A. K., G. J. Kuperman, J. M. Teich, L. Leape, B. Shea, E. Rittenberg, E. Burdick, D. L. Seger, M. Vander Vliet, and D. W. Bates. 1998. Identifying adverse drug events: Development of a computer-based monitor and comparison with chart review and stimulated voluntary report. *J Am Med Inform Assoc* 5 (3):305–314.

Joustra, A. C. 2003. *Concept of Dual Pathways.* Personal communication to Institute of Medicine's Committee on Data Standards for Patient Safety.

Kaplan, H. 2002. *Alertness to Danger When Rates of Injury Are Low.* Personal communication to Institute of Medicine's Committee on Data Standards for Patient Safety.

Lucas, D. A. 1987. Human performance data collection in industrial systems. In: *Human Reliability in Nuclear Power.* London: IBC Technical Services.

Perrow, C. 1984. *Normal Accidents: Living with High-Risk Technologies.* New York, NY: Basic Books.

Reason, J. 1990. *Human Error.* Cambridge, UK: Cambridge University Press.

Roberts, K. H. 2002. *Highly Reliable Systems.* Presentation to IOM Committee on Data Standards for Patient Safety on September 23, 2002. Online. Available: http://www.iom.edu/includes/DBFile.asp?id=10916 [accessed February 6, 2004].

Skiba, R. 1985. *Taschenbuch Arbeitssicherheit (Occupational Safety Pocket Book).* Bielefeld, Germany: Erich Schmid Verlag.

Van der Schaaf, T. W. 1992. *Near Miss Reporting in the Chemical Process Industry.* Eindhoven, Netherlands: Technische Universiteit Eindhoven.

Van der Schaaf, T. W., and L. Kanse. 2000. Errors and Error Recovery. Pp. 27-38 *Human Error in System Design and Management (Lecture Notes in Control and Information Sciences, 253).* eds. P. F. Elzer, R. H. Kluwe, and B. Boussoffara. London, England: Springer Verlag.

Van der Schaaf, T. W., D. A. Lucas, and A. R. Hale. 1991. *Near Miss Reporting as a Safety Tool.* Oxford: Butterworth-Heinemann.

Wright, L. B. 2002. *The Analysis of UK Railway Accidents and Incidents: A Comparison of Their Causal Patterns.* Glasgow: University of Strathclyde.

Part III

Streamlining Patient Safety Reporting

Concerns about patient safety have led to increased use of reporting systems. Part III of the report examines the different types of patient safety data applications (Chapter 8) and the development of a common report format and set of data standards for use with patient safety reporting systems (Chapter 9).

PATIENT SAFETY DATA APPLICATIONS

Clinical performance data can be used for many purposes—for example, by regulators for accountability purposes, by individual and organizational consumers for making purchasing decisions, and by care providers for designing improved care processes. Each group has different data requirements. Accountability-based applications, on the one hand, generally focus on individual health care providers and the health care delivery institutions in which they work. Learning-based approaches, on the other hand, generally focus on health care delivery processes. Chapter 8 outlines the many uses of clinical performance data and the pitfalls associated with each. The chapter concludes by emphasizing the need to invest more in approaches that can lead to system redesign and improvement.

STANDARDIZED REPORTING

To learn from adverse event and near-miss data, researchers need to aggregate the data to formulate research priorities, identify trends, and compare various approaches to patient safety. To carry out these data aggregations, researchers need standard, nationally accepted ways of defining, classifying, and characterizing adverse events and near misses. There has been some cross-fertilization among the various reporting systems; to address local needs, however, each system has been developed largely independently of others. Thus one finds across state reporting systems many different definitions for such key patient safety terms as adverse event, many different classifications of adverse events,[1] and diverse approaches to collecting and coding data relevant to adverse events and near misses.

At the moment, each institution that wants to implement a patient safety reporting system must invent its own system. This effort involves deciding on a process for collecting and analyzing the salient data and then identifying and defining what events are to be reported on; what data elements are to be collected; and how each data element should be defined, classified, and coded.

A standardized report format would reduce the burden on providers of complying with outside requests for patient safety information. Today, for example, an adverse event that has been detected in an institution in New York State must, potentially, be reported to the institution's own system and possibly to voluntary systems such as MedMARX. If the adverse event is serious, it may need to be reported to the New York Patient Occurrence Reporting and Tracking System (NYPORTS), a federal system, and the Joint Commission on Accreditation of Healthcare Organizations. Each of these systems has very different definitions of reportable events and data reporting requirements. This lack of standardization imposes unnecessary burdens and is a major disincentive to reporting adverse events. Chapter 9 addresses the steps needed to establish a standardized reporting format.

Recommendation 7. AHRQ should develop an event taxonomy and common report format for submission of data to the national patient safety database. Specifically:

- **The event taxonomy should address near misses and adverse events, cover errors of both omission and commission, allow for the designation of primary and secondary event types for cases in which**

---

[1]There is some movement toward consensus. SAFER (State Alliance for Error Reporting), a workgroup of states, is considering whether the National Quality Forum's list of Serious Reportable Events can be developed into a core set of reportable events that each state could adopt (National Quality Forum, 2002).

more than one factor precipitated the adverse event, and be incorpo-
rated into SNOMED CT.
- The standardized report format should include the following:
  - A standardized minimum set of data elements.
  - Data necessary to calculate a risk assessment index for deter-
    mining prospectively the probability of an event and its severity.
  - A free-text narrative of the event.
  - Data necessary to support use of the Eindhoven Classification
    Model—Medical Version for classifying root causes, including
    expansions for (1) recovery factors associated with near-miss
    events, (2) corrective actions taken to recover from adverse
    events, and (3) patient outcome/functional status as a result of
    those corrective actions.
  - A free-text section for lessons learned as a result of the event.
  - Clinical documentation of the patient context.
- The taxonomy and report format should be used by the federal
reporting system integration project in the areas for basic domain,
event type, risk assessment, and causal analysis but should provide
for more extensive support for patient safety research and analysis
(Department of Health and Human Services, 2002).

REFERENCES

Department of Health and Human Services. 2002. *HHS Moves Forward to Establish New
    System for Collecting Patient Safety Data.* Online. Available: http://www.hhs.gov/
    news/press/2002pres/20021125.html [accessed August 18, 2003].
National Quality Forum. 2002. *Serious Reportable Events in Patient Safety: A National
    Quality Forum Consensus Report.* Washington, DC: National Quality Forum.

8

Patient Safety Reporting Systems and Applications

CHAPTER SUMMARY

Patient safety performance data may be used in support of many efforts aimed at improving patient safety: regulators may use the data for accountability purposes such as licensure and certification programs; public and private purchasers may use the data to offer financial or other incentives to providers; consumers may use comparative safety performance data when choosing a provider; and clinicians may use the data when making referrals. Most important, patient safety data are a critical input to the efforts of providers to redesign care processes in ways that will make care safer for all patients. Applications in all of these areas are currently hampered by inadequate patient safety data systems. Although all applications along the continuum from accountability to learning contribute to a safer health care environment, the committee believes that applications aimed at fundamental system redesign offer particular promise for achieving substantial improvements in safety and quality across the entire health care sector.

High-quality health care is, first, safe health care. Patients should be able to approach health professionals free of fear that seeking help could lead to harm. If safety is to be a core feature of health care delivery systems, clinicians, administrators, and patients will need tools, based on reliable clinical data, to build and assure a safe care environment. Health professionals must be able to identify safety problems, test solutions, and determine whether their solutions are working. Patients and their representatives need to know what risks exist and how they might be avoided. Data on clinical performance are one key building block for a safe health care delivery system.

Clinical performance data can serve a full range of purposes, from accountability (e.g., professional licensure, legal liability) to learning (e.g., the redesign of care processes, testing of hypotheses). Different purposes necessitate differences in data collection methods, analytic techniques, and interpretation of results. An ideal clinical performance reporting system should be able to function simultaneously along the entire continuum of applications, but such broad use requires careful data system design, automated systems that link directly to care delivery, and explicit data standards.

There are many legitimate applications of clinical performance data, each having its own historical underpinnings and approaches. All of these applications are intended to improve the safety of patient care. The interactions of clinicians and patients are influenced by the environment (e.g., legal liability, purchasing and regulatory policies); the education and training of health professionals (e.g., multidisciplinary training); the health literacy and expectations of individuals (e.g., patients' understanding of chronic condition and the importance of healthy behaviors); and the organizational arrangements or systems that support care delivery (e.g., internal reporting systems, the availability of computer-aided decision support systems). The greatest gains in patient safety will come from aligning incentives and activities in each of these four areas.

This chapter provides an overview of the many applications of clinical performance data and a discussion of their likely impact. A case study is used to illustrate some of the undesirable consequences that can come from the use of various applications if the data, performance measures, and approaches are not chosen carefully, and if too much emphasis is placed on accountability as opposed to learning applications. Finally, the importance of investing more in approaches targeted directly at fundamental system redesign is briefly discussed. Such approaches offer the greatest potential to improve patient safety but require a far more sophisticated data infrastructure than currently exists in most health care settings.

Although much of the discussion in this chapter presumes the availability of computerized clinical information systems, the collection and analysis of clinical performance data can be carried out without computerized clinical information systems. Such collection and analysis would, however, be greatly facilitated by computerized clinical information systems and the national health information infrastructure (NHII).

THE CONTINUUM OF APPLICATIONS

The many applications of clinical performance data are illustrated in Figure 8-1. To the left of the spectrum are applications used by public-sector legal and regulatory bodies that are intended to hold health care professionals and organizations accountable (e.g., professional and institutional licensure and legal liability). To the right of the spectrum are applications that focus on learning, both for organizations and for professionals. The feedback of performance data to clinicians for continuing education purposes falls into this category, as does the redesign of care processes by health care organizations based on analysis of data collected in near-miss and adverse event reporting systems. Falling between these two extremes are applications intended to encourage health care providers to strive for excellence by rewarding those who achieve the highest levels of performance with higher payments and greater demand for their services.

Virtually all applications of clinical performance data are intended to produce improvements in safety and quality. However, their immediate aims—accountability, incentives, and system redesign—are quite different.

Aim defines the system—W. E. Deming (1988)

Accountability

Health care policy makers have long argued that there is an inherent imbalance in access to and understanding of health care information between health care providers and health care consumers (Arrow, 1963; Haas-Wilson, 2001; Robinson, 2001). To help redress this imbalance, health care overseers—federal, state, and county governments; health professional groups; and other patient representatives—have sought to guarantee a minimum level of health care delivery performance on behalf of the general health-consuming public. In recent years, some consumer-driven approaches have been adopted, such as state-level reporting of serious medical errors and the publication of health outcome data.

Health care overseers have carried out their accountability role through licensing programs for health care professionals and certification and accreditation programs for provider institutions and health plans. Traditionally, these oversight processes have focused on the establishment of "market entry" requirements (e.g., medical doctors must graduate from an accred-

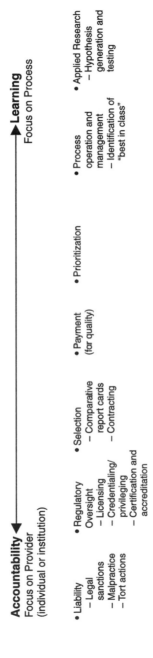

FIGURE 8-1 A continuum of possible uses and mechanisms of action for patient safety data.

ited school and have completed a 1-year internship) and the ongoing identification of substandard performers through such mechanisms as peer review of individual cases (quality assurance), review of patient complaints, and routine inspections of practice settings.

In recent years, many states have established adverse event reporting systems. Health care oversight officials at the state level report that such systems are a useful tool for facility oversight, providing an additional window into facility operations that might otherwise not be available (Rosenthal et al., 2001). Consumers look to government to ensure that facilities are safe and providers are competent. In one survey, nearly 75 percent of respondents said that government should require health care providers to report all serious medical errors (The Henry J. Kaiser Family Foundation and Agency for Healthcare Research and Quality, 2000). In some instances, health outcome data (e.g., hospital mortality rates, mortality rates associated with cardiac surgery) have been used for accountability purposes as well (see the discussion below).

For the most part, legal liability and regulatory oversight processes focus on identifying very poor performers—the "bad apples" (see Figure 8-2) (Berwick, 1989). These processes set a minimum performance standard that is used to assess care providers. For those providers who fail to meet the minimum standard, sanctions (e.g., fines, termination of license) are levied, or reeducation programs and more stringent oversight are demanded.

Incentives

Previous Institute of Medicine (IOM) reports reveal a U.S. health care system that routinely fails to achieve the safest and highest quality of care for Americans who seek its services (Institute of Medicine, 2000, 2001). The vast majority of providers are not negligent, incompetent, or impaired, yet the services they provide are clearly inadequate, suggesting that minimum performance standards alone cannot achieve generally excellent care delivery (James, 1992).

Applications along the middle of the continuum are intended to bridge this gap by providing incentives (e.g., financial payments, public esteem or disgrace) and tools (e.g., comparative data on quality) that will motivate many providers to improve safety and quality. Selection refers to the use of comparative data by group purchasers or individuals to choose health plans and providers. In a quality-driven marketplace, purchasers (through contracting) and patients choose providers that deliver the safest and most effective care (see Figure 8-3). In theory, such selection should motivate all

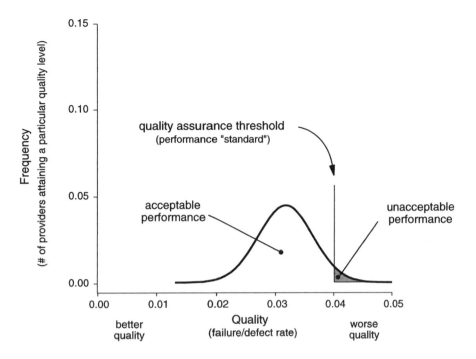

FIGURE 8-2 Use of safety data for accountability, licensing, or legal action (focus on the lower tail).

providers to improve so they will rank better on comparative safety and quality reports and gain more business in the future. The provision of higher payments to providers that deliver safer and more effective care works in a similar fashion by making it attractive to all providers to strive to achieve a high ranking (Berwick et al., 2003).

These types of applications require certain data and information to be "transparent," a term denoting the situation in which those involved in health care choices at any level—including patients, health professionals, and purchasers—have sufficiently complete, understandable information about clinical performance to make wise decisions (Institute of Medicine, 2001). Choices involve not just the selection of a health plan, a hospital, or a physician but also the series of testing and treatment decisions that patients face as they work their way through a health care delivery interaction. Transparency changes the focus of accountability, shifting both control and responsibility from clinical professionals and health care overseers to patients.

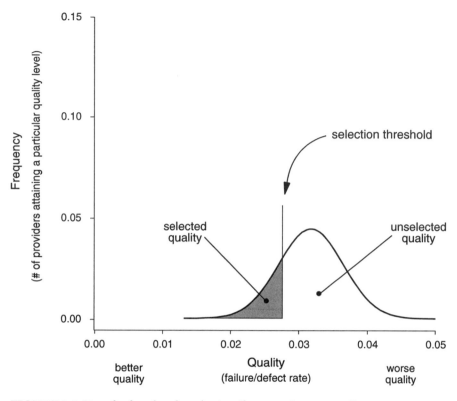

FIGURE 8-3 Use of safety data for selection (focus on the upper tail).

True transparency necessitates detailed and complete performance data that are valid, reliable, and relevant to the types of decisions an individual must make. For example, a patient about to undergo bypass surgery (or the general internist acting as the patient's representative) must first select a hospital and a surgeon. In a transparent world, all participants would have access to hospital- and surgeon-specific performance datasets including a rich set of process and outcome measures, satisfaction reports, and other information.

To date, public reporting of performance data has been limited, but experience is growing (Agency for Healthcare Research and Quality, 2001; Baumgarten, 2002; California HealthCare Foundation, 2003; Centers for Medicare and Medicaid Services, 2003; Department of Health and Human Services, 2002a, b; Dudley et al., 2002; McCormick et al., 2002; National Committee for Quality Assurance, 2002a, b). Most public reporting has focused on organizations (i.e., hospitals and nursing homes) and, to some degree, surgical interventions (Schauffler and Mordavsky, 2001). Very limited information has been reported on medical groups or physicians. Early reporting efforts focused on outcome data (e.g., mortality), while more recent comparative reports have tended to include process-of-care measures, patient perceptions of care, and accreditation status (McGlynn and Adams, 2001).

Studies suggest that public reporting of comparative performance information has had little if any impact on consumer decision making (Schauffler and Mordavsky, 2001). For example, report cards on health plans and hospitals have had a minimal effect on consumers' selection of health plans (Gabel et al., 1998; Thompson et al., 2003), and simple, easy-to-understand mortality statistics at the level of hospitals and individual physicians do not affect patients' choices of hospitals or physicians (Chassin et al., 1996, 2002; Mennemeyer et al., 1997; Schneider and Epstein, 1996).

Many factors likely contribute to this lack of response on the part of consumers, including a lack of awareness of the existence of performance information, limitations placed on the choice of health plans and providers by employee benefits or insurance plan design, the presentation of performance information in a manner that is overly complex and fails to capture those aspects of performance of particular interest to consumers, reports not being produced by a trusted source, and questionable validity and reliability of the measures selected and underlying data sources (Hibbard et al., 2001; Hibbard, 1998, 2003; Institute of Medicine, 2001; McGlynn and Adams, 2001; Schauffler and Mordavsky, 2001; Simon and Monroe, 2001). Finally, individual patients are accustomed to choosing specialists and hospitals mainly on the advice of their primary care provider (referring physician), rather than on the basis of performance statistics (Mennemeyer et al., 1997). To date, the use of performance data by patients' referring physicians has not been widespread enough to influence market dynamics.

Health care delivery organizations and professionals have a great deal to gain from a balanced system of public reporting. To the extent that safer care produces fewer injuries, it can significantly reduce legal exposure, as evidenced by the malpractice experience of surgical anesthesiologists following successful profession-wide improvement efforts (Joint Commission on Accreditation of Healthcare Organizations, 1998; Chassin, 1998; Cohen et al., 1986; Cooper et al., 2002; Duncan and Cohen, 1987; Gaba, 1989; Pierce, 1996). Public reporting creates a level playing field where competitors share equal incentives to invest in better care.

The greatest benefit of public reporting may come not from influencing patient behavior but from causing health providers to set priorities and goals and motivating them to achieve those goals. Motivation operates through both explicit rewards and the public exposure of shared professional and organizational commitments. It recognizes that change is inherently difficult and that the health care system may need an external goad to drive internal change. Most health care organizations do express a genuine desire to deliver the best possible care to their patients, but they are beset by a host of competing demands. Explicit external expectations, implemented through public reporting balanced across institutions by independent auditing of underlying data systems, can establish shared priorities and parallel investment in the necessary data infrastructure.

Many efforts now under way are aimed at providing financial rewards to providers based on either their relative performance ranking compared with their peers or improvements in their individual performance over time (Bailit Health Purchasing, 2002a; Bailit Health Purchasing, 2002b; Kaye, 2001; Kaye and Bailit, 1999; National Health Care Purchasing Institute, 2002; White, 2002). These payment-for-performance programs focus on health plans, hospitals, clinicians, or some combination of these and utilize many different models of compensation. In addition, a limited number of programs are experimenting with the provision of financial rewards (e.g., lower premiums or copayments) to consumers who select higher-performing providers (Freudenheim, 2002; Salber and Bradley, 2001). Information is not yet available for assessing the impact of financial incentives on the behavior of consumers or providers and ultimately on the safety and quality of care.

The IOM has identified a set of 20 priority areas for the U.S. health care system, and the Department of Health and Human Services will soon be releasing the first annual National Healthcare Quality Report, focused on many of these priority areas (Agency for Healthcare Research and Quality, 2002; Institute of Medicine, 2003). These efforts are intended to stimulate actions to improve quality on the part of health care professionals and organizations. The aim is to encourage complementary and synergistic efforts at the national and community levels and on the part of many stakeholders (e.g., purchasers, regulators, providers, and consumers) to improve safety and quality in a few key areas.

System Redesign

On the far right of the continuum of applications is what might be described as learning approaches. Health care providers' internal safety and quality improvement programs fall into this category, as do voluntary reporting programs in which providers share information on near misses and adverse events or comparative performance data. The work of many health care oversight organizations routinely extends far beyond their core public accountability responsibilities to the use of performance data and the organization's expertise in improvement methods to help health care providers learn, change systems, and improve performance.

Figure 8-4 illustrates the difference between accountability and learning approaches. While accountability sets a minimum performance standard and directly addresses health care providers whose performance falls below that standard (i.e., the far right tail of the distribution), learning approaches attempt to (1) eliminate inappropriate variation (making the distribution tall and narrow) and (2) document continuous improvement (move all participants in the process to the left in the direction of better quality).

Historically, many learning approaches have relied extensively on comparative performance data, often using the same types of data included in public report cards or provided to purchasers in payment-for-quality programs. These data may not be the most appropriate for setting priorities. A substantial body of evidence has identified a very large gap in overall health care performance, implying that average care may be quite poor (Institute of Medicine, 2001; McGlynn et al., 2003). Comparisons against theoretical "best performance," combined with assessments of readiness for change (e.g., available leadership, data systems), may be more effective in identifying improvement opportunities. For example, successful benchmarking strategies do not use average performance as a starting point. Instead, initial efforts are made to identify the "best in class," and extensive analysis is then undertaken to understand and share the processes that achieve top-level performance (American Productivity and Quality Center, 2003). Even excellent organizations can show significant improvement through such an approach. Focusing on the average performer will likely result in a tighter distribution, while a "best in class" focus will not only tighten but dramatically shift the distribution toward higher quality levels.

Shifting the distribution significantly may also have the effect of exposing true "bad apple" performers (represented by the black dot in Figure 8-4), thus enhancing accountability. While rare within the overall health care system, such poor performers do exist and demand a response. They often hide within the tail of the distribution, relying upon chance events among colleagues to obscure their own consistently poor performance. Successful learning and system redesign can shift the tail of the distribution, clearly exposing such individuals for appropriate professional intervention.

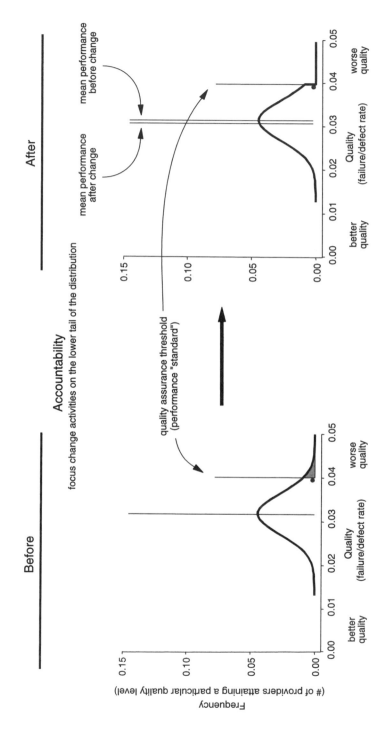

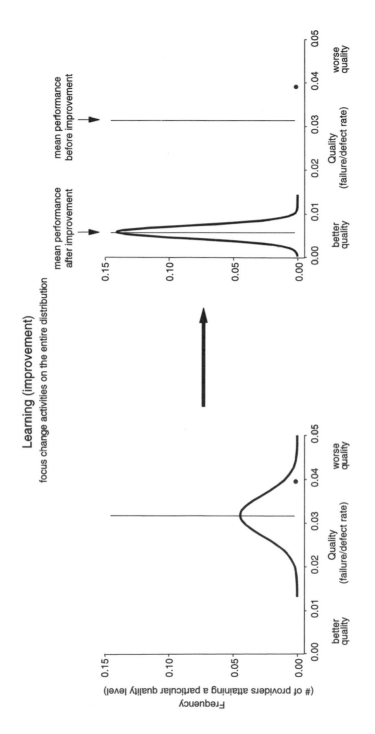

FIGURE 8-4 Use of patient safety data: Accountability versus system redesign.

ACCOUNTABILITY VERSUS LEARNING: UNDERSTANDING THE CONTINUUM

There are clearly many important applications of patient safety data and many different users. When called upon to respond to the most egregious performance failures, legal and regulatory programs appropriately aim to bar substandard providers from practice and to provide compensation to the injured. Incentive-based approaches aim to create an environment that rewards safety and quality and, in so doing, to encourage providers to pursue system redesign.

Although the three broad categories of applications—accountability, incentives, and system redesign—have quite different immediate aims and operate independently, they are intertwined in several important ways. First, depending upon how well they are crafted, the approaches pursued by legal and regulatory bodies and by purchasers and consumers in the marketplace can have either a positive or a negative effect on the efforts of providers to create a learning environment. Second, applications in all three categories rely to a great extent on the same underlying safety data systems and will do so increasingly in the future. Finally, all three consume scarce health care resources (e.g., dollars, provider time and attention), making an appropriate balance of activities imperative. This section presents a case study involving the use of mortality reports for accountability purposes and then uses this case study to illustrate key points related to issues surrounding the use of patient safety data, including the selection of measures, the risk that the use of performance data will instill fear and provoke defensive behavior on the part of providers, and the concept of preventability. The section ends with a discussion of the implications of the range of applications for patient safety data systems.

CASE STUDY

Between 1986 and 1992, the Health Care Financing Administration (HCFA) released a series of annual reports assessing mortality outcomes across approximately 5,500 hospitals that treated Medicare patients in the United States (Health Care Financing Administration, 1987). A team of HCFA researchers and statisticians developed risk adjustment models for mortality following hospital discharge and improved and refined those tools over time. Within the reports, the highest 5 percent of hospitals in terms of risk-adjusted death rates were labeled "high mortality outliers," while the bottom 5 percent were labeled "low mortality outliers." The news media distributed the resulting raw and risk-adjusted mortality rates, as well as the rankings, widely. HCFA's aims in publishing comparative mortality performance data were to assist peer review organizations in targeting their Medicare quality oversight activities, to inform health care consumers so they could make better choices about their own care, and to help health care professionals improve the quality of the care they delivered (Krakauer et al., 1992).

A series of studies, including one analysis performed by the HCFA statistical team itself, evaluated the HCFA mortality reports against various gold-standard clinical measures (Green et al., 1990, 1991; Krakauer et al., 1992; Rosen and Green, 1987). Positive predictive value (Weinstein and Fineberg, 1980) for the HCFA mortality reports ranged from 25 to 64 percent. In other words, for every 12 hospitals labeled as "high mortality outliers," at least 4 and as many as 9 were falsely identified. Among those hospitals judged to demonstrate excellent outcomes, as many as 3 in 5 were miscategorized (Green et al., 1991).

In 1993, Bruce Vladek, HCFA's administrator, halted release of the Medicare mortality reports. He judged that the reports were having little impact on care delivery performance while continuing to generate controversy and consume significant resources (Vladek, 1991).

Over a decade has passed since HCFA (now the Centers for Medicare and Medicaid Services) produced the annual mortality reports described in this case study. The intervening years have allowed dispassionate reflection on the reasoning, methods, barriers, effects, and limitations associated with a national attempt to use clinical data to drive change in health care delivery. The Medicare mortality reports, updated by parallel consideration of similar, more recent efforts, can serve as a useful case study for understanding issues surrounding data standards for patient safety.

Selection of Measures

Outcome measures, although of keen interest to regulators, purchasers, and individuals, are particularly difficult to use for accountability purposes since they do not necessarily measure competence (Trunkey and Botney, 2001). The outcomes individuals experience are influenced by multiple factors, many of which are outside the control of the health care provider. Given the pejorative nature and potential professional and business consequences of outcome-based accountability systems, health care providers demand accurate, reliable rankings. Patients and patient representatives also require reliable comparisons. In many circumstances, current clinical data systems and risk adjustment strategies are technically incapable of meeting those reasonable expectations.

There are many potential sources of variation in measured health outcomes (see Box 8-1), and risk adjustment methods can account only for differences in known patient factors. For example, Eddy estimates that all major factors proven to explain infant mortality rates (race, maternal alcohol consumption, maternal tobacco smoke exposure, altitude, and differences in prenatal care delivery performance) account for only about 25 percent of documented variation in patient outcomes (Eddy, 2002). The other 75 percent of outcomes are beyond the reach of risk adjustment strategies.

Geographic aggregation (e.g., variation in hospital programs and local referral patterns) can also play a defining role. A recent evaluation of hospital quality outcome measures found that most produced statistically reliable results when aggregated to the level of a metropolitan area, state, or multistate region, but only a few measures produced valid results at the level of individual hospitals (Bernard et al., 2003). The fact that an outcome mea-

---

BOX 8-1
Possible Sources of Variation in Measured Outcomes

- Differences in clinical performance
- Differences in individual patients
  - Known factors
    - Physiologic/anatomic disease expression and response (severity)
    - Comorbid illnesses (complexity)
    - Patient compliance
    - Patient values, preferences, and resources
  - Unknown factors
- Differences in the structure of the care delivery system (data aggregation)
  - Unreliable attribution of performance among professionals and organizations within complex care delivery collaborations
  - Risk-associated referral patterns, undetected by individual patient measures
- Differences in measurement (data collection and analysis)
  - Completeness of data collection (extraction of manual or electronic data)
    - Case finding
    - Level of clinical assessment (e.g., was the test performed and recorded?)
    - Field finding (e.g., was the clinical result extracted?)
  - Accuracy of data collection
    - Consistent and complete field definitions
    - Accuracy of data entry
  - Pertinent details of data collection (e.g., administrative vs. clinical system)

sure demonstrates statistical significance overall, at an aggregated level, does not mean that it will reliably distinguish performance at a detailed individual level (Andersson et al., 1998; Hixson, 1989; Silber et al., 1995). Consequently, many hospital and physician ranking systems based on outcome measures perform poorly (Blumberg and Binns, 1989; Green et al., 1997; Greenfield et al., 1988; Jollis and Romano, 1998; Krumholz et al., 2002; Marshall et al., 2000).

Comparisons of risk-adjusted quality outcomes, when applied for purposes of accountability, work best when they are narrowly focused (e.g., on a single clinical entity); when the underlying patient factors that affect outcomes are well understood; and when those performing the comparisons can access accurate, complete, standardized patient data at a high level of clinical detail. For example, several measurement systems for risk-adjusted mortality outcomes for open heart surgery can account for more than 60 percent of all observed variation in those outcomes (Hannan et al., 1998; O'Connor et al., 1998).

Most health care settings lack the necessary data to support accurate risk adjustment and ranking of providers. Standardized clinical data are not captured as part of the care delivery process. The HCFA mortality reports were produced from Medicare claims data, which lack important clinical detail. Accuracy is also a problem in claims data (Green and Wintfeld, 1993).

On the other hand, learning systems exhibit a high tolerance for imperfect data and an ability to use such data productively. When used for process improvement, risk adjustment removes variation arising from patient factors that are beyond the care delivery system's control and makes the effects of process changes more clearly identifiable (i.e., it improves the signal-to-noise ratio), an aim quite different from that of accountability systems of improving predictive value. For example, a risk adjustment model that accounts for only 25 percent of outcome variability (by modeling out the contribution of known cofactors) can significantly improve a team's ability to see structure in the data or determine more accurately whether a process change has improved outcomes. The same risk adjustment likely would not improve comparative outcome data to the point where they could reliably rank care providers for accountability.

The Cycle of Fear

All efforts to improve safety and quality through the use of performance data run the risk of instilling fear and provoking defensive behavior on the part of providers. Scherkenbach outlines three sequential factors in that response, labeling them the "cycle of fear" (see Figure 8-5) (Scherkenbach, 1991, p. 98).

Knowledge of predictable human responses to accountability data is a key factor in the design of an effective patient safety reporting system. It is also an important consideration in deciding how much emphasis to place on accountability versus learning applications because the former applications run a much higher risk of instilling fear than do the latter.

Reaction 1: Kill the Messenger

Accountability data inherently focus on individual health professionals or care delivery organizations. Upon being flagged as an outlier, most humans react defensively. They perceive a negative evaluation as a direct attack. In response, they raise defensive barriers that make positive communications difficult.

Under the philosophy that the best defense is a good offense, they often counterattack (shift the blame). They challenge the measurement system, analytic methods, and accuracy of the evaluation. They question the competence and motives of those conducting the assessment. Most important, they try to block access to data that could contribute to similar criticism in the future. For example, Berwick and Wald conducted a survey of hospital leaders' reactions to the release of the HCFA mortality data in 1987. They found

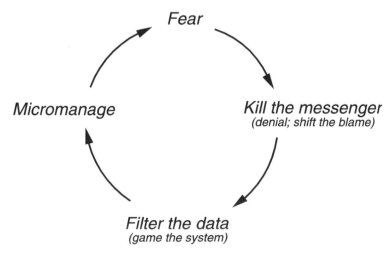

FIGURE 8-5 Scherkenbach's cycle of fear.
SOURCE: Scherkenback, 1991.

that all hospitals, regardless of mortality rate, shared an extremely negative view of the accuracy, usefulness, and interpretability of the data (Berwick and Wald, 1990).

Reaction 2: Filter the Data (Game the System)

Many of the data used in outcome analyses are generated by the individuals and institutions who are the focus of the evaluation. In such circumstances, even among conscientious, honest observers, the sentinel effect can significantly alter the data that are recorded and affect comparative outcome rankings. Some such data manipulation may be neither unconscious nor honest: when confronted by outcome measurement for accountability, it is often far easier to look good by gaming the data system than to be good by managing and improving clinical processes.

Anecdotal accounts of "filtering the data" are common in health care. For example, a hospital in the western United States was found to be a high mortality outlier for acute myocardial infarct (AMI) on an early HCFA mortality report. Upon internal review, the hospital discovered that almost all AMI patients were being coded as admissions from their community-based physician's office, even though many had come through the hospital's emergency department. Upon realizing that source of admission was an important element in the HCFA risk adjustment model, the hospital began coding *all* AMI patients as having entered the hospital through the emergency department. By the following year, the hospital had gone from being a high mortality outlier to being a low mortality outlier on the HCFA AMI mortality report without introducing any change in clinical care (James, 1988).

The extent of systematic data manipulation in health care is not known. However, in one study 39 percent of physicians reported falsifying insurance records to obtain payment for care they believed was necessary even though it was not covered by the patient's policy (Wynia et al., 2000). There is also evidence that voluntary injury detection systems underreport events, although this may be attributable in part to the burden of reporting (Evans et al., 1998).

Industries outside of health care have repeatedly demonstrated that a safe reporting environment is critical to robust failure detection and that robust failure detection is essential to the design of safe systems that significantly reduce failure rates (Institute of Medicine, 2000). Such experience suggests that, whenever possible, accountability for patient safety should focus at the level of an organization rather than the level of individual health professionals working within the organization. Unfortunately, most health care is delivered outside hospitals and nursing homes by clinicians in small practice settings who lack any strong tie to an organization.

Reaction 3: Micromanage

Most health care delivery consists of complex processes and systems involving many interacting factors that are usually summed by performance metrics. As a result, such summary measures will exhibit a component of apparently random variation (Berwick, 1991). The use of data for accountability can lead health professionals to attempt to focus on tracking and responding to minute, random fluctuations in their process data, whereas careful analysis and redesign of work processes are needed to improve performance. Indeed, micromanagement can lead to worse outcomes, causing overseers to demand more rigorous inspection and oversight, which will likely lead to another iteration of the cycle of fear.

The Concept of Preventability

The most effective patient safety strategies rest upon a broad definition of preventable adverse events. As defined in this report, an adverse event is any unintended harm to a patient caused by medical management rather than by the underlying disease or condition of the patient. Some adverse events are unavoidable. Patients and their caregivers are sometimes forced to knowingly accept adverse secondary consequences to achieve a more important primary treatment goal. The concept of preventability separates care delivery errors from such recognized but unavoidable treatment consequences.

Providers seeking to improve safety generally focus on preventable adverse events. Members of the health care professions, who often associate the term "error" with professional neglect or incompetence or fear that others will do so, may seek to define preventability very narrowly, greatly limiting the scope and impact of patient safety improvement.

For example, a hospital team developed a data-based clinical trigger tool to identify adverse drug events (ADEs), increasing the ADE detection rate by almost two orders of magnitude. The team then analyzed and prioritized causes for the ADEs detected. The single largest category, accounting for 28 percent of events, was allergic and idiosyncratic drug reactions among patients with no previous history of reaction. Thinking at the level of individual health professionals, all members of the team initially agreed that such injuries were outside clinicians' control and accountability and that the topic thus was not worthy of further exploration. However, the team ultimately took a systems approach, noting that there is often a range of medications available to address a particular clinical need and that those medications may pose different risks for allergic reaction. The team created computerized alerts that recommended a safer alternative if a physician ordered a medication with a high allergy risk. In addition, the team implemented immediate review of a developing ADE by a pharmacist, under the theory that early intervention might abort the event before it progressed to more serious levels. When implemented, the team's intervention reduced serious allergic and idiosyncratic drug reactions within the hospital by more than 50 percent (Evans et al., 1994; Pestotnik et al., 1996).

Another good example of a problem previously thought to be largely unpreventable (after standardizing sterile measures) is that of bloodstream infections with central venous lines. While they have important advantages (e.g., the ability to administer large volumes of fluid), short-term vascular catheters are associated with serious complications, particularly infections. Central venous catheters impregnated with rifampin and minocycline have been shown to reduce the incidence of catheter-related bloodstream infection (Darouiche et al., 1999).

It is also important to recognize that current beliefs concerning preventability may be quite limited. Many events presently judged not to be preventable may be so with careful investigation and creative thought. Finally, even if a class of injuries is not presently preventable, a broad focus can generate and prioritize a research agenda that can improve patient safety over time.

Patient safety data systems should cast a wide net, focusing on all types of adverse events, not just those that are preventable based on current understanding and current systems of care delivery. Achieving this broad focus will require careful use of the term "error," with clear recognition of its linkage to system-level solutions and attention to its pejorative connotations for health professionals. Using the term "injuries" may even be preferable and might make it possible to avoid the type of negative behavior described by the cycle of fear.

Implications for Patient Safety Data Systems

Patient safety data systems must be able to support the full range of applications, from accountability to learning. If they are to do so, they must be carefully designed to capture all relevant data and comply with national data standards. It will also be important to establish an external auditing process to certify the integrity of patient safety data reported externally for purposes of regulation, public reporting, or payment.

Data System Design

Efficient patient safety data systems that can span a continuum of uses will require careful design. Accountability measures usually report high-order, summary data (James, 1994a, b, 2003). Process management and improvement, on the other hand, require detailed decision-level data (Berwick et al., 2003).

Patient safety data systems should be designed to capture, as part of the patient care process, the data needed for learning applications. While data systems designed for learning can supply accountability data, the opposite is not true; summary data collected for accountability usually lack sufficient detail for learning-based uses (James, 2003). In the absence of careful planning, a health care delivery organization with limited resources may find that all of its measurement resources are consumed by special data collection to comply with external reporting requirements, with none remaining for learning and system redesign (Casalino, 1999). By contrast, a carefully designed data system that captures detailed decision-level data for improvement will be able to comply with external reporting requirements through a concept known as "data reuse" (see Chapter 2).

Learning depends on profound knowledge of key work processes. Process and outcome measures provide insight on what fails, how often and how it fails, what works, how it works, and how to make it work better. Data systems designed for learning can integrate data collection directly into work processes. Integrated data collection is usually more timely, accurate, and efficient. More important, properly designed learning data are immediately useful to front-line workers for process management, so that the burden of data collection is less likely to be perceived as an unfunded mandate (Langley et al., 1996).

Standardized Data

Patient safety data systems should adhere to national data standards. Many external applications of patient safety data, including accountability, the provision of incentives, and priority setting, make use of comparative data. Standardized data definitions are necessary to make such comparisons. Comparative data also serve learning purposes when used to identify "best in class" providers.

Standardized data are important as well for the identification of infrequently occurring safety issues. Many patient injuries occur at such low rates that any single organization will not be able to generate sufficient data within a reasonable length of time for organizational learning to take place. Data rates will be too low to permit recognizing patterns, testing possible solutions, and developing effective preventive actions. Without data standards, moreover, it is difficult for different care delivery organizations to share injury reports, compare results, benchmark processes, and learn from one another's experience.

Patient Safety Data Audits

When patient safety data are used for external performance reporting, it is important that the data be audited. When performance data are used for licensure or payment purposes or to support purchaser or consumer decisions, providers have an incentive to "look their best." Audits are necessary to assure all stakeholders that the reporting system is fair. They also provide useful feedback to providers on ways to redesign and strengthen their patient safety data systems.

A data audit conducted by an independent reviewer is intended to ascertain that (1) the data sources used by a health care organization to identify individual adverse events or derive aggregate performance measures (e.g., mammography rate) are complete and accurate, and (2) aggregate measures have been properly calculated (e.g., the denominator includes only women over the age of 50). As discussed further in Chapter 4, an audit process for adverse event reporting may involve review of a provider's processes for case finding (e.g., individual reports, automated triggers), evaluation (i.e., conduct of root-cause analyses), and classification.

A data audit is different from a patient safety program audit. The primary aim of a data audit is to provide assurance that the numbers reported are reasonably complete, accurate, and reproducible and thus useful for shared analysis and comparison. By design, such an audit does not address how a health care organization responds to an injury or makes decisions for accountability for safety performance. A program audit is much broader than a data audit and focuses on organizational elements that influence safety (e.g., whether a culture of safety exists; whether adequate attention is paid to safety issues at the level of the governing board and managerial and clinical leadership; whether adequate decision supports, such as drug–drug interaction alerts, are available to assist clinicians). The critical elements of an effective patient safety program are discussed in Chapter 9.

In light of the increased emphasis on the public reporting of performance data, it is particularly important that such data be valid and reliable. The assurance provided by an external audit is an essential element of transparency and a potent antidote to misrepresentation, cheating, and corruption. With sufficient reliable, complete, and understandable information, patients are better prepared to participate in health care decisions, and accountability becomes an inherent feature of the care delivery system. Over the long term, the role of health care oversight may narrow, focusing to a great extent on the integrity of the data system used to generate public reports.

Auditing is used extensively outside the health care sector. For example, the American financial markets are driven to a great extent by the information contained in standardized financial statements released by publicly traded companies. The Securities and Exchange Commission oversees (1) the establishment of accounting standards (i.e., generally accepted accounting principles) by the Federal Accounting Standards Board, (2) the establishment of explicit standards describing how an acceptable audit will be conducted (Generally Accepted Audit Standards) by the Audit Standards Board, and (3) the conduct of audits by certified auditors (certified public accountants) (Financial Accounting Standards Board, 2003).

Experience with auditing is far more limited in the health care sector. The National Committee for Quality Assurance (NCQA), a private-sector accrediting and performance reporting organization, oversees an auditing process to assure the integrity of aggregate-level performance data reported by about 460 health plans on 60 performance measures in the Health Plan Employer Data and Information Set (National Committee for Quality Assurance, 2003). The performance measurement data are used to produce comparative performance reports for health care purchasers, employers, and consumers. The data are also required as part of NCQA's health plan accreditation program. To ensure the integrity of the data reported by health plans, NCQA has auditing criteria (National Committee for Quality Assurance, 2001) that include a program to license audit organizations and certify auditors. There are currently 11 licensed organizations and 71 certified auditors. The auditing criteria address such areas as data completeness, data integrity, thoroughness of system processes, and accuracy of medical record review.

In light of the many types of patient safety applications involving many different users, the health care sector would benefit from national data audit criteria for assessing the integrity of patient safety data systems used to generate reports in support of the full continuum of patient safety applications.

AHRQ, in collaboration with private-sector entities, should assume a lead role in the development of national audit criteria for patient safety data.

THE NEED TO INVEST MORE RESOURCES IN LEARNING APPROACHES

The committee believes that the health system has underinvested by a large margin in learning approaches. The American health care system will continue to lack sufficient capacity to deliver excellent care to all patients without fundamental change in the overall level of performance of the system as a whole.

It is imperative that all health care providers develop comprehensive patient safety systems that promote learning. Learning systems relentlessly redesign care processes in pursuit of "best in class." They attempt to change the shape of the performance distribution by improving all parts of the process, regardless of initial standing (Berwick et al., 2003). And learning approaches are far less susceptible to barriers arising from the cycle of fear. Chapter 5 provides a discussion of comprehensive patient safety systems in health care organizations.

REFERENCES

Agency for Healthcare Research and Quality. 2001. *Annual Report of the National CAHPS Benchmarking Database 2000: What Consumers Say About the Quality of Their Health Plans and Medical Care.* Rockville, MD: Westat.

———. 2002. *National Healthcare Quality Report.* Online. Available: http://www.ahcpr.gov/qual/nhqrfact.htm [accessed August 18, 2003].

American Productivity and Quality Center. 2003. *Benchmarking.* Online. Available: http://www.apqc.org/portal/apqc/site/generic2?path=/site/benchmarking/free_resources.jhtml [accessed August 18, 2003].

Andersson, J., K. Carling, and S. Mattson. 1998. Random ranking of hospitals is unsound. *Chance* 11 (3):34–37, 39.

Arrow, K. J. 1963. Uncertainty and the welfare economics of medical care. *Am Econ Rev* 50 (5):941–973.

Bailit Health Purchasing. 2002a. *Ensuring Quality Health Plans: A Purchaser's Toolkit for Using Incentives.* Washington, DC: National Health Care Purchasing Institute.

———. 2002b. *Provider Incentive Models for Improving Quality of Care.* Washington, DC: National Health Care Purchasing Institute.

Baumgarten, A. 2002. *California Managed Care Review 2002.* Oakland, CA: California HealthCare Foundation.

Bernard, S. L., L. A. Savitz, and E. R. Brody. 2003. *Validating the AHRQ Quality Indicators: Final Report.* Rockville, MD: Agency for Healthcare Research and Quality.

Berwick, D. M. 1989. Continuous improvement as an ideal in health care. *N Engl J Med* 320 (1):53–56.

———. 1991. Controlling variation in health care: A consultation from Walter Shewart. *Med Care* 29 (12):1212–1225.

Berwick, D. M., and D. L. Wald. 1990. Hospital leaders' opinions of the HCFA mortality data. *JAMA* 263 (2):247–249.

Berwick, D. M., B. James, and M. J. Coye. 2003. Connections between quality measurement and improvement. *Med Care* 41 (1 Supplement):I30–I38.

Blumberg, M. S., and G. S. Binns. 1989. *Risk-Adjusted 30-Day Mortality of Fresh Acute Myocardial Infarctions: The Technical Report.* Chicago, IL: Hospital Research and Educational Trust (American Hospital Association).

California HealthCare Foundation. 2003. *New Web Site Helps Californians Choose a Quality Nursing Home.* Online. Available: http://www.chcf.org/print.cfm?itemID =20148 [accessed August 19, 2003].

Casalino, L. P. 1999. The unintended consequences of measuring quality on the quality of medicare. *N Engl J Med* 341 (15):1147–1150.

Centers for Medicare and Medicaid Services. 2003. *Dialysis Facility Compare.* Online. Available: http://www.medicare.gov/Dialysis/Home.asp [accessed August 19, 2003].

Chassin, M. R. 1998. Is health care ready for six sigma quality? *Milbank Q* 764:565–591.

———. 2002. Achieving and sustaining improved quality: Lessons from New York State and cardiac surgery. *Health Aff* (Millwood) 21 (4):40–51.

Chassin, M. R., E. L. Hannan, and B. A. DeBuono. 1996. Benefits and hazards of reporting medical outcomes publicly. *New Engl J Med* 334 (6):394–398.

Cohen, M. M., P. G. Duncan, W. D. Pope, and C. Wolkenstien. 1986. A survey of 112, 000 anaesthetics at one teaching hospital (1975–1983). *Can Anaesth Soc J* 33:22–31.

Cooper, J. B., R. S. Newbower, C. D. Long, and B. McPeek. 2002. Preventable anesthesia mishaps: A study of human factors. *Qual Saf Health Care* 11(3):277–282. [Reprint of a paper that appeared in *Anesthesiology*, 1978, 49:399–406.]

Darouiche, R. O., I. I. Raad, S. O. Heard, J. I. Thornby, O. C. Wenker, A. Gabrielli, J. Berg, N. Khardori, H. Hanna, R. Hachem, R. L. Harris, and G. Mayhall. 1999. A comparison of two antimicrobial-impregnated central venous catheters: Catheter study group. *N Engl J Med* 340 (1):1–8.

Deming, W. E. 1988. *System definition.* Personal communication to Brent James.

Department of Health and Human Services. 2002a. *HHS Launches National Nursing Home Quality Initiative: Broad Effort to Improve Quality in Nursing Homes Across the Country.* Online. Available: http://www.dhhs.gov/news/press/2002pres/ 20021112.html [accessed August 19, 2003].

———. 2002b. *Secretary Thompson Welcomes New Effort to Provide Hospital Quality of Care Information.* Online. Available: http://www.dhhs.gov/news/press/2002pres/ 20021212.html [accessed August 19, 2002].

Dudley, R. A., D. Rittenhouse, and R. Bae. 2002. *Creating a Statewide Hospital Quality Reporting System: The Quality Initiative.* San Francisco, CA: Institute for Health Policy Studies.

Duncan, P. G., and M. M. Cohen. 1987. Postoperative complications: Factors of significance to anaesthetic practice. *Can J Anaesth* 34:2–8.

Eddy, D. 2002. *Summarizing Analyses Performed on Behalf of the National Committee for Quality Assurance, While Evaluating Infant Mortality Rates as a Possible Measurement Set.* Personal communication to Institute of Medicine's Committee on Data Standards for Patient Safety.

Evans, R. S., S. L. Pestotnik, D. C. Classen, T. P. Clemmer, L. K. Weaver, J. F. Orme Jr., J. F. Lloyd, and J. P. Burke. 1998. A computer-assisted management program for antibiotics and other antiinfective agents. *N Engl J Med* 338 (4):232–238.

Evans, R. S., S. L. Pestotnik, D. C. Classen, S. D. Horne, S. B. Bass, and J. P. Burke. 1994. Preventing adverse drug events in hospitalized patients. *Ann Pharmacother* 28 (4):523–527.

Financial Accounting Standards Board. 2003. *FASB Facts.* Online. Available: http://www.fasb.org/facts/ [accessed August 4, 2003].

Freudenheim, M. 2002. June 26. Quality goals in incentives for hospitals. *New York Times.* Section Late Edition-Final, Section C, Page 1, Col. 5.

Gaba, D. M. 1989. Human error in anesthetic mishaps. *Int Anesthesiology Clin* 27 (3):137–147.

Gabel, J. R., K. A. Hunt, and K. Hurst. 1998. When employers choose health plans do NCQA accreditation and HEDIS data count? *Health Care Quality.* Online. Available: http://www.cmwf.org/programs/health_care/gabel_ncqa_hedis_293.asp [accessed December 15, 2003].

Green, J., and N. Wintfeld. 1993. How accurate are hospital discharge data for evaluating effectiveness of care? *Med Care* 31 (8):719–731.

Green, J., L. J. Passman, and N. Wintfeld. 1991. Analyzing hospital mortality: The consequences of diversity in patient mix. *JAMA* 265 (14):1849–1853.

Green, J., N. Wintfeld, M. Krasner, and C. Wells. 1997. In search of America's best hospitals: The promise and reality of quality assessment. *JAMA* 277 (14):1152–1155.

Green, J., N. Wintfeld, P. Sharkey, and L. J. Passman. 1990. The importance of severity of illness in assessing hospital mortality. *JAMA* 263 (2):241–246.

Greenfield, S., H. U. Aronow, R. M. Elashoff, and D. Watanabe. 1988. Flaws in mortality data: The hazards of ignoring comorbid disease. *JAMA* 260 (15):2253–2255.

Haas-Wilson, D. 2001. Arrow and the information market failure in health care: The changing content and sources of health care information. *J Health Polit Policy Law* 26:Part 3.

Hannan, E. L., A. J. Popp, B. Tranmer, P. Fuestel, J. Waldman, and D. Shah. 1998. Relationship between provider volume and mortality for carotid endarterectomies in New York State. *Stroke* 29:2292–2297.

Health Care Financing Administration. 1987. *Medicare Hospital Mortality Information, 1986.* HCFA Pub. No. 01-002. Washington, DC: U.S. Government Printing Office.

Hibbard, J. H. 1998. Use of outcome data by purchasers and consumer: New strategies and new dilemmas. *Int J Quality Health Care* 10 (6):503-508.

———. 2003. Engaging health care consumers to improve the quality of care. *Med Care* 41 (1-Supplement):161–170.

Hibbard, J. H., E. Peters, P. Slovic, M. L. Finucane, and M. Tusler. 2001. Making health care quality reports easier to use. *Jt Comm J Qual Improv* 27 (11):591–604.

Hixson, J. S. 1989. *Efficacy of Statistical Outlier Analysis for Monitoring Quality of Care.* Chicago, IL: American Medical Association Center for Health Policy Research.

Institute of Medicine. 2000. *To Err Is Human: Building a Safer Health System.* Washington, DC: National Academy Press.

————. 2001. *Crossing the Quality Chasm: A New Health System for the 21st Century.* Washington, DC: National Academy Press.

————. 2003. *Priority Areas for National Action: Transforming Health Care Quality.* Washington, DC: The National Academies Press.

James, B. C. 1988. *IHC Health Services.* Personal communication to Institute of Medicine's Committee on Data Standards for Patient Safety.

————. 1992. Good enough? Standards and measurement in continuous quality improvement. In: *Bridging the Gap Between Theory and Practice.* Chicago, IL: Hospital Research and Educational Trust (American Hospital Association). Pp. 1–24.

————. 1994a. Outcomes measurement. In: *Bridging the Gap Between Theory and Practice: Exploring Outcomes Management.* Chicago, IL: Hospital Research and Educational Trust (American Hospital Association). Pp. 1–37.

————. 1994b. Breaks in the outcomes measurement chain. *Hosp Health Netw* 68 (14):60.

————. 2003. Information system concepts for quality measurement. *Med Care* 41 (1 Supplement):I71–I79.

Joint Commission on Accreditation of Healthcare Organizations. 1998. Sentinel events: Approaches to error reduction and prevention. *Jt Comm J Qual Improv* 24 (4):175–186.

Jollis, J. G., and P. S. Romano. 1998. Pennsylvania's focus on heart attack: Grading the scorecard. *N Engl J Med* 338 (14):983–987.

Kaye, N. 2001. *Medicaid Managed Care: A Guide for the States.* Portland, ME: National Academy for State Health Policy.

Kaye, N., and M. Bailit. 1999. *Innovations in Payment Strategies to Improve Plan Performance.* Portland, ME: National Academy for State Health Policy.

Krakauer, H., R. C. Bailey, K. J. Skellan, J. D. Stewart, A. J. Hartz, E. M. Kuhn, and A. A. Rimm. 1992. Evaluation of the HCFA model for the analysis of mortality following hospitalization. *Health Serv Res* 27 (3):317–335.

Krumholz, H. M., S. S. Rathore, J. Chen, Y. Wang, and M. J. Radford. 2002. Evaluation of a consumer-oriented Internet health care report card: The risk of quality ratings based on mortality data. *JAMA* 287 (10):1277–1287.

Langley, G. J., K. M. Nolan, C. L. Norman, L. P. Provost, and T. W. Nolan. 1996. *The Improvement Guide: A Practical Approach to Enhancing Organizational Performance.* San Francisco, CA: Jossey-Bass.

Marshall, M. N., P. G. Shekelle, S. Leatherman, and R. H. Brook. 2000. The public release of performance data: What do we expect to gain? A review of the evidence. *JAMA* 283 (14):1866–1874.

McCormick, D., D. U. Himmelstein, S. Woolhandler, S. M. Wolfe, and D. H. Bor. 2002. Relationship between low quality-of-care scores and HMOs' subsequent public disclosure of quality-of-care scores. *JAMA* 288 (12):1484–1490.

McGlynn, E., and J. Adams. 2001. Public release of information on quality. In: R. Anderson, T. Rice, and G. Kominksi, eds. *Changing the U.S. Health Care System: Key Issues in Health Services Policy and Management*, 2nd Edition. San Francisco, CA: Jossey-Bass, Inc. Pp. 183–202.

McGlynn, E. A., S. M. Asch, J. Adams, J. Keesey, J. Hicks, A. DeCristofaro, and E. A. Kerr. 2003. The quality of health care delivered to adults in the United States. *N Engl J Med* 348 (26):2635–2645.

Mennemeyer, S. T., M. A. Morrisey, and L. Z. Howard. 1997. Death and reputation: How consumers acted upon HCFA mortality information. *Inquiry* 34 (2):117–128.

National Committee for Quality Assurance. 2001. *HEDIS Compliance Audit: Volume 5*. Washington, DC: National Committee for Quality Assurance.

———. 2002a. *NCQA Report Cards*. Online. Available: http://hprc.ncqa.org/menu.asp [accessed May 6, 2002].

———. 2002b. *The State of Health Care Quality: Industry Trends and Analysis*. Washington, DC: National Committee for Quality Assurance.

———. 2003. *HEDIS Technical Specifications: Volume 3*. Washington, DC: National Committee for Quality Assurance.

National Health Care Purchasing Institute. 2002. *Rewarding Results*. Online. Available: http://www.nhcpi.net/rewardingresults/index.cfm [accessed April 22, 2002].

O'Connor, G. T., J. D. Birkmeyer, L. J. Dacey, H. B. Quinton, C. A. Marrin, N. J. Birkmeyer, J. R. Morton, B. J. Leavitt, C. T. Maloney, F. Hernandez, R. A. Clough, W. C. Nugent, E. M. Olmstead, D. C. Charlesworth, and S. K. Plume. 1998. Results of a regional study of modes of death associated with coronary artery bypass grafting. *Northern New England Cardiovascular Disease Study Group* 66 (4):1323–1328.

Pestotnik, S. L., D. C. Classen, R. S. Evans, and J. P. Burke. 1996. Implementing antibiotic practice guidelines through computer-assisted decision support: Clinical and financial outcomes. *Ann Intern Med* 124 (10):884–890.

Pierce, E. C. Jr. 1996. The 34th Rovenstine lecture 40 years behind the mask: Safety revisited. *Anesthesiology* 84 (4):965–975.

Robinson, J. C. 2001. The end of asymmetric information. *J Health Polit Policy Law* 26:Part 3.

Rosen, H. M., and B. A. Green. 1987. The HCFA excess mortality lists: A methodological critique. *Hosp Health Serv Adm* 32 (1):119–127.

Rosenthal, J., M. Booth, L. Flowers, and T. Riley. 2001. *Current State Programs Addressing Medical Errors: An Analysis of Mandatory Reporting and Other Initiatives*. Portland, ME: National Academy for State Health Policy.

Salber, P., and B. Bradley. 2001. *Perspective: Adding Quality to the Health Care Purchasing Equation*. Online. Available: http://www.healthaffairs.org/WebExclusives/index.dtl?year=2001 [accessed February 20, 2004].

Schauffler, H. H., and J. K. Mordavsky. 2001. Consumer reports in health care: Do they make a difference? *Annu Rev Public Health* 22:69–89.

Scherkenbach, W. 1991. *The Deming Route to Quality and Productivity: Road Maps and Road Blocks, 11th Edition*. Washington, DC: CEE Press Books, George Washington University.

Schneider, E. C., and A. M. Epstein. 1996. Influence of cardiac-surgery performance reports on referral practices and access to care. *N Engl J Med* 335 (4):251–256.

Silber, J. H., P. R. Rosenbaum, and R. N. Ross. 1995. Comparing the contributions of groups of predictors: Which outcomes vary with hospital rather than patient characteristics? *J Am Statistical Assoc* 90 (429):7–18.

Simon, L. P., and A. F. Monroe. 2001. California provider group report cards: What do they tell us? *Am J Med Qual* 16 (2):61–70.

The Henry J. Kaiser Family Foundation and Agency for Healthcare Research and Quality. 2000. *National Survey on Americans as Health Care Consumers: An Update on the Role of Quality Information*. Online. Available: http://www.kff.org/content/2000/ 3093/ [accessed August 11, 2003].

Thompson, J. W., S. D. Pinidiya, K. W. Ryan, E. D. McKinley, S. Alston, J. E. Bost, J. B. French, and P. Simpson. 2003. Health plan quality data: The importance of public reporting. *Am J Prev Med* 24 (1):62–70.

Trunkey, D. D., and R. Botney. 2001. Assessing competency: A tale of two professions. *J Am Col Surg* 192 (3)385–395.

Vladek, B. C. 1991. *Letter to Hospital Administrators: Accompanying Fiscal Year 1991 Medicare Mortality Information*. Baltimore, MD: U.S. Department of Health and Human Services, Health Care Financing Administration.

Weinstein, M. C., and H. V. Fineberg. 1980. *Clinical Decision Analysis*. Philadelphia, PA: W.B. Saunders Company. Pp. 86–88.

White, R. 2002, January 14. A shift to quality by health plans. *Los Angeles Times*. Section C-1.

Wynia, M. K., D. S. Cummins, J. B. VanGeest, and I. B. Wilson. 2000. Physician manipulation of reimbursement rules for patients: Between a rock and a hard place. *JAMA* 283 (14):1858–1865.

9

Standardized Reporting

CHAPTER SUMMARY

Effective and efficient patient safety reporting systems within the context of an integrated health information infrastructure are essential to the creation of a new standard of care for evidence-based medicine and the ongoing improvement of clinical practice. However, many of the existing reporting systems vary in a number of design features (Institute of Medicine, 2000) and approaches to patient safety (e.g., voluntary, mandatory, internal, external). The data standards used within these systems also vary widely, rendering the data incomparable across systems for more extensive research and analysis.

This chapter develops a framework for the standardized collection and codification of those report data most important to detecting, analyzing, understanding, and learning from patient safety-related events. The first section emphasizes the need for a standardized report format and outlines its essential elements. The second section discusses a common set of data standards for patient safety reporting that can enable the aggregation of data from voluntary and state reporting systems, as well as support the establishment of a national patient safety database first called for in To Err Is Human *(Institute of Medicine, 2000). Next, the chapter reviews factors affecting the implementation of the report format and issues of deidentification and data protection. Lastly, the chapter provides examples of primary and secondary uses of the report data.*

THE NEED FOR A STANDARDIZED REPORT FORMAT

At present, there is no agreement on a common set of data elements for representing patient safety information, much less specification of allowable values for those elements. Each entity self-determines the content of its reports; some even develop their own terminology to represent the information. At the state level, for example, New York and Florida are 2 of 21 states with mandatory requirements for reporting adverse events. The data elements they collect for the most serious adverse events have some areas of commonality:

- Similar patient information is collected.
- Similar information is collected on the time/location of the incident.
- Each requires a description of the occurrence and analysis of its root causes.
- Each requires a description of the corrective actions taken.
- Only one health care data standard, the International Classification of Diseases, Ninth Edition (ICD-9), Clinical Modification (CM), is used by each to identify the diagnosis and procedures associated with the event (Rosenthal et al., 2000).

However, each state has developed its own taxonomy for classifying actual events. The New York Patient Occurrence Reporting and Tracking System (NYPORTS) works within the broad categories of statutorily defined reportable incidents. The system makes use of a detailed list of 54 reportable codes with "includes" and "excludes," organized by type of event, to promote greater consistency among state hospitals (Rosenthal et al., 2001). Florida, on the other hand, divides the events into two categories—those that must be reported within 15 days and on an annual basis (Rosenthal et al., 2001). Each category includes four or five broad types of events to be reported. Another important difference is that the New York system has a set of questions designed specifically for medication errors, a known major adverse event category; the Florida system does not. The differences among the 15 state patient safety systems are even more pronounced.

The following "real world" example further illustrates the problem with numerous disparate data elements for documenting an adverse event. If an individual suffered a serious adverse drug event (ADE) while in a New York hospital, the clinician would first file a report internally for review by the designated hospital representative. A second report would be filed with the New York State Department of Health through NYPORTS. Another third report could be voluntarily submitted to the Food and Drug Administration (FDA), either through the FDA MedWatch reporting system or through private-sector organizations such as the United States Pharmacopia (USP), to inform the FDA of potential serious problems with the drug. Adding further to the burden of disparate and multiple methods for representing an ADE are the voluntary reporting requirements of the hospitals' accrediting organization, the Joint Commission for Accreditation of Healthcare Organizations (JCAHO), whose proposed taxonomy provides yet another dataset for classifying and reporting such events. Already this example involves four different reports with varying data elements for the same ADE.

In the case of the FDA, reports are submitted to support the agency's regulatory obligations for postmarket surveillance of drugs marketed in the United States, particularly those associated with ADEs. To this end, the organization needs the capability to analyze and compare the ADEs occurring during the clinical trial process with those experienced in clinical practice. However, the FDA uses one terminology, MedDRA, for representation of ADEs experienced by patients during clinical trials and documentation in the manufacturer's dossier for regulatory approval, and another in its MedWatch reporting system. The agency also accepts data from private-sector organizations using different data standards. Thus, for the FDA alone, the data related to one particular ADE is represented by three different data sources. More importantly, the data from clinical trials and postmarket surveillance cannot be compared without costly mapping of the terms among the different taxonomies.

An additional consideration relates to the ability to share and compare data in integrated systems. For example, a clinician who wanted to conduct an analysis of or research on ADE reports compared with events detected and/or prevented with various decision support systems (e.g., pharmacy systems, computerized physician order entry, bar-code medication administration) could not do so without common methods for representing the most basic ADE data (e.g., drug involved, type of event, route of administration, dosage). The ability to compare the factors contributing to an ADE among systems would add to the knowledge and understanding of events. It would also provide a common reference point for classifying event data derived from other sources (e.g., malpractice claims, complaints, claims attachments) and different health care settings (e.g., primary care, inpatient, nursing home). However, such analysis cannot be undertaken without a common language.

The remedy for the disparate scenario described above is the development of a common reporting format of domain areas, data elements, and terminologies that would serve as a common language for reporting, research, and analysis on patient safety. The format would be able to accommodate the rich text of narrative reports that will likely remain the mainstay of patient safety reporting. Common data standards would be used to make the information comparable to the patient safety data extracted from clinical information systems and electronic health record systems (EHRs) such as that from automatic trigger systems. With the common format, health care organizations would experience less burden in fulfilling both data capture and reporting requirements.

New knowledge obtained from the reports could be fed back into clinical information systems and care processes in a standardized manner and thereby be applied for preventing and detecting future adverse events. The standard report format could be employed for a number of purposes: populating a national patient safety database; meeting the functional requirements for the establishment of patient safety organizations in the private sector as proposed in pending legislation; providing a format easily implemented by those states that have not yet established patient safety reporting systems; and serving as a common format for mapping data across established state reporting systems, as well as to a national database. The data protection and legal considerations that arise in the generation of numerous reports from shared data elements are addressed later in this chapter.

During the development process to establish a high-functioning model for the aviation industry, Farrier (1997) voiced many concerns about standardized reporting. Although there will always be discussions about how and why the present state of affairs came to pass and which entities hold the key to correcting any problems, the obstacles, complications, and objections to broad-based information flow can be distilled down to essentially four principal issues: disagreement over the proper form and content of databases, ambiguities in the terminology used in reports, proper versus improper involvement of investigative models in the data collection process, and competition among end users of safety information. The incident reporting systems of the aviation industry have been in operation for quite some time, yet the limitations of coded data remain in several areas: data retrieval is only as good as the original coding; databases are often incomparable because of proprietary language, architecture, or other features; and judgments about what data should be captured and how they should be indexed are subjective and change over time, constraining the study of different events in the same code-based system (Farrier, 1997). The chief barriers to coding event data have been a lack of standardization and the ambiguity of descriptive terms among investigators, as well as the perceived requirement that investigators draw conclusions about an event instead of limiting themselves to informed assessments for learning and improvement purposes (Farrier 1997).

The committee took these concerns into consideration in developing its recommendations on data standards to support patient safety. Data standards, including the standardized report format, should be dynamic and respond to new knowledge in an evolutionary manner while adhering to the basic principles and purposes of standardization. As stated in *To Err Is Human*, a standardized report format can (1) permit data to be combined and tracked over time, (2) lessen the burden on health care organizations that operate in multiple states or are subject to the reporting requirements of multiple agencies and/or private oversight processes and group purchasers, and (3) facilitate communication with consumers and purchasers about patient safety (Institute of Medicine, 2000).

A common report format could also augment the recent effort by the federal government to integrate its numerous patient safety reporting systems. Specifically, the Department of Health and Human Services (DHHS) has planned a three-phased integration of the federal systems at the Agency for Healthcare Research and Quality (AHRQ), the Centers for Disease Control and Prevention (CDC), the Centers for Medicare and Medicaid Services (CMS), and the Food and Drug Administration (FDA). Phase I, currently being carried out by the Kevric Company, involves designing a common database, incorporating a common user interface, and linking the six primary FDA and CDC reporting systems. Phase II involves integrating the database and the remaining DHHS reporting systems, while Phase III encompasses integrating the reporting systems of other government agencies (i.e., Department of Defense [DOD], Veterans Health Administration [VHA]), the states that have reporting systems, and data provided by other countries. Appendix C provides detailed examples of selected federal, state, and private sector reporting systems. Use of a standardized report format among these patient safety systems would facilitate its dissemination and widespread adoption across the health sector.

ESSENTIAL ELEMENTS OF A STANDARDIZED REPORT FORMAT

Several reporting formats currently in use or in development can serve as a foundation and reference point for the establishment of a common format and taxonomy for patient safety events. Systems of interest include AHRQ's proposed taxonomy for the integration of all DHHS patient safety reporting systems, the VHA system, and the Australian Patient Safety Foundation's (APSF) Advanced Incident Monitoring System (AIMS). Other reporting systems—such as that of United States Pharmacopeial Convention, Inc., the Medical Event Reporting System for Transfusion Medicine (MERS TM), and the systems used by medical specialties (e.g., anesthesia, emergency room)—have many characteristics that should also be incorporated into certain domain areas of the common reporting format.

The committee believes the format should be designed to support the full range of reporting systems (e.g., federal, state, internal/external institutional, paper, electronic) and multiple detection methods (e.g., chart review, electronic surveillance, administrative reports). It should also be flexible enough to meet local data collection needs and accommodate evolving views of what constitutes the appropriate data to collect. The quality of adverse event reporting itself is contingent on many factors, each influenced by the cognitive and social characteristics of the participants (Cook, 2003). Formulation of a classification and assessment process for the reporting format must be accomplished in a manner that supports feedback from the reporting system, to research and analysis on patient safety, and back to the organizational system, providing new knowledge for learning and improvement. Research on and analysis of patient safety events require that reporting systems supply a steady flow of the data needed for continuous quality improvement, in much the same way that other industries utilize data for hazard analysis (Cook, 2003). The reporting format must also be capable of providing information that leads to a greater understanding of the nature of adverse events—for example, why such events occur, how they are recognized, what the critical control points are along the care continuum, what types of recovery or corrective actions are taken, and the effect on patient outcomes (Cook, 2003).

In an effort to develop a prototype for reporting events related to transfusion medicine, Battles et al. undertook a study in 1997 to assess the ideal attributes of a medical event reporting system. The study tapped a group of experts in the fields of aviation safety, nuclear power, cognitive psychology, industrial engineering, artificial intelligence, education and training, and transfusion medicine from the United States, the United Kingdom, and Australia (Battles et al., 1998). The result was a set of system design parameters for overall features and for system input, data collection, the analytical process, and interventions (see Box 9-1). The VHA chartered its National Cen-

BOX 9-1
Desirable Parameters of a Medical Event
Reporting System Adapted for General Use

Overall
- Collect and analyze reports of adverse events and interpret results.
- Institute a nonreprisal system in which no adverse consequences are attributed to the reporter.
- Report all events, including no harm/near misses.
- Solicit input from anyone with firsthand information about an event.

System input
- Identify the specific procedures involved.
- Indicate whether there was misidentification of [blood sample], patient, or product.
- Indicate the location of failures in the [transfusion] treatment process.
- Identify any equipment malfunctions involved in the event.

Data collection
- Allow further contact with reporters for data clarification while maintaining anonymity.
- Make blank report forms available to all who might wish to report events.
- Emphasize narrative descriptions of events, in which the usefulness of reports resides.
- Use an adaptable online interactive computer system for easy reporting.
- Have a trained system operator with knowledge of the domain to receive reports.

Analytical process
- Have the ability to track back from the reported event to the root cause.
- Look beyond a single event to the entire [blood] system.
- Categorize events as to where the failure(s) occurred in the process.
- Identify links between active human errors and latent system failures.
- Categorize events as [slips] no harm, mistakes/errors, or system design errors.
- Identify common problem areas across institutions.

Interventions
- Identify underlying system failures through analysis of all events.
- Make recommendations based on event analysis to decision makers at appropriate levels.
- Target problem areas prone to events for additional study.
- Track implemented corrective actions to determine their effectiveness.
- Develop intervention strategies through multidisciplinary groups.

SOURCE: Battles et al., 1998.

ter for Patient Safety (NCPS) in 1998 and began operations in 1999, building the system according to many of these basic principles. However, the VHA system, like others, does not include "nonreprisal" treatment for intentionally unsafe acts. The parameters shown in Box 9-1 are directly applicable to the development of a generic reporting format for the wide range of adverse events, medical errors, and near misses. The committee has incorporated these principles into its recommended design for a standard reporting format.

Basic Domains

At the time of the MERS TM study, most existing incident reporting systems described only what happened and paid little attention to why the event occurred; root-cause analyses were often cursory and incomplete (Battles et al., 1998). Historically, all reporting systems contained the most basic elements of a reporting format, regardless of the type of report—itemized, computerized, or narrative text. The reports typically included the following:

- Who discovered the incident, classified according to role in the health system (e.g., physician, nurse)
- How the incident was discovered
- What happened—the type of event
- Where in the care process the incident was discovered or occurred
- When the incident occurred
- Why—preliminary delineation by the most dominant cause, with the seriousness of the event determining whether a detailed investigation would be conducted.

The inability to produce patient safety data that were meaningful enough to create change in the care process can be attributed mainly to a failure to recognize that causal analysis is the most important element of the report. The best source of data for the causal analysis is the report's narrative text. While the what, where, when, who, and why of an event are necessary components of any report, detailed causal analysis gets to the heart of the circumstances that led to the event and informs the process for system improvement.

The Australian system incorporates an innovative approach to address this need. AIMS is structured to differentiate between two levels of detail: (1) a minimum dataset of initial information about the event reflective of the basic domain areas—where, when, and to whom the event occurred, what happened, and the severity of the incident (with automatic generation of a risk matrix), and (2) a detailed dataset of comprehensive information for events that caused harm to the patient or that pose a major future risk (Australian Patient Safety Foundation, 2003). The detailed dataset expands the data collection beyond the minimum dataset to include information on the mechanism of the incident, root causes, contributing factors, actions taken, outcome, and consequences to the organization (Australian Patient Safety Foundation, 2003).

Event-Type Taxonomy

Event types are used to classify events in a taxonomy (e.g., medication or surgical event). Such taxonomies are generally hierarchical to distinguish events within a category. For example, a medication event might be further differentiated in the taxonomy as a "right medication/wrong dose" event or a "wrong medication" event. It is also important to note that the terms "event," "occurrence," and "incident" are synonymous and used according to preference in different patient safety systems. For example, NYPORTS uses "occurrence," AIMS uses "incident," and most other systems (and the IOM) use "event." However, the terms all represent the same concept—that an adverse event or near miss has happened. All three terms also represent the totality of the mishaps that occurred along the chain of clinical processes leading to the outcome, rather than a single mishap.

Currently, no single taxonomy comprehensively represents all event types. Instead, over the past decade, several different taxonomies have been developed by health care organizations, medical specialties (e.g., anesthesia, trauma), and state and federal regulatory agencies to accommodate their particular interests in patient safety. Although organizations and regulatory agencies accept reports on all types of events, their structured taxonomies were developed as distinct and independent sets to reflect the most common types of serious events of importance to them, rather than a comprehensive set embodying the universe of events and injuries that can occur. Most terms represented are errors of commission, excluding errors of omission and near misses. If an event occurs that is not represented in the taxonomy, it is placed in an ambiguous "other" or "miscellaneous" category. One example of an overall approach is the National Quality Forum's (NQF) "short list" of 27 reportable events that result in serious harm to or death of the patient, such as wrong-site surgery, wrong drug administration, or falls. The NQF list reflects the states' efforts to standardize the types of events that are most often reported to the state government with a narrow focus on events in which serious harm or death occurred. Standardization of even a "short list" can be considered progress. However, from an organizational perspective, it is necessary to evolve from a primary focus on sentinel events to the broader issues of adverse events and near misses. For this purpose, a safety event that would have a high impact on quality improvement needs to be captured, classified, and coded.

Because the inherent rules or conditions for classifying events differ for each patient safety taxonomy or organization, the taxonomies lack the capacity for comparison. The 21 state-based reporting systems vary significantly in how events are defined, classified, and coded. The Massachusetts Department of Health uses 17 broad categories (e.g., falls, medication, neglect) to organize 137 different types of incidents (e.g., fall-fracture, fall-laceration) (New York Patient Occurrence Reporting and Tracking System, 2001). NYPORTS has 8 major categories for 54 types of incidents, differentiated according to "includes" and "excludes" (New York Patient Occurrence Reporting and Tracking System, 2002). Tennessee's taxonomy is very similar to that of NYPORTS, yet it uses different code numbers and has modified some of the term definitions (Tennessee Department of Health, 2003). The end result is a number of disparate, incomplete taxonomies that are beset by inconsistencies and vagueness (Nebeker et al., 2002).

The National Academy for State Health Policy has attempted to address this issue among the states by facilitating the establishment of a workgroup, the State Alliance for Error Reporting, to review and seek clarity on the NQF list of serious reportable events, identify similarities and differences between this list and existing state reporting systems, and discuss strategies for ensuring consistent implementation of the NQF list. After conducting its assessment, the State Alliance developed a crosswalk of the NQF event list and the systems of the states that had mandatory reporting requirements at the time, supplemented by a user's guide to assist with implementation. This effort represents a significant step toward a common language among state reporting systems; however, it remains far too limited, and maintaining the operational crosswalks will prove costly in both time and resources, particularly when more events are added to the list.

Because of their public availability, the current most commonly used terminologies for representing adverse events are the ICD-9/10 CM External Causes and Injury Codes (E-codes) for diagnoses and procedures and Logical Observation Identifiers, Names and Codes (LOINC) for representing laboratory and other types of data that support surveillance for infectious diseases and biological threats. Most adverse events today are detected through multiple sources and generally documented according to the ICD–9/10 CM E-Codes (Bates et al., 2003). Those codes provide direct and indirect evidence of the clinical state of the patient, comormid conditions, and the patient's progress during hospitalization or a visit (Bates et al., 2003). However, the codes lack temporal information and clinical content (Campbell, 2002), cannot differentiate events that occurred prior to hospitalization from those that occurred during hospitalization, lack the ability to categorize degree of harm, are unable to capture near misses (Williams, 2003), and cannot be linked to a complication or E-Code from the ICD–9/10 CM procedure codes. Despite their limitations, the ICD–9/10 CM E-Codes are useful as one mechanism for detecting adverse events. The committee recommends additional investment to expand them and to enhance their capacity to capture patient safety information. Doing so would also facilitate international collaboration, given the work being done by the World Health Organization in this area.

For example, the Utah Department of Health has been studying the potential value of the E-Codes for patient safety event reporting and has recommended several improvements to enable the terminology to function as part of a statewide patient safety tracking information network that would feed into a national database: (1) add yes/no fields or an additional digit associated with each code to indicate whether a condition was present on admission (note that some states have developed a method in their taxonomies or discharge data requirements for this purpose); (2) improve the codes for degree of harm with additional fields delineating temporary harm, permanent harm, or death; (3) improve the codes for intentionality; (4) allow codes for multiple similar adverse events; and (5) improve the ability to code events documented only by nonphysicians (e.g., notes from pharmacists or nurses) (Williams, 2003). In addition, population-specific extensions should be made available for more accurate representation of patient data.

While the ICD codes have been applied in several studies for successful identification of ADEs involving chart reviews, pharmacy and laboratory data can also provide direct evidence of adverse events, such as dosing errors, antidotes, and clinical values out of range (Bates et al., 2003), and are important to automated surveillance systems. LOINC is the primary terminology for laboratory databases, providing data designed to identify and name test results (Laboratory LOINC) and/or clinical observations (Clinical LOINC), including information about the amount, route, and timing of physiologic challenges (e.g., oral glucose tolerance test) (Regenstrief Institute, 2001). Laboratory LOINC is also vital to CDC's public health surveillance activities aimed at identifying the presence of nosocomial infections, biological threats, infectious diseases, and the like within the American population. Clinical LOINC's extensiveness and flexibility for multiple purposes render significant potential for representing adverse events. Columbia University, which has developed and maintained the MERS TM terminology for blood transfusion–related events, has undertaken research to extend the terminology for application in general therapeutic areas (MERS TH) and to create LOINC codes for aspects of root-cause analysis (e.g., antecedent events, contributing factors, and outcomes) (Kaplan, 2003).

Medical specialty groups have developed event-type taxonomies that are more specific to their particular domain area and often have more granularity in term definitions. For example, MERS TM divides events into two primary sections—those related to the blood center (15 categories, such as initial donor suitability, testing, and labeling) and those related to the transfusion service (13 categories, such as order entry, sample handling, and unit issue). Transfusion service events are specified in 97 event codes (e.g., for sample testing, computer warning overridden, and sample tubes mixed up) (Westat, 2001). The greater specificity of the event-type definitions allows for a more directed analysis and comparison of the critical control points related to a particular event. Key event types in the expanded version, MERS TH, have been assigned codes in the LOINC system. The complexity of drug and medical device events also requires a more comprehensive terminology, for example, when utilizing the more sophisticated decision support tools.

As with the problems posed by the disparate taxonomies used by state systems, anesthesia specialists have long been frustrated by the inability to collect and analyze uniform data elements across departments and institutions. Disparate data has been a barrier to improving anesthesia care, reducing errors, and identifying opportunities to reduce health care costs (Anesthesia Patient Safety Foundation, 2003). Adding to the complexity of the anesthesia domain are the technological demands associated with real-time monitoring of patients both electronically and physically using any number of devices simultaneously, such as those for electrocardiography, pulse oximetry, and capnography and infusion pumps (Gaba, 2000), each employing different data standards depending on the organization and vendor. In 2000, the Anesthesia Patient Safety Foundation (APSF) established an overall effort to create a common data dictionary and a Distributed Anesthesia Terms and Mapping System so that the different systems would have a common reference point. As in other domains, having common terms allows for the automated collection and comparison of large volumes of clinical data from multiple institutions for outcome research and benchmarking (Anesthesia Patient Safety Foundation, 2003). To facilitate the use of common anesthesia terms in clinical information systems, patient safety terms in the data dictionary have been incorporated into Systemized Nomenclature of Human and Veterinary Medicine, Clinical Terms (SNOMED CT). This example emphasizes the need for an integrated approach to patient safety encompassng all clinical care.

Patient safety terminology should be incorporated into the National Committee on Vital and Health Statistics (NCVHS) core terminology group. In particular, a terminology and taxonomy for patient safety events should be developed and included in SNOMED CT (e.g., the anesthesia model). As stated in Chapter 4, the committee supports incorporating the Universal Medical Device Nomenclature System (UMDNS) as the medical device terminology and normalized notations for clinical drugs (RxNORM) as the clinical drug terminology in the core group. Patient safety terms in the core terminology group should be mapped through aggregation logic to important supplemental terminologies, such as MedDRA and the Global Medical Device Nomenclature (GMDN), to facilitate automated report generation. Finally, efforts should be undertaken by the National Library of Medicine (NLM) to create and maintain the patient safety terminology mappings and disseminate them publicly for widespread adoption.

To further efforts toward data standardization, the committee believes that the best method of satisfying the terminology requirements for Phase I of the federal patient safety data integration project is the use of the designated NCVHS core terminology group with mappings to supplemental terminologies. This approach would support research and analysis of data from the national patient safety database and federal reporting systems.

Australia's AIMS takes a similar approach by leveraging the term/concept capabilities of a relational database that relies on a Generic Reference Model (GRM). The Health Incident Type taxonomy of event categories (e.g., falls, pressure ulcers, medication), plus a number of specialty areas (e.g., anesthesia, intensive care, surgery), were created as the entry point into the system. Once an incident type has been determined, the GRM is used to elicit more detail about the factors contributing to the incident (Australian Patient Safety Foundation, 2002). For example, while the Health Incident Types are at the highest level (e.g., medical devices), when one clicks on that domain, the information system shifts to the highly detailed clinical taxonomy/terminology for devices—UMDNS. The system then can request from the reporter more clinical detail in terms appropriate to that type of medical device event. Appendix G provides a listing of the health incident types (Australian Patient Safety Foundation, 2002).

Once the basic domain areas for an event have been documented, the next important step is assessment of the event's seriousness (i.e., severity) to determine what further action should be taken.

Risk Assessment Index

As the study of patient safety systems has progressed, more sophisticated systems have begun to emphasize the collection of more detailed information for the causal analysis and investigation of serious incidents. To improve the systems' organization, most have incorporated a risk assessment index to help gauge whether a full investigation of the incident is warranted. Risk assessment can be used to estimate the effect of a particular disease or patient safety incident on the physiological integrity of the patient (Iezzoni, 1997) and can include an evaluation of functional status. For patient safety, explicit criteria for assessing the degree of risk can be expressed as a risk matrix that enables the severity of the outcome of an incident to be plotted against the likelihood of the incident recurring (Australian Patient Safety Foundation, 2003). The risk assessment is used as a tool to set priorities and identify which areas require root-cause analysis or further attention (Australian Patient Safety Foundation, 2003).

In its simplest form, a risk matrix can be a one-dimensional scale for determining the range of severity from near miss to death. USP's MedMARx system uses a nine-tier approach[1] to rank medication events, see Table 9-1. Definitions of severity are clearly set to minimize confusion by clinicians using the system.

The VHA requires prioritization scoring for both close calls and adverse events for (1) the actual or potential severity of the event and (2) the probability of occurrence according to specific definitions (Eldridge, 2001). For severity, the scale is catastrophic, major, moderate, and minor; for probability, it is frequent, occasional, uncommon, and remote (Department of Veterans Affairs, 2001). The parameters are organized in a 4 × 4 matrix. Once these two parameters have been established, the prioritization score is available from the Safety Assessment Code (SAC) Matrix of 3 = highest risk, 2 = intermediate risk, and 1 = lowest risk (Eldridge, 2001). The SAC is then

---

[1]The USP risk assessment index is based on that developed by the National Coordinating Council for Medication Error Reporting and Prevention.

TABLE 9-1 USP MedMARx Error Outcome Categories (severity scale)

Category	Definition
No error	
Category A	Circumstances or events that have the capacity to cause error
Error, No Harm	
Category B	An error occurred, but the error did not reach the patient
Category C	An error occurred that reached the patient but did not cause the patient harm
Category D	An error occurred that reached the patient and required monitoring to confirm that it resulted in no harm to the patient and/or required intervention to preclude harm
Error, Harm	
Category E	An error occurred that may have contributed to or resulted in temporary harm to the patient and required intervention
Category F	An error occurred that may have contributed to or resulted in temporary harm to the patient and required initial or prolonged hospitalization
Category G	An error occurred that may have contributed to or resulted in permanent patient harm
Category H	An error occurred that required intervention necessary to sustain life
Error, Death	
Category I	An error occurred that may have contributed to or resulted in the patient's death

SOURCE: U.S. Pharmacopeia, 2003.

used to determine what action must be taken (Department of Veterans Affairs, 2001). The AIMS risk assessment index is based on the VHA model but extends the matrix to 5×5, as seen in Table 9-2.

MERS TM has developed an even more sophisticated risk assessment index (RAI), outlined in Table 9-3 for comparison, using four axes for classification of events—severity and probability as in the VHA and AIMS models, but on a 5×6 axis, with two adjustment factors applied to the severity/probability calculation—product issued and unplanned recovery. In contrast with the other systems, MER TM assigns numerical values to the matrix panels, and the RAI is calculated as a product of severity multiplied by probability. If the blood product was issued, 0.2 is added to the RAI, and/or if there was an unplanned recovery, 0.1 is added to the RAI (Westat, 2001). A root-cause analysis is recommended if the RAI is greater than or equal to

TABLE 9-2 AIMS Risk Assessment Index

Likelihood	Insignificant	Minor	Moderate	Major	Catastrophic
Almost Certain	Yellow	Orange	Orange	Red	Red
Likely	Yellow	Yellow	Orange	Red	Red
Possible	Green	Yellow	Yellow	Orange	Red
Unlikely	Green	Green	Yellow	Orange	Orange
Rare	Green	Green	Yellow	Orange	Orange

SOURCE: Australian Patient Safety Foundation, 2003.

0.5, or if it is less than 0.5 but the risk is high for the organization (Westat, 2001). Organizational risk is considered an effect that may result in financial loss or damaged reputation (Westat, 2001).

AHRQ has specifically stated that a risk assessment scale will be included in its DHHS integration project. The committee believes a risk assessment scale should be included in the common patient safety report format. In addition to an RAI, the committee believes that differentiating between probability and preventability is important to the analysis of events. Therefore, a method for assessing and a taxonomy for representing preventability should also be agreed upon and implemented. For example, if the event in question is a medication error that resulted from a mixup of medi-

TABLE 9-3 MERS TM Risk Assessment Index

Qualified Estimate of Severity of Patient Harm		Quantified Estimate of Probability of Recurrence					
		Extremely High	Very High	High	Medium	Low	Very Low
		0.99	0.90	0.75	0.50	0.25	0.10
Extremely High	0.99	1.0	0.90	0.70	0.50	0.2	0.1
Very High	0.90	0.9	0.80	0.70	0.40	0.2	0.1
High	0.75	0.7	0.70	0.60	0.40	0.2	0.1
Medium	0.50	0.5	0.40	0.40	0.20	0.1	0.05
Low	0.25	0.2	0.20	0.20	0.10	0.1	0.02
Very Low	0.10	0.1	0.10	0.10	0.05	0.02	0.01

SOURCE: Westat, 2001.

cations spelled and pronounced similarly, there is a definite way to prevent recurrences: change the name of one of the medications. This type of event would be rated highly preventable. From another perspective, the probability of recurrence would be high if the name of a medication is not changed. The preventability is based on the anticipated frequency of one medication again being accidentally substituted for the other. In this case, the cause might relate to poor handwriting and other similarities between the medications (e.g., dosing regimen).

Causal Analysis

Once it has been determined that an event is or could have been serious, a root cause analysis (RCA) should be performed. An RCA is considered mandatory for serious events by JCAHO and state regulatory agencies. The VHA, AIMS, MERS TM, several states, and other organizations have well-developed models for root cause analysis. To date, methodologies for RCA have been guided by the pioneering work of Jens Rasmussen in assessing system, environmental, and human aspects of errors and James Reason in understanding the dynamics of human factors and latent conditions that lead to error (Reason, 1990).

The VHA's NCPS uses narrative text for causal analysis based on the principles surrounding human, organizational, and technical factors identified by Rasmussen and Reason, but employing an interpretation for VHA facilities focused on six areas (Bagian et al., 2001):

- Human factors communication
- Human factors training
- Human factors fatigue/scheduling
- Environment and equipment
- Rules, policies, and procedures
- Barriers (safeguards)

Each area has a series of specific questions to guide reporters in their documentation (Bagian et al., 2001). The RCA occurs at each hospital and includes the narrative, the analysis, proposed remedies, and a plan for implementation and follow-up (Gosbee, 2003). Information is extracted from the report of the analysis (usually in narrative form) and recorded in a relational database. The goal of NCPS is to analyze system vulnerabilities in hospitals, find and implement solutions, and provide support to the facilities (McKnight and Gosbee, 2002). Maintaining the information in a relational database facilitates the discovery of commonalities or trends among RCA reports that can lead to the identification of similar system failures/issues (McKnight and Gosbee, 2002). In fact, NCPS has instituted the Primary Analysis and Categorization project to synthesize information from each RCA narrative text report into coded keywords with definitions (i.e., a glossary) to facilitate the identification of commonalities among events (McKnight and Gosbee, 2002). The initial scope of the project involves categorizing each RCA into five domain areas (McKnight and Gosbee, 2002):

- Location of event
- Activities or processes surrounding the event
- Activity or process outcomes characterizing the event
- Actions taken to prevent a similar event from happening in the future
- Outcomes that measure whether the actions were effective

At VHA, each director signs the RCA plans for change and system improvements resulting from the root cause analysis. If the patient safety manager believes that learning from the RCA would have VHA-wide or worldwide application, a secondary analysis is performed that results in a clearly defined nationwide alert or advisory, a newsletter or monthly meeting item, a change to national policy (such as VHA's correct-surgery directive), and/or work with medical device companies on a product redesign (Gosbee, 2003).

AIMS has incorporated into its GRM (with permission) an adaptation of the model developed by VHA. The GRM encompasses a system that represents the contributing factors of an event as determined in the causal analysis. In AIMS, these contributing factors are called component factors. The GRM provides a framework that defines relationships among the component factors of the classification system and a set of terms describing the attributes of each component. These definitions vary by type of incident and classification, with permutations currently exceeding 500,000 in number (Australian Patient Safety Foundation, 2003). Figure 9-1 is a diagram of the GRM.

AIMS also includes data on outcomes and consequences of events, which the committee believes to be an important part of the causal analysis. Two sets of data are collected: (1) patient outcome as related to the duration, severity, and resource impact of the disease type, injury type, suffering, disability, or death; and (2) consequences for the organization, including immediate and subsequent actions taken, impact in terms of cost, and legal liability (Australian Patient Safety Foundation, 2003). Outcome data in relation

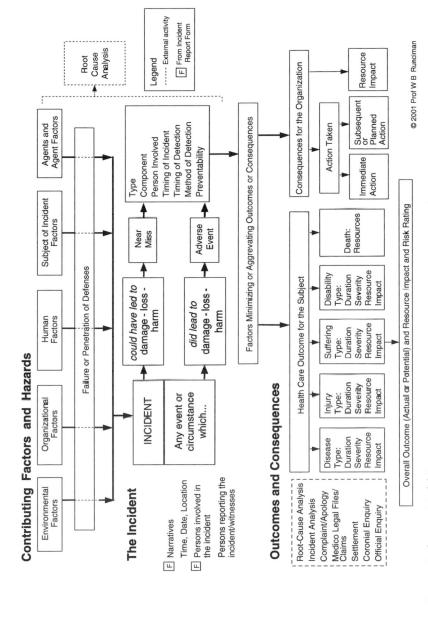

FIGURE 9-1 Generic Reference Model Diagram.
SOURCE: Australian Patient Safety Foundation, 2002.

to actions taken can help clinicians better understand the recovery aspect of adverse events.

Other health care organizations have been involved in further research on causal analysis methodologies employed successfully by other sectors and have adapted those models to meet their needs. The Eindhoven Classification Model, developed at Eindhoven University of Technology in the Netherlands, is often used in the chemicals sector and other high-risk industries and was chosen as the RCA model for the TM study; it incorporates the earlier work of Rasmussen and Reason (Battles et al., 1998). Using the Eindhoven Classification Model: Medical Version, investigators examine the root causes of an incident from three perspectives (Battles et al., 1998):

- Technical factors—equipment, software, forms
- Organizational factors—policies, procedures, and protocols
- Human factors—knowledge-based (familiar procedures applied to frequent decision-making situations), rule-based (routine tasks requiring little conscious effort), and skill-based (problem solving activities often in new situations) (Battles et al., 1998)

For ease of application, the model incorporates a causal tree that is useful for displaying critical activities and decisions in both logical and chronological order (Battles et al., 1998) as the investigation is undertaken. The event is diagrammed using all possible causes and recoveries gathered during the investigation, revealing the event's underlying root causes (see Figure 9-2); the codes used in the model are defined in Table 9-4.

Of particular importance in the RCA is the ability to discover points of recovery and prevention (i.e., critical control points) to minimize future events. Recovery is the distinguishing factor between an accident and a near miss. Van der Schaff defines human recovery as the feature of the human system component to detect, localize, and correct earlier component failures (Van der Schaaf, 1992). These component failures may be either one's own previous errors, those of a colleague, or technical factors. Use of the Eindhoven model to assess near misses is vital to the identification of causal and recovery factors, providing the new knowledge that can be integrated at the front line of care to develop a more highly reliable system. AHRQ has designated the Eindhoven model as the causal analysis taxonomy for the federal patient safety integration project. The committee supports the adoption of the Eindhoven model, with the following additions to the taxonomy:

- Classification for recovery factors associated with near-miss events, as stated in Chapter 4

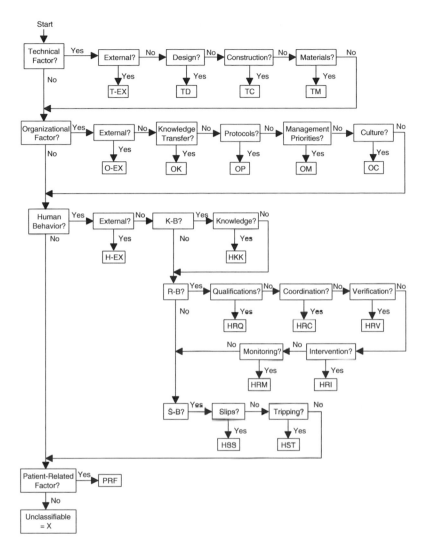

FIGURE 9-2 Eindhoven Classification Model: Medical Version.
SOURCE: Eindhoven Safety Management Group, 1997.

  • Representation of corrective actions that were taken to recover from
actual incidents, as stated in the functional requirements set forth in Chapter 3
  • Representation of patient outcome/functional status (outcome) as a
result of corrective actions taken

TABLE 9-4 Codes Used in Eindhoven Classification Model, Medical Version

Category	Description	Code
Latent errors	Errors that result from underlying system failures	
Technical	Refers to physical items, such as equipment, physical installations, software, materials, labels, and forms	
External	Technical failures beyond the control and responsibility of the investigating organization	TEX
Design	Failures due to poor design of equipment, software, labels, or forms	TD
Construction	Correct design was not followed accurately during construction	TC
Materials	Material defects not classified under TD or TC	TM
Organizational		
External	Failures at an organizational level beyond the control and responsibility of the investigating organization	OEX
Transfer of knowledge	Failures resulting from inadequate measures taken to ensure that situational or domain-specific knowledge or information in transferred to all new or inexperienced staff	OK
Protocols/procedures	Failures related to the quality and availability of the protocols within the department (too complicated, inaccurate, unrealistic, absent, or poorly presented)	OP
Management priorities	Internal management decisions in which safety is relegated to an inferior position in the face of conflicting demands or objectives. This is a conflict between production needs and safety (e.g., decisions about staffing levels)	OM
Culture	Failures resulting from collective approach to risk and attendant modes of behavior in the investigating organization	OC

Continued

TABLE 9-4 *Continued*

Category	Description	Code
Active errors (human)	Errors or failures resulting from human behavior	
External	Human failures originating beyond the control and responsibility of the investigating organization	HEX
Knowledge-based behaviors		
Knowledge-based errors	The inability of an individual to apply existing knowledge to a novel situation	HKK
Rule-based behaviors		
Qualifications	Incorrect fit between an individual's qualifications, training, or education and a particular task	HRQ
Coordination	Lack of task coordination within a health care team in an organization	HRC
Verification	Failures in the correct and complete assessment of a situation, including relevant conditions of the patient and materials to be sued, before starting the intervention	HRV
Intervention	Failures that result from faulty task planning (selecting the wrong protocol) and/or execution (selecting the right protocol but carrying it out incorrectly)	HRI
Monitoring	Failures during monitoring of process or patient status during or after intervention	HRM
Skill-based behaviors		
Slips	Failures in performance of fine motor skills	HSS
Tripping	Failures in whole-body movements	HST
Other		
Patient-related factor	Failures related to patient characteristics or conditions that influence treatment and are beyond the control of staff	PRF
Unclassifiable	Failures that cannot be classified in any other category	X

SOURCE: Battles et al., 1998.

Lessons Learned

Evaluation of the RCA should seek to document the lessons learned from the event and a process for eliminating or controlling its causes. Documentation of lessons learned has been a key reason for the success of other high-risk industries in identifying and maintaining a record of actions that can prevent events or help in recovering from them.

Summary of Domain Areas for a Common Report Format

This section has described those elements of a common report format that the committee believes would be most productive in the aggregation and evaluation of adverse events and near misses within the context of a partially or fully integrated health information system. The information to be input into this report format can be derived from the original narratives provided by the reporters of the events and supplemental information from causal analysts. The report format consists of core domain areas for which appropriate taxonomies need to be developed where none exist or refined where they do exist. Given the concept of data reuse and the interconnectedness of the NHII, health information systems should be able to capture common data elements for the generation of multiple reports without redundant data entry. Likewise, all report generation should meet the privacy and security requirements outlined in the Health Insurance Portability and Accountability Act of 1996 (HIPAA). Box 9-2 summarizes the domain areas that the committee believes to be most important to the establishment of standards for more comprehensive reporting of patient safety events.

The patient safety report can be made available electronically using the Health Level Seven (HL7) Clinical Document Architecture (CDA) standard. The form can be printed for those who prefer documentation on paper or completed electronically by those comfortable with doing so. At this early stage, reporting should focus on the collection of narrative free text from the reporter. Taxonomies for the common report format can be developed and employed by the patient safety representative to classify the report. A more structured report format can be available that utilizes both designated domains for areas for reporting and narrative text. The taxonomies to classify the report data should evolve over time as clinicians and researchers gain new knowledge and a better understanding of the nature, causes, and recovery aspects of events.

BOX 9-2
Domain Areas for a Common
Patient Safety Reporting Format

The discovery
- Who discovered/reported the event—role, not names
- How discovered

The event itself
- What happened—type of event
- Where in the care process the event was discovered and/or occurred
- When the event occurred
- Who was involved—functions, not names
- Why—the most dominant cause based on a preliminary analysis
- Risk assessment
  - Severity of the event
  - Preventability of the event
  - Likelihood of recurrence of a similar event

Narrative of the event—includes contributing factors

Ancillary information
- Product information (blood, devices, drugs) if involved in the event
- Patient information (including age, gender, ethnicity, diagnoses, procedures, comorbid conditions)

Detailed causal analysis—On the basis of the above information, a decision should be made on whether a formal root-cause analysis should be carried out. The analysis should include examination of the following:
- Technical, organizational, and human factors associated with the Eindhoven model to document what happened and why in detail
- Recovery factors that can occur at each point for near misses
- Corrective actions that were taken to recover from actual incidents
- Patient outcome/functional status as a result of the corrective actions taken
- Whether a similar case has recently been investigated

Lessons learned

As stated earlier in this chapter, there is no comprehensive patient safety taxonomy for representing adverse event and near-miss data in the United States, although JCAHO has expressed interest in this concept and has been working on the development of a taxonomy framework. Because growing international awareness of the importance of patient safety to quality care, the World Health Organization (WHO) has contracted with JCAHO to evaluate the methods used in countries around the world to define and classify patient safety data; develop a framework for analyzing the strengths and weaknesses of different patient safety classification and reporting systems; and develop a common dictionary of patient safety terms and a taxonomy for patient safety reporting that could be used for cross-country, cross-organizational comparisons. JCAHO will guide the development of the international taxonomy in consultation with WHO and its partners, including the Australian Patient Safety Foundation.

The committee believes this is an important step toward more comprehensive and standardized reporting on patient safety; however, we also emphasize that it is just as important that JCAHO's work on a taxonomy framework meet the requirements for comprehensive reporting in each domain area outlined throughout this report, and particularly in this chapter. Ultimately, the methods JCAHO employs to develop its taxonomy framework should also reflect the work being undertaken by AHRQ in its project to integrate all federal safety-related reporting systems. The committee believes AHRQ should commission a group of stakeholders to fully develop the patient safety event taxonomy.

IMPLEMENTATION OF THE REPORT FORMAT

This chapter has provided a detailed set of recommendations on the elements of a patient safety report format that are important to the establishment of high-functioning patient safety systems and the generation of meaningful data to support quality improvement. Initially, a preliminary short-term pilot study should be undertaken to evaluate the cost and accuracy of the proposed report format. Adjustments to the committee's recommendations can be made based on the results of this research. Next, a sound process is necessary for the format's implementation.

Commitment to use of the report format is essential. AHRQ should play a leadership role in the implementation of the standardized format. To facilitate its adoption, AHRQ could require that the report format and associated data standards be utilized in the agency's ongoing patient safety programs and for population of the national patient safety database. All forthcoming legislation related to the establishment of voluntary patient safety organizations could require use of the standardized format as a condition for certification of compliance with federal regulations. Population of the national patient safety database will be accomplished using submissions from both voluntary patient safety organizations and state regulatory agencies; therefore, state organizations that do not have established reporting systems can implement and use the standardized format for dual purposes (with de-identification of the data forwarded to the national database). States that do have reporting systems in place can initially map their current format to the standardized format, with plans to migrate to the latter over time for simplification. From the perspective of health care providers, particularly for physicians who operate independently out of small group offices, use of a common report format should ease the incorporation of a safety program for documenting adverse events and near misses. Likewise, clinicians who operate in various settings with different reporting formats (e.g., nursing homes and home care) will be able to map their data to the standardized format for analysis and comparison of their event detection and prevention with the efforts of other settings. Finally, larger health care organizations will have a reliable method for assessing patient safety and quality with other organizations inside and outside their network.

The second requirement for adoption of the common report format is the provision of adequate support for its implementation in the form of tools, guides, and technical assistance. State agencies may also require financial assistance. From a technical standpoint, HL7 can play an important role. At HL7's May 2003 meeting, formation of a Patient Safety Special Interest Group was proposed to the Technical Steering Committee; sponsorship of the group would fall under the Regulated Clinical Research Information Management Technical Committee. Formation of this group was approved at HL7's September 2003 meeting.

The group's mission is to create the message components required for the exchange of patient safety information and clinical documents for the reporting of adverse events. Specific immediate tasks include the following:

- Create scenarios to define the requirements for identifying and reporting medical errors, adverse events, and near misses.
- Identify the set of trigger events to initiate the transmission of such data.
- Develop the messages, message segments, and data fields necessary to support the reporting of medical errors.
- Create clinical documents for reporting medical errors.
- Identify and promote the required terminology to support the reporting of medical errors.
- Coordinate and cooperate with other groups interested in using these messages and documents.
- Enable and promote the use of these standards and make them as widely available as possible.

Along with definition of the technical specifications for implementing the report format, other tools, guides, and assistance are needed. For example, as part of its project to integrate federal patient safety reporting systems, AHRQ has required that the contractor develop a user version of the front-end data entry system and the prototype data warehouse that can serve as a local institution's own event reporting system and database (Agency for Healthcare Research and Quality, 2002). Having a software program available to users at nominal or no cost is an important component of AHRQ's implementation plan. Training materials will be developed and workshops provided to enable hospital staff and other users to utilize the system (Agency for Healthcare Research and Quality, 2002).

The committee believes that AHRQ should also extend a request for proposals for the development of a generic software application of the report format employing the terminologies and data standards presented in this chapter. A built-in reporting capacity for physicians' offices and small hospitals would ease the burden of their migration to information systems. Further, it is unlikely that these entities will be able to begin that migration without financial and technical assistance. The software application for reporting will help generate standardized reports as a baseline for patient safety systems. Providing the software to these small entities will help address two of the main barriers to adoption of the report format: (1) per physician cost and operating costs and (2) culture and readiness.

The Australian AIMS provides a suite of software tools to facilitate use of the reporting system; similar tools should be developed and included in AHRQ's package for standardized patient safety reporting. The high functionality of the AIMS database is a direct result of this software suite, which facilitates the implementation and use of the reporting system. The AIMS interface is downloadable to the health care provider's computer, along with the suite of tools (Australian Patient Safety Foundation, 2003):

- Data Manager, to manage incident reports
- Analyzer, to generate standard and user-defined reports from the database
- Administrator, to set up and maintain the AIMS software and generate audit trails
- Database Administrator, for downloading updates to AIMS and applying them to the database; for importing unclassified data from third-party systems; for archiving audit trails; and for uploading de-identified, classified data

- Workflow Manager, for informing staff when incidents are reported and for managing action plans (including multiple timelines and persons responsible) and allowing administration to access the status of each project
- Risk Register, for managing ongoing risks either linked to or independent of particular incidents or events

DE-IDENTIFICATION AND DATA PROTECTION

Internal and external patient safety reports serve different yet overlapping purposes. Whereas internal reports must contain highly detailed and often identifiable information, most external reports need contain only de-identified data. For both internal and external reports, standardized report formats would facilitate reuse of the data contained in clinical care systems, use of standardized analysis techniques, and comparative analysis of aggregate data. Although internal and external patient safety reports will not be identical, they will share many common elements, some of which must be de-identified for external reporting.

The key challenge to patient safety reporting system development is determining how to design the systems in a manner that addresses the needs of all stakeholders while encouraging reporting of medical errors and providing public access to reports of preventable errors. Consumers, payers, trial attorneys, and other groups demand open and public disclosure of adverse events that result in death or serious harm. Health care providers and malpractice carriers insist on confidentiality and legal protection for reported errors. Fear of legal liability in a punitive environment can dampen providers' willingness to generate information about errors and thus limit what can be learned about how, when, and where medical mistakes occur. Underreporting of medical errors due to provider anxieties about legal exposure can undermine the effectiveness of patient safety reporting systems.

Generally, disclosures to external organizations should not include identifiable information, with the exception of specific public health activities required by law. However, concern about potential discoverability and fear of retaliation against those who report safety incidents are major impediments to effective reporting programs. Traditionally, the proceedings of quality management reviews are protected from discoverability by state laws regarding peer review protections and reporting system authorizing statutes. Many states are evaluating whether data from patient safety reports should be conclusively protected under these statutes or publicly available to afford transparency and accountability to the public. Current legislative proposals address solely the protection of voluntary reporting systems by strengthening peer review statutes at the national level. Enhanced protection could facilitate the establishment of voluntary reporting systems and willingness to populate a national patient safety database of de-identified data. The committee believes that adequate legal protection of voluntarily reported data is essential for the integrity and effectiveness of patient safety learning systems. The committee also believes that further study is needed to define the appropriate conditions for disclosure and protection of data from patient safety reports in all systems.

Under these conditions, clinical information can be reused to generate reports on an ADE to government regulatory agencies (e.g., FDA) and state public health regulatory agencies (e.g., NYPORTS). If patient safety initiatives are explicitly defined to be a part of quality initiatives, a hospital may choose to participate with USP in a program to monitor medication errors under the terms of a business associate agreement. In accordance with terms of that agreement, USP could accept patient safety reports with identifiable information and create de-identified reports to the national patient safety database. To meet the requirements for JCAHO's sentinel event policy, the hospital could submit de-identified data containing an RCA of the event and an action plan of corrective measures. Integrated health information systems would automatically screen the data elements for each report requirement in accordance with the established legal protections. Further research is needed on how information systems can be leveraged in this manner.

PRIMARY AND SECONDARY USES OF REPORT DATA

Information stemming from the proposed patient safety reports, particularly the causal analysis, has both primary and secondary applications in improving the care processes. Most primary uses relate to the feedback loop that supplies data for refining care processes and enhancing decision support tools, while secondary uses include database research into the epidemiology of occurrences, public health surveillance, drug safety surveillance, and other studies (Lowrance, 2002). Several organizations that currently have patient safety reporting systems are using the data for safety and quality improvement purposes. This section provides brief descriptions of selected programs implemented by these organizations.

VHA has instituted a solid flow of information for primary applications involving both short- and long-term system improvements. The data flow from the reporter to the patient safety manager, from the manager to the RCA team, and again between the reporter and the RCA team to provide feedback and add to the findings. The feedback to the reporter is relatively immediate to demonstrate the meaningfulness of the reporter's efforts, as well as to ensure reinforcement for learning. For example, VHA's directive *Ensuring Correct Surgery* relies on patient safety data as primary feedback to address surgical events. The directive provides specific information on what steps must be taken to ensure that a surgical procedure is performed on the right patient, at the correct site, and if applicable with the correct implant (Department of Veterans Affairs, 2002). Review and analysis of patient safety reports on surgical events have led to the development of a specific set of minimum preoperative procedures to be completed days to 1 hour before surgery (i.e., consent form validating the site, laterality, name, and reason for the procedure, plus marking of the site soon before the surgery); a set of minimum procedures to be carried out just before or when the patient enters the operating room, 1 hour or less before surgery (i.e., staff must ask the patient to state his or her name, social security number, and location on body of procedure); and a set of minimum operating room procedures for completion minutes to seconds before surgery (i.e., a designee is responsible for ensuring that all procedures are in place that require verification—patient, procedure, site, implant—by operating room personnel) (Department of Veterans Affairs, 2002). Procedures are listed on posters and placed at strategic points to assist VHA staff in remembering them at each stage and are also included in brochures provided to patients who register for surgery. From January through June 2003, VHA experienced no reported cases of an incorrect surgery when the procedures required by the *Ensuring Correct Surgery* directive were followed (Eldridge, 2003).

Another example, related to the needs of special populations, is associated with the Child Health Accountability Initiative (CHAI) undertaken by the Child Health Corporation of America. CHAI has established a three-track approach to quality: Track I—clinical improvement in the areas of medication safety, patient safety, pain management, and clinical research; Track II—building bridges among key organizations to establish national priorities and share vital data on pediatric quality and safety improvement measures; and Track III—informing the field by disseminating information to policy makers and the public (Payne and Throop, 2002). The initiative's work on medication safety began with an intense investigation of all medication orders written at participating hospitals, followed by an analysis of the types and patterns of events and the creation of site-specific improvement plans (Payne and Throop, 2002). The first phase of this effort laid the groundwork for the subsequent phases of study and resulted in a 24.7 percent decrease in prescribing errors, a 73.9 percent increase in intercepted errors, and a 49.2 percent reduction in prescribing errors not intercepted

(Payne and Throop, 2002). For the second phase, the hospitals focused on a specific type of adverse event related to two high-risk areas for pediatric patients—sedation and analgesia—and one hospital in particular developed and tested a trigger system methodology for identifying and resolving ADEs. Several CHAI hospitals achieved a 75 percent reduction in medication errors (Payne and Throop, 2002). Using the modified trigger tools first developed by David Classen, ADE identification per 100 hospital days was 40 percent higher than with hospital-wide reporting mechanisms (Payne and Throop, 2002). Table 9-5 provides an overview of the CHAI medication safety project.

The most common secondary use of patient data is to satisfy needs for public health surveillance. Epidemiological methods for scientific data analysis are necessary to identify and track health threats, assess population health, create and monitor programs and services, and conduct research, particularly given the new threat of bioterrorism. Incident reports and surveillance with trigger tools enable public health authorities to screen efficiently for emerging diseases or epidemics (National Committee on Vital and Health Statistics, 2001). Common data standards related to patient safety and public health events are vitally important to the cross-dimensional communications across local, regional, and national entities of the NHII.

Other secondary uses of data are being employed by payers. For example, Blue Cross of California, owned by Wellpoint, Inc., has initiated an award of bonuses to physicians who meet certain quality-of-care measures, including childhood immunization rates; screening rates for breast, cervical, and colorectal cancers; and quality indicators related to asthma, diabetes, and depression (Desmarais, 2002). Another program in development by employers and health plans will provide financial incentives to physicians who establish the following: clinical information programs, such as an EHR, in their offices; a system for regularly following up on the care of chronically ill patients; or patient education programs (Desmarais, 2002). All programs are designed according to evidence-based medicine and evaluate patient outcomes as part of the criteria for the award. At present, however, many providers lack the technologies and data standards needed to engage in these programs. The ability to reuse patient data, including safety data, for quality improvement purposes would ease providers' transition to electronic systems while at the same producing immediate gains and reinforcement for collection of the data and follow-up on patient care. Wellpoint recently joined with the RAND Corporation on a grant from the Robert Wood Johnson Foundation to assess payer-oriented incentive programs.

CONCLUSIONS

Improving patient safety requires the determination and dissemination of best safety practices and systemic improvements derived through rigorous scientific analysis of data collected from numerous sources on the wide range of adverse events and near misses that can occur within a health care organization. The analysis should encompass multiple comparability studies of abundant patient safety report data available at the organizational, state, and/or federal level, as well as other valuable sources of patient safety data within the context of an integrated health information infrastructure (e.g., chart reviews, malpractice data, surveillance of trigger data, patient safety reports, quality measures, disease registries). To this end, safety reporting systems should incorporate commonly defined data elements that can meet the needs of multiple agencies and purposes within the context of integrated systems and the NHII.

The purpose of this chapter has been to develop a framework, summarized in Box 9-2, for the collection and codification of the report data most important to the discovery, analysis, and understanding of and learning from patient safety events. This framework should produce a strong evidence base of specific safety measures that can lead to safer care, the prevention of events from occurring in the first place, and facilitated recovery when they do occur. Maintaining the value of rich narrative data from free-text reports, the framework provides a model from which to initiate codification of these narrative data to resolve conflicts and relieve burdens resulting from the current state of overly complex and disparate reporting requirements. The framework includes domains for basic event data (who, what, when, where, why, how), ancillary product and patient information, a risk assessment model, a causal analysis model, recovery factors, outcome, and lessons learned. The appropriate taxonomies need to be developed or refined to fully represent each domain area. These taxonomies should encompass the core terminologies identified by NCVHS as central to the NHII and those identified for the AHRQ sponsored project to integrate federal patient safety reporting systems. As organizations migrate to fully integrated health information systems, it should be possible to generate multiple reports automatically using common data elements compatible with the NHII.

The committee believes the achievement of a safety culture is a national imperative. To this end, health care organizations, state and federal regulatory agencies, and research organizations must move forward in the near term to adopt the common patient safety data standards proposed in this

TABLE 9-5 Overview of Child Health Accountability Initiative (CHAI) Medication Safety Project

Year	1999	2000
Area of emphasis	Pediatric Intensive Care Unit	Sedation and Analgesia
Description of CHAI projects	Formed multidisciplinary teams centered on rapid improvement in medication errors Developed new medication error tracking tools Investigated all medication orders written at participating hospitals Analyzed types and patterns of errors Developed and implemented site-specific improvement plans	Implemented new reporting form Developed standardized data dictionary Created medication usage process maps Completed (IHI) Breakthrough Series for ADEs Participated in IHI Idealized Design for the Medication System
Result	24.7 percent decrease in the pediatric ICU medical prescribing error rate 73.9 percent increase in intercepted errors 49.2 percent reduction in prescribing errors that were not intercepted	75 percent reduction in medication errors in sedation and analgesia Systems that are safer by a factor of 10 New clinical processes shown to reduce errors Identification of automation as essential in reducing errors Trigger system concept for identifying and resolving ADEs in pediatrics

SOURCE: Payne and Throop, 2002.

2001	2002	
Trigger System Methodology	Trigger System and Technology	
Adapted and tested a trigger chart review tool for the pediatric population Implemented the trigger system across CHAI hospitals	Identified and defined a collection of medication rule sets for the top 100 drugs used for pediatrics Implemented personal digital assistant (PDA) technology for data collection using nine pediatric triggers Tested five to seven new pediatric-specific triggers Compared methodology with other methods of ADE reporting	The Child Health Accountability Initiative (CHAI) medication safety project has created the foundation for national safety measures in pediatrics. CHAI is working toward a goal of national adoption of the CHAI pediatric trigger methodology and integration of the triggers into computerized physician order entry as the industry standard.
A highly effective, new method of reducing errors; triggers had a higher rate of ADE identification than any other method Identification of nine triggers that have the greatest number of ADEs in pediatric hospital settings Realization that most trigger- and nontrigger-identified ADEs are attributable to prescribing/ordering errors		Through its Informing the Field and Building Bridges tracks, CHAI is collaborating with health care providers and national quality and safety organizations to reduce medication errors for the youngest health care consumers.

report. Doing so will make it possible to streamline and simplify the mechanisms for research, analysis, and learning with regard to adverse events in our health care system, as has been done in the aviation industry and other high-risk sectors. Standardization of data will enable the evolution of a new knowledge base of patient safety information and system improvements that can be readily incorporated into the practice of evidence-based medicine.

REFERENCES

Agency for Healthcare Research and Quality. 2002. *Patient Safety Database: Request for Proposal No. AHRQ-02-0015.* Online. Available: http://www.ahcpr.gov/fund/rfp02015.htm [accessed June 2002].

Anesthesia Patient Safety Foundation. 2003. *Data Dictionary Task Force Unveils DATAMS.* Online. Available: http://www.apsf.org/dictionary/DATAMS/datams.html [accessed August, 2003].

Australian Patient Safety Foundation. June 3, 2002. *Briefing Book: Australian Incident Monitoring System.* Adelaide, South Australia: Australian Patient Safety Foundation.

———. 2003. *Australian Incident Monitoring System: Collect, Classify, Analyze, Learn.* Adelaide, South Australia: Australian Patient Safety Foundation.

Bagian, J. P., C. Lee, J. Gosbee, J. DeRosier, E. Stalhandske, N. Eldridge, R. Williams, and M. Burkhardt. 2001. Developing and deploying a patient safety program in a large health care delivery system: You can't fix what you don't know about. *Jt Comm J Qual Improv* 27 (October) (10):522–532.

Bates D. W., R. S. Evans, H. Murff, P. D. Stetson, and G. Hripcsak. 2003. *Detecting Adverse Events Using Information Technology.* Boston, MA: Division of General Medicine and Primary Care, Brigham and Women's Hospital.

Battles, J. B., H. S. Kaplan, T. W. Van der Schaaf, and C. E. Shea. 1998. The attributes of medical event-reporting systems: Experience with a prototype medical event-reporting system for transfusion medicine. *Arch Pathol Lab Med* 122 (3):231–238.

Campbell, J. R. August 22, 2002. *Presentation and Testimony on Converging the Clinical Care Model.* National Committee on Vital and Health Statistics, Subcommittee on Standards and Security. Washington, DC.

Cook, R. I. 2003. *Prospects for Using Adverse Event Reporting to Improve Patient Safety.* Commissioned paper for the Institute of Medicine Committee on Data Standards for Patient Safety.

Department of Veterans Affairs. 2001. *National Center for Patient Safety Triage Cards for Root Cause Analysis.* Ann Arbor, MI: Veterans Health Administration.

———. 2002. *National Center for Patient Safety: Ensuring Correct Surgery Directive.* Ann Arbor, MI: Veteran Health Administration.

Desmarais, H. November 25, 2002. *Presentation to the IOM Committee on Data Standards for Patient Safety. Health Insurance Association of America on Patient Safety and Quality Initiatives.* Washington, DC.

Eindhoven Safety Management Group. 1997. *The Development of an Incident Analysis Tool for the Medical Field.* Report EUT/BDK/85. Netherlands: Eindhoven University of Technology.

Eldridge, N. 2001. *Presentation on the Veterans Health Administration National Center for Patient Safety to the National Committee on Vital and Health Statistics, Subcommittee on Populations, Workgroup on Quality.* Washington, DC.

———. 2003. *Veterans Health Administration National Center for Patient Safety.* Personal communication to Institute of Medicine's Committee on Data Standards for Patient Safety.

Farrier, T. A. 1997. *Breaking the Codes: Barriers to Effective Collection and Retrieval of Safety Data.* Proceedings at the International Society of Air Safety Investigators.

Gaba, D. M. 2000. Anaesthesiology as a model for patient safety in health care. *BMJ* 320 (7237):785–788.

Gosbee, J. 2003. *Veterans Health Administration National Center for Patient Safety.* Personal communication to Institute of Medicine's Committee on Data Standards for Patient Safety.

Iezzoni, L. I., ed. 1997. *Risk Adjustment for Measuring Healthcare Outcomes.* Chicago, IL: Foundation of the American College of Healthcare Executives.

Institute of Medicine. 2000. *To Err Is Human: Building a Safer Health System.* Washington, DC: National Academy Press.

Kaplan, H. 2003. Meeting with the Institute of Medicine Staff to Committee on Data Standards for Patient Safety Regarding MERS TH.

Lowrance, W. W. 2002. *Learning from Experience: Privacy and the Second Use of Data in Health Research.* London, UK: The Nuffield Trust for Research and Policy Studies in Health Services.

McKnight, S., and J. Gosbee. 2002. *Improved Searching and Analysis of RCS Data. Veteran Health Administration National Center for Patient Safety.* White paper.

National Committee on Vital and Health Statistics. 2001. *Information for Health: A Strategy for Building the National Health Information Infrastructure.* Online. Available: http://ncvhs.hhs.gov/nhiilayo.pdf [accessed April 18, 2002].

Nebeker, J. R., J. F. Hurdle, J. M. Hoffman, B. Roth, C. R. Weir, and M. H. Samore. 2002. Developing a taxonomy for research in adverse drug events: Potholes and signposts. *J Am Med Inform Assoc* 9:80–85.

New York Patient Occurrence Reporting and Tracking System. 2001. *NYPORTS User's Manual. Version 2.1.* Albany, NY: New York State Department of Health.

———. 2002. *NYPORTS: Includes/Excludes Occurrence List.* Albany, NY: New York State Department of Health.

Payne, D., and C. Throop. November 25, 2002. *The Patient Safety and Quality Initiatives of Child Health Corporation of America: A Briefing for the Institute of Medicine.* Presentation to the Institute of Medicine Committee on Data Standards for Patient Safety. Washington, DC.

Reason, J. 1990. *Human Error.* Cambridge, UK: Cambridge University Press.

Regenstrief Institute. 2001. *Logical Observation Identifiers, Names and Codes: User's Guide.* Indianapolis, IN: Regenstrief Institute.

Rosenthal, J., T. Riley, and M. Booth. 2000. *State Reporting of Medical Errors and Adverse Events: Results of a 50-State Survey.* Portland, ME: National Academy for State Health Policy.

Rosenthal, J., M. Booth, L. Flowers, and T. Riley. 2001. *Current State Programs Addressing Medical Errors: An Analysis of Mandatory Reporting and Other Initiatives.* Portland, ME: National Academy for State Health Policy.

Tennessee Department of Health. 2003. *Hospital Fax Reporting of Incidents and Abuse.* Provided by J. Rosenthal to Institute of Medicine Staff to Committee on Data Standards for Patient Safety.

U.S. Pharmacopeia. 2003. *Summary of Information Submitted to MedMARx in the Year 2002: The Quest for Quality.* Rockville, MD: The United States Pharmacopeial Convention, Inc. Provided by Diane Cousins on December 2003.

Van der Schaaf, T. W. 1992. Near Miss Reporting in the Chemical Process Industry. Eindhoven, Netherlands: Technische Universiteit Eindhoven.

Westat. 2001. *MERS-TM: Medical Event Reporting System for Transfusion Medicine Reference Manual.* In support of Columbia University under a grant from the National Heart, Lung, and Blood Institute, National Institutes of Health (Grant RO1 HL53772, Harold S. Kaplan, MD., Principal Investigator). Version 3.0. New York, NY: Trustees of Columbia University.

Williams, S. D. January 8, 2003. *Comments on Using ICD-9-CM and ICD-10-CM Codes to Identify Medical Errors or Adverse Events.* Letter to the Institute of Medicine Committee on Data Standards for Patient Safety.

Appendixes

A

Biographies of
Committee Members

Paul C. Tang, M.D., M.S., *Chair,* is Chief Medical Information Officer at the Palo Alto Medical Foundation and Associate Clinical Professor at the University of California, San Francisco. He received his B.S. and M.S. in Electrical Engineering from Stanford University and his M.D. from the University of California, San Francisco. He is a practicing, board-certified physician in Internal Medicine. His responsibilities include implementing an electronic medical record system and directing an eHealth initiative. His research interests include medical informatics, computer-based patient record systems, clinical decision support, and Internet-based health care services. Previously, Dr. Tang was Medical Director of Information Systems at Northwestern Memorial Hospital and Associate Professor of Medicine at Northwestern University Medical School. Dr. Tang has served on several Institute of Medicine (IOM) committees and is currently a member of the IOM Health Care Services Board. He is a Fellow of the American College of Medical Infomatics, the American College of Physicians, the College of Healthcare Information Management Executives, and the Healthcare Information and Management Systems Society. He is Past Chair of the Computer-based Patient Record Institute and serves on the Board of Directors of the American Medical Informatics Association.

Molly Joel Coye, M.D., M.P.H., *Vice-Chair,* is the Founder and Chief Executive Officer of the Health Technology Center, a nonprofit organization dedicated to advancing the use of beneficial technologies for healthier people and communities. Until 2000, Dr. Coye was the director of the west coast office for The Lewin Group, a leader in health care policy, strategic planning, and management consulting. She previously directed product development for HealthDesk Corporation, a developer of consumer software for interactive health communication and disease management and was Executive Vice President for Managed Care in the Good Samaritan Health System, a nonprofit integrated health care system and the largest provider system in the Santa Clara Valley. From 1991 to 1993, Dr. Coye was the Director of the California Department of Health Services, managing a budget of more than $16 billion, 5,000 employees, and 160 branch and field offices throughout the state. Dr. Coye also directed the Division of Public Health at the Johns Hopkins School of Hygiene and Public Health and served as Commissioner of Health for the State of New Jersey from 1986 to 1990. Dr. Coye is a member of the Institute of Medicine, was a member of the IOM Committee on the Quality of Healthcare in America, and chaired the IOM Committee on Access to Insurance for Children. A former trustee of The California Endowment and the China Medical Board, Dr. Coye is currently a member of the Board of Trustees of the Program for Appropriate Technology in Health (PATH). She received her M.D. and M.P.H. from Johns Hopkins University.

Suzanne Bakken, R.N., D.N.Sc., F.A.A.N., is Alumni Professor of Nursing and Professor of Biomedical Informatics at Columbia University. She received her B.S.N. from Arizona State University in 1974; her M.S. in Critical Care from the University of California, San Francisco (UCSF) in 1980; and her D.N.Sc. in Nursing Informatics from UCSF in 1989. She was a Post-Doctoral Fellow in Medical Informatics at Stanford University. Her primary professional interests are evidence-based advanced practice nursing, medical informatics, and HIV/AIDS. Dr. Bakken is a Fellow for both the American Academy of Nursing and the American College of Medical Informatics. She has worked actively in the area of data standards for the past decade. previously serving as the American Nurses Association Liaison to Health Level 7 and Chair of the Convergent Terminology Group for Nursing of the SNOMED International Editorial Board. She is currently a member of the Clinical LOINC Committee and leads the work item task force for an International Standards Organization standard for a reference terminology model for nursing.

E. Andrew Balas, M.D., Ph.D., is the Director of the Center for Health Care Quality, a health policy think tank at the University of Missouri. He also serves as the Director of the European Union Center of Missouri, a multidisciplinary initiative to explore the policy implications of emerging new technologies. He holds the Thomas P. Weil Distinguished Professorship at the Department of Health Management and Informatics, School of Medicine, University of Missouri. He received his M.D. in 1977 from Semmelweis University School of Medicine, his M.S. in Applied Mathematics from Eotvos University of Science in 1983, and his Ph.D. in Medical Informatics from the University of Utah School of Medicine. Dr. Balas, as a Congressional Health Policy Fellow, worked for the Public Health Subcommittee of the U.S. Senate. He has also served on several review panels of the National Institutes of Health and the Agency for Health Care Research and Quality. He is an elected Fellow of the American College of Medical Informatics. In addition, Dr. Balas served on the Quality of Health Care in America Technical Panel 3: Using Information Technology to Improve Quality in Health Care.

David W. Bates, M.D., M.Sc., is Chief of the Division of Internal Medicine at the Brigham and Women's Hospital in Boston and Associate Professor at Harvard Medical School. He is also the Medical Director of Clinical and Quality Analysis for Partner's Healthcare Systems, where he evaluates the impact of information systems across the Partner's network. Dr. Bates's primary interest has been the use of computer systems to improve care, and he has conducted extensive work on evaluating the incidence and preventability of adverse drug events. At the national level, Dr. Bates is one of two science advisors to the SCRIPT project, which is charged with developing medication indicators that may be adopted by the Centers for Medicare & Medicaid Services. In addition, he serves as an advisor to the Leapfrog Group and is the editor of *Journal of Clinical Outcomes Management*. Dr. Bates received his M.D. from Johns Hopkins University School of Medicine in 1983 and his M.Sc. from the Harvard School of Public Health in 1990. He is a practicing, board-certified physician in Internal Medicine.

John R. Clarke, M.D., is a Professor of Surgery at Drexel University, an Adjunct Professor of Computer and Information Science at the University of Pennsylvania, and an Adjunct Senior Fellow of the Leonard Davis Institute of Health Economics. Dr. Clarke is a member of several regional, national, and international professional societies, including the American Association for Artificial Intelligence, the American Medical Informatics Association, and the Society for Medical Decision Making. He is a Governor of the American College of Surgeons. He has been involved in many activities involving patient safety. He has also conducted research in the area of medical errors using large databases and computer-based decision support. He has published extensively in the areas of clinical decision making. He received his B.A. from Wesleyan University in 1965 and his M.D. from the University of Pennsylvania in 1968.

David C. Classen, M.D., M.S., is a Vice President at First Consulting Group (FCG) and leads FCG's quality of health care initiatives consulting practice in this area. Dr. Classen is also an Associate Professor of Medicine at the University of Utah and a Consultant in Infectious Diseases at the University of Utah School of Medicine. Previously, he served as Chief Medical Resident at the University of Connecticut and was the chair of Intermountain Health Care's Clinical Quality Committee for Drug Use and Evaluation. He received his M.D. from the University of Virginia School of Medicine and his M.S. in Medical Informatics from the University of Utah School of Medicine. Dr. Classen's research interests are in the computer applications of epidemiologic techniques to investigate clinical outcomes. He is also involved in the development of expert system technologies to provide decision support in the monitoring and prescribing of medications. Dr. Classen has lectured and consulted, nationally and internationally, on clinical process improvement, computer-assisted decision support, and information system technology in health care. He is the author and coauthor of numerous scientific publications and book chapters on the use of decision support and epidemiologic techniques to improve the use and safety of medications.

Simon P. Cohn, M.D., M.P.H., is the National Director of Health Information Policy for the Kaiser Permanente Medical Care Program, Oakland, California. He has been a leader in Kaiser Permanente's efforts to develop comprehensive health information systems to support both the delivery of health care and health research. Dr. Cohn is a nationally recognized expert on issues related to HIPAA Administrative Simplification, health care data management, clinical classifications, and electronic transmission of health care data. He is a member of the National Committee on Vital and Health Statistics and chairs its Subcommittee on Standards and Security. He is also a member of the National Uniform Claims Committee and the AMA CPT Editorial Panel. Dr. Cohn is board certified in Emergency Medicine and continues an active clinical practice. He is a Fellow of the American College of Emergency Physicians and American College of Medical Informatics.

Carol Cronin, M.S.W., M.S.G., is currently serving as a Senior Technical Advisor to the Delmarva Foundation, where she is assisting with hospital performance public reporting. In addition, she has worked as an independent consultant on consumer health information and Medicare to a number of foundations and nonprofits, including the Atlantic Philanthropies, AARP, the Markle Foundation, the National Health Council, and the Robert Wood Johnson Foundation. Previously, she served as the first Director of the Center for Beneficiary Services at the Health Care Financing Administration (HCFA; now the Centers for Medicare & Medicaid Services), where she was responsible for planning, implementing, and evaluating the National Medicare Education Program (NMEP) from 1998 to 2000. She also served as chief HCFA spokesperson on beneficiary issues to the media, Congress, and national aging, consumer, and health industry organizations. From 1984 to 1994, she worked in leadership positions in Washington, DC, for the employer-based Washington Business Group on Health and the Managed Health Care Association on issues related to health outcomes measurement, accreditation, and consumer satisfaction. She holds an A.B. from Smith College and a Master's of Social Work and Master's of Gerontology from the University of Southern California.

Jonathan S. Einbinder, M.D., M.P.H., is Corporate Manager for Quality Data Management in the Clinical Informatics Research & Development group at Partners HealthCare System. He is responsible for facilitating the use of information systems for quality measurement and improvement at Partners. He also has appointments at Harvard Medical School and in the Department of Medicine at Brigham and Women's Hospital, where he practices as a general internist. Dr. Einbinder is a graduate of the Columbia University College of Physicians & Surgeons. After residency training in Internal Medicine at Brigham and Women's Hospital and Harvard Community Health Plan, he completed fellowships in Clinical Computing and General Medicine at Beth Israel Deaconess Medical Center, receiving an M.P.H. from the Harvard School of Public Health. Prior to joining Partners, Dr. Einbinder was Assistant Professor in the Department of Health Evaluation Sciences at the University of Virginia, where he directed the Clinical Data Repository project and taught in the department's M.S. degree program.

Larry D. Grandia, M.E., is currently Chief Technology Officer and Executive Vice President for Premier, Inc., in San Diego. His responsibilities include fee-for-service areas such as performance services, comparative data and decision support, benchmarking, information technology consulting, and Premier's internal information technology management systems. Prior to joining Premier in 2000, Mr. Grandia was President and Chief Executive Officer of DAOU Systems, Inc., a publicly traded health care information technology (IT) professional services company. Before that, he led IT functions for Intermountain Health Care, Inc., a leading not-for-profit health care system based in Salt Lake City, for more than two decades. He has also held positions at IBM and at a regional health care management engineering and consulting firm. He is a frequent health care industry speaker and has been active in industrywide professional groups. Mr. Grandia earned a Master's in Engineering Administration, with honors, at the University of Utah following an undergraduate degree in general engineering and industrial management at the University of Wyoming.

W. Ed Hammond, Ph.D., is Professor Emeritus in the Departments of Community and Family Medicine and Biomedical Engineering at Duke University. Dr. Hammond shares responsibility for the medical informatics courses taught at the Duke University medical center and for graduate studies in medical informatics in the Department of Biomedical Engineering. Dr. Hammond brings to the program a unique combination of engineering, computer science, administration, education, and medical background. He is experienced in networking (hardware and software), in databases and database design, in programming languages, in decision support, and in the computer-based medical record. Dr. Hammond has taught courses and given tutorials in these areas for many years. For nearly 30 years, he has been developing the internationally known computer-based medical record system, The Medical Record (TMR). Dr. Hammond's research has focused on producing medical informatics products that can be used in the real world. He has been a member of the Board of Directors of the American Medical Informatics Association and now serves as Treasurer of that organization; he has served twice as Chairman of the Health Level 7 standards group; he is immediate past president of the American College of Medical Informatics; and he is a former chair of the Association for Computing Machinery's Special Interest Group on Biological Engineering. Past activities include participation in the Summit Task Force for restructuring the aims and goals of the American Medical Record Association and coleader of a workshop on Current Topics in Medical Informatics. He is a member of the International Medical Informatics Association's Working Group 10 on Hospital Information Systems.

Brent C. James, M.D., M.Stat., is the Vice President for Medical Research and Continuing Medical Education and Executive Director of the Institute for Health Care Delivery Research at Intermountain Health Care, Inc., which is widely recognized for its work in clinical quality improvement and electronic clinical decision support systems. He received his M.D. in 1978 and his M.Stat. in Biostatistics in 1984 from the University of Utah. He currently holds Adjunct Professorships in the University of Utah's Department of Family and Preventive Medicine and Department of Medical Informatics. He is a Visiting Lecturer in the Department of Health Policy and Management at the Harvard School of Public Health and Adjunct Professor in the School of Public Health at Tulane University. He also sits on the boards of several not-for-profit health care institutions with missions directed at measuring and improving the quality and availability of health care services. Dr. James was a member of the Institute of Medicine's National Roundtable on Health Care Quality and the Quality of Health Care in America Committee.

Kevin B. Johnson, M.D., M.S., is an Associate Professor and Vice Chair of Biomedical Informatics, with a joint appointment in the Department of Pediatrics at Vanderbilt University Medical School. He received his M.D. from Johns Hopkins University School of Medicine and his M.S. in Medical Informatics from Stanford University. He served as a Pediatric Chief Resident at Johns Hopkins. He was a member of the faculty in both Pediatrics and Biomedical Information Sciences at Johns Hopkins until 2002. He is a practicing, board-certified physician in Pediatrics. His research areas are clinical information systems development; the uses of advanced computer technologies, including the World Wide Web, personal digital assistants, and pen-based computers in medicine; and the development of computer-based documentation systems for the point of care. Dr. Johnson is the author of numerous publications and has served on several editorial boards, including the journal of the Ambulatory Pediatrics Association and the *Journal of American Informatics Association* (JAMIA), for which he is an Assistant Editor. He recently was appointed as the Director of JAMIA's Student Editorial Board. He has been an active participant in the informatics efforts of many national organizations, including the American Medical Informatics Association; the American Board of Pediatrics; the Medical Informatics Special Interest Group of the Ambulatory Pediatrics Association, which he chairs; the American Academy of Pediatrics National Electronic Medical

Record Committee, which he chaired; and the Steering Committee on Clinical Information Technologies, which he cochairs.

Jill Rosenthal, M.P.H., is a program manager at the National Academy for State Health Policy (NASHP). Ms. Rosenthal provides policy analysis and technical assistance in emerging state health policy issues, focusing primarily on patient safety. Other issues she has addressed include the Children's Health Insurance Program (CHIP), health disparities, and health care cost containment. While at NASHP she has coauthored a series of reports that focus primarily on state initiatives to address medical errors and patient safety. She has 12 years of experience in public health and health planning, primarily in the areas of health promotion and health policy development, analysis, and advocacy. Prior to joining NASHP, Ms. Rosenthal spent 8 years in West Virginia as Program Manager for the West Virginia Center for Rural Health Development and as Field Director for the West Virginia Bureau for Public Health's Tobacco Control Program. Ms. Rosenthal earned a Bachelor's in Psychology from Colgate University and a Master's in Public Health from the University of North Carolina, Chapel Hill.

Tjerk W. van der Schaaf, Ph.D., has been a staff member of the Department of Technology Management at the Eindhoven University of Technology in the Netherlands since 1985. He is currently serving as an Associate Professor of Human Factors in Risk Control and as the coordinator of the Eindhoven Safety Management Group. His main research areas are human behavior (errors and error recovery) and industrial safety, based on organizational learning from (reported) incidents and near misses. Transfer of these experiences in industry and transportation to the medical domain is a major focus, with patient safety projects in the United States, United Kingdom, and the Netherlands. He has coauthored several papers on medical event reporting with James Battles, who is currently a Senior Service Fellow at the Agency for Healthcare Research and Quality, Center for Quality Improvement & Patient Safety. Dr. van der Schaaf received his Ph.D. in 1992 from the Eindhoven University of Technology in safety management based on near-miss reporting in the chemical process industry.

B

Glossary and Acronym List

GLOSSARY

Adverse event. An event that results in unintended harm to the patient by an act of commission or omission rather than by the underlying disease or condition of the patient.

Adverse event triggers. Clinical data related to patient care indicating a reasonable probability that an adverse event has occurred or is occurring. An example of trigger data for an adverse drug event is a physician order for an antidote, a medication stop, or a dose decrease.

Alert message. A computer-generated output that is created when a record meets prespecified criteria; for example, receipt of a new laboratory test result with an abnormal value (Shortliffe et al., 2001).

Assertional knowledge. Primitive knowledge that cannot be defined from other knowledge.

Authentication. A process for positive and unique identification of users, implemented to control system access (Shortliffe et al., 2001).

Case-based reasoning. A decision support system that uses a database of similar cases (van Bemmel, 1997).

Causal continuum assumption. The assumption that the (failure) causal factors of consequential accidents are similar to those of nonconsequential near misses.

327

Chart review. The retrospective review of the patient's complete written record by an expert for the purpose of a specific analysis. For patient safety, to identify possible adverse events by reviewing the physician and nursing progress notes and careful examination for certain indicators.

Classification. A taxonomy that arranges or organizes like or related terms for easy retrieval (National Committee on Vital and Health Statistics, 2000).

Clinical data repository. Clinical database optimized for storage and retrieval for information on individual patients and used to support patient care and daily operations (Shortliffe et al., 2001).

Clinical Document Architecture. A document markup standard that specifies the structure and semantics of "clinical documents" for the purpose of exchange (Van Hentenryck, 2001).

Clinical domain. A clinical area of interest that might be modeled for a clinical information system. (van Bemmel, 1997)

Clinical event monitor. Rule-based programs that sit atop a clinical data repository, supporting real-time error prevention.

Clinical information systems. The components of a health care information system designed to support the delivery of patient care, including order communications, results reporting, care planning, and clinical documentation (Shortliffe et al., 2001).

Close call. An event or situation that could have resulted in an adverse event but did not, either by chance or through timely intervention (U.S. Department of Veterans Affairs, 2002).

Code. A numeric or alphanumeric representation assigned to a term so that it may be more readily processed (National Committee on Vital and Health Statistics, 2000).

Comparability. Ability to compare similar data held in different computer systems. Comparability requires that the meaning of data is consistent when shared among different parties (National Committee on Vital and Health Statistics, 2000).

Computer detection rules. Boolean combinations of medical events, for example, new medication orders and laboratory results outside certain limits that suggest an adverse drug event might be present.

Computerized physician order entry (CPOE). Clinical systems that utilize data from pharmacy, laboratory, radiology, and patient monitoring systems to relay the physician's or nurse practitioner's diagnostic and therapeutic plans and alert the provider to any allergy or contraindication that the patient may have so that the order may be immediately revised at the point of entry prior to being forwarded electronically for the targeted medical action (First Consulting Group, 2003).

Concept orientation. Elements of the terminology are coded concepts, with possibly multiple synonymous text representations and hierarchical or definitional relationships to other coded concepts. No redundant, ambiguous, or vague concepts exist (Sujansky, 2003).

Concept permanence. The meaning of each coded concept in a terminology remains forever unchanged. If the meaning of a concept needs to be changed or refined, a new coded concept is introduced. No retired codes are deleted or reused (Sujansky, 2003).

Conceptual model. A model of the main concepts of a domain and their relationships (van Bemmel, 1997).

Consistency of views. Consistency of views says that concepts in multiple classes have the same appearance in each context (e.g., corticosteroid as hormone or antiinflammatory agent has the same attributes and descendant concepts).

Data acquisition. The input of data into a computer system through direct data entry, collection from a medical device, or other means (Shortliffe et al., 2001).

Data element. The basic unit of information having a unique meaning and subcategories of distinct units or values (van Bemmel, 1997).

Data interchange standards. Syntactic and semantic rules for defining data elements and which govern the seamless communication between computer systems while preserving the meaning of the data and intended functions.

Data mining. The use of a basic set of tools to extract patterns from the data in a data warehouse (van Bemmel, 1997).

Data set. A group of data elements specifically selected for a particular clinical purpose, such as clinical quality measurement, patient safety reporting, etc.

Data type. Defines how a data element is formatted or expressed. Simple data types include date, time, numeric, string, blob (large binary objects, such as images), currency, or coded element; complex data types include a structure for names, addresses, etc. (Hammond, 2002).

Data warehouse. Database optimized for long-term storage, retrieval, and analysis of records aggregated across patient populations, often serving the longer term business and clinical analysis needs of an organization. (Shortliffe et al., 2001).

Decision support systems. A system consisting of a knowledge base and an inference engine that is able to use entered data to generate advice (van Bemmel, 1997).

Decision trees. A diagrammatic representation of the outcomes associated with chance events and voluntary actions (Shortliffe et al., 2001).

Default reasoning. Drawing of plausible inferences on the basis of less than conclusive evidence in the absence of information to the contrary.

Definitional knowledge. Knowledge that can be defined or constructed from other knowledge.

Domain completeness. Domain completeness must not restrict terminology size through presuppositions about ultimate dimensions (e.g., no preset coding system that restricts depth or breadth of the hierarchy).

Electronic health record. A repository of electronically maintained information about an individual's health care and corresponding clinical information management tools that provide alerts and reminders, linkages with external health knowledge sources, and tools for data analysis (Shortliffe et al., 2001).

Encryption. The process of encoding (scrambling) data such that a specific key is needed to decode the data. Most methods are based on the use of prime numbers (van Bemmel, 1997).

Error. The failure of a planned action to be completed as intended (i.e., error of execution), and the use of a wrong plan to achieve an aim (i.e., error of planning) (Institute of Medicine, 2000). It also includes failure of an unplanned action that should have been completed (omission).

Evidence. Scientific evidence is a replicable and generalizable observation that can be experienced nearly identically by independent people from different places and at different times.

Evidence-based guidelines. Consensus approaches for handling recurring health management problems aimed at reducing practice variability and improving health outcomes. Guideline development emphasizes using clear evidence from the existing literature, rather than expert opinion alone, as the basis for advisory materials (Shortliffe et al., 2001).

Explicit relationships. The relationships between concepts in a hierarchy are clearly defined (e.g., relationship between staphylococcal pneumonia and pneumonia is differentiated from relationship between staphylococcal pneumonia and staphylococcus, where the former is a class relation and the latter is an etiologic relation).

Extensible markup language (XML). A specification designed specifically for Web documents. It allows designers to create their own customized tags to provide functionality not available with HTML (Newton, 2001).

Health care terminology. A collective term used to describe the continuum of code set, classification, and nomenclature (vocabulary) (National Committee on Vital and Health Statistics, 2000).

Iatrogenic injury. Injury originating from or caused by a physician (*iatros*, Greek for "physician"), including unintended or unnecessary harm or suffering arising from any aspect of health care management, including problems arising from acts of commission or omission.

Informatics. The science that studies the use and processing of data, information, and knowledge (van Bemmel, 1997).

Interoperability. The ability of one computer system to exchange data with another computer system such that, at a minimum, the message from the sending system can be placed in the appropriate place in the receiving system (National Committee on Vital and Health Statistics, 2000).

Interpreter. A component of production rule system deciding which rule to execute on each selection execute cycle.

Judgment. A discriminating or authoritative appraisal, opinion, or decision, based on sound and reasonable evaluation.

Knowledge base. A collection of systematically stored facts, heuristics, and models that can be used to make decisions or solve problems (Shortliffe et al., 2001).

Knowledge representation. Expresses medical knowledge in computer-tractable form.

Knowledge representation formalism. Formalism used to express knowledge. Also known as knowledge representation language.

Knowledge representation language. Formalism used to express knowledge. Also known as knowledge representation formalism.

Levels of evidence. It is widely recognized that various scientific methodologies produce various levels of evidence, that is, chances of identical experience when replicated by independent observers. In the testing of presumably beneficial health care interventions, the multicenter randomized controlled clinical trial is widely regarded as the top-quality source due to the demonstrable weaknesses of alternative methodologies. Randomized trials are central to Food and Drug Administration drug approval, strongly preferred information sources by most clinical practice guidelines, and prominently featured by the international Cochrane collaboration. When randomization is not possible or randomized controlled trial results are not available, original research data from controlled observations represent the next best choice (e.g., linking risky behaviors to adverse effects).

Links. Components of semantic nets representing relationships between objects.

Mandatory reporting. Those patient safety reporting systems that by legislation and/or regulation require the reporting of specified adverse events, generally events of serious harm and death.

Mapping. The process of cross-linking terms from different terminologies so that comparisons and analyses can be undertaken.

Multiple classification. Multiple classification must not restrict terminology such that a concept is prevented from being assigned to as many classes as required (e.g., "viral pneumonia" can be in classes "pneumonia" and "viral diseases").

National Health Information Infrastructure (NHII). A set of technologies, standards, applications, systems, values, and laws that support all facets of individual health, health care, and public health (National Committee on Vital and Health Statistics, 2001).

Natural language processing (NLP). Accessing data in the narrative form or free text and creating machine-understandable interpretations of those data (van Bemmel, 1997).

Near miss. An error of commission or omission that could have harmed the patient, but serious harm did not occur as a result of chance (e.g., the patient received a contraindicated drug but did not experience an adverse drug reaction), prevention (e.g., a potentially lethal overdose was prescribed, but a nurse identified the error before administering the medication), or mitigation (e.g., a lethal drug overdose was administered but discovered early and countered with an antidote).

Neural networks. A system in hardware or software of interconnected nodes developed in analogy with the human brain (van Bemmel, 1997).

Nodes. Components of semantic nets representing objects or classes of objects.

Nomenclature. A nomenclature, or vocabulary, is a set of specialized terms that facilitate precise communication by eliminating ambiguity (National Committee on Vital and Health Statistics, 2000).

Nonambiguity. Nonambiguity says that concepts must have exactly one meaning and, where a common term has two or more associated meanings (homonymy), they must be disambiguated into distinct concepts (e.g., "Paget disease" must be split into "Paget disease of the bone" and "Paget disease of the breast") (Cimino, 1998).

Nonredundancy. Nonredundancy says that a mechanism must exist that can help prevent multiple terms for the same concept from being added to the terminology as unique concepts.

Nonvagueness. Nonvagueness says that concepts in the terminology must be complete in meaning (e.g., "ventricle" is not usually considered a fully described concept, nor does it represent some generic class of anatomic terms, i.e., it means neither "heart ventricle" nor "brain ventricle" when taken out of context).

Notational aspect of knowledge representation language. The way in which information is stored in an explicit format. Also known as syntactic aspect of knowledge representation language.

Patient safety. The prevention of harm caused by errors of commission and omission.

Procedural knowledge. Knowledge of *how* other than *that*.

Proof theory. A component of logic system that is a formal specification of the notion of correct inference.

Recovery. An informal set of human factors that lead to a risky situation being detected, understood, and corrected in time, thus limiting the sequence to a near-miss outcome, instead of it developing further into possibly an adverse event.

Reference terminology. Concept-oriented terminologies possessing characteristics such as a grammar that defines the rules for automated generation and classification of new concepts as well as combination of atomic concepts to form molecular expressions (Spackman et al., 1997).

Reporting formats. Sets of data elements required for reporting purposes.

Root-cause analysis. A process for identifying the basic or causal factors that underlie variation in performance, including the occurrence or possible occurrence of a sentinel event. Typically, the analysis focuses primarily on systems and processes, not individual performance (Joint Commission on Accreditation of Healthcare Organzizations, 2003).

Rule base. A component of production rule system that represents knowledge as "if-then" rules.

Safe care. Safe care involves making evidence-based clinical decisions to maximize the health outcomes of an individual and to minimize the potential for harm. Both errors of commission and omission should be avoided.

Safety incident. Defined by the National Research Council as an event that, under slightly different circumstances, could have been an accident.

Semantics. Components of logic system that specify the meanings of the well-formed expressions of the logical language.

Slots. Components of the frame system that describe objects.

Soundness. A property of logic system that every sentence derived from a set of sentences is also a valid consequence of that set of sentences.

Standards. A set of characteristics or quantities that describes features of a product, process, service, interface, or material. The description can take many forms, such as the definition of terms, specification of design and construction, detailing of procedures, or performance criteria against which a product, process, and other factors can be measured (National Research Council, 1995).

Surveillance. Routine collection and review of data to examine the extent of a disease, to follow trends, and to detect changes in disease occurrence, such as infectious disease surveillance, postmarketing surveillance, etc. (van Bemmel, 1997).

Synonomy. Synonomy supports multiple nonunique names for concepts.

Syntactic aspect of knowledge representation language. The way in which information is stored in an explicit format. Also known as notational aspect of knowledge representation language.

Syntax. The rules (grammar) for the description, storage, and transmission of messages or for the composition of a program statement (van Bemmel, 1997). The rules that specify the legal symbols and constructs of a language (Shortliffe et al., 2001).

Terminologies. Terminologies define, classify, and in some cases code data content.

User interface. A conceptual layer of a system architecture that insulates the programs designed to interact with users from the underlying data and the applications that process those data (Shortliffe et al., 2001).

Voluntary reporting. Those reporting systems for which the reporting of patient safety events is voluntary (not mandatory). Generally, reports on all types of events are accepted.

Working memory. A component of production rule system containing information that the system has gained about the problem thus far.

ACRONYM LIST

ADE	adverse drug event
AE	adverse event
AERS	Adverse Event Reporting System
AHRQ	Agency for Healthcare Research and Quality
AIMS	Australian Incident Monitoring System
AMI	acute myocardial infarction
ANSI	American National Standards Institute
ASC	Accredited Standards Committee
ASR	Alternative Summary Reporting—Medical Devices
ASTM	American Society for Testing and Materials
BPD	Blood Product Deviation Reporting System
CDA	Clinical Document Architecture
CDC	Centers for Disease Control and Prevention
CEN	Comité Européan Normalisation
CHF	congestive heart failure
CHI	Consolidated Health Informatics
CHIP	Children's Health Insurance Program
CIS	clinical information systems
CMS	Centers for Medicare and Medicaid Services
COPD	chronic obstructive pulmonary disease
CORAS	Risk Assessment of Security Critical Systems
CPOE	computerized physician order entry
CPT	Current Procedural Terminology
CQI	continuous quality improvement
CQuIPS	Center for Quality Improvement and Patient Safety
DHHS	Department of Health and Human Services
DICOM	Digital Imaging and Communications in Medicine
DoD	Department of Defense

DQIP	Diabetes Quality Improvement Project
DSM	Diagnostic and Statistical Manual
DSN	Dialysis Surveillance Network
E-Codes	External Causes and Injury Codes
EPC	Evidence-based Practice Center
ESRD	end-stage renal disease
FACCT	Foundation for Accountability
FCG	First Consulting Group
FDA	Food and Drug Administration
FMEA	failure mode and effect analysis
GELLO	Guideline Expression Language, Object Oriented
GLIF	Guideline Interchange Format
GP	general practitioner
GRM	Generic Reference Model
HACCP	hazard analysis and critical control points
HAZOP	hazard and operability studies
HCFA	Health Care Financing Administration
HCPCS	Health Care Financing Administration Common Procedure Coding System
HFMEA	Healthcare failure mode and effect analysis
HHCC	Home Health Care Classification
HIMSS	Healthcare Information Management Systems Society
HIPAA	Health Insurance Portability and Accountability Act of 1996
HL7	Health Level Seven
ICD–9 CM	International Classification of Diseases, Ninth Edition, Clinical Modification
ICD–10	International Classification of Diseases, Tenth Edition
ICD–O	International Classification of Diseases, Oncology
ICF	International Classification of Functioning, Disability and Health
ICNP	International Classification of Nursing Practice
ICPC	International Classification of Primary Care
IEEE	Institute of Electrical and Electronics Engineers
IHE	Integrating the Healthcare Enterprise

IOM	Institute of Medicine
ISMP	Institute for Safe Medication Practice
ISO	International Organization for Standardization
IT	information technology
JAMIA	*Journal of American Informatics Association*
JCAHO	Joint Commission on Accreditation of Healthcare Organizations
LOINC	Logical Observation Identifiers, Names and Codes
MAUDE	Manufacture and User Data Experience-Medical Devices
MDS	Minimum Data Set for Nursing Home Care
MedDRA	Medical Dictionary for Drug Regulatory Affairs
MedSun	Medical Product Surveillance Network
MER	Medication Errors Reporting
MERS TM	Medical Event Reporting System for Transfusion Medicine
MeSH	Medical Subject Headings
MHS PSP	Military Health System Patient Safety Program
MPSMS	Medicare Patient Safety Monitoring System
MRI	magnetic resonance imaging
NANDA	North American Nursing Diagnosis Association
NASA	National Aeronautics and Space Administration
NaSH	National Surveillance System for Health Care Workers
NASHP	National Academy for State Health Policy
NCHS	National Center for Health Statistics
NCPDP	National Council for Prescription Drug Programs
NCPS	National Center for Patient Safety
NCQA	National Committee for Quality Assurance
NCVHS	National Committee on Vital and Health Statistics
NDC	National Drug Code
NDF RT	National Drug File Clinical Drug Reference Terminology
NEDSS	National Electronic Disease Surveillance System
NEMA	National Equipment Manufacturers Association
NHII	national health information infrastructure
NHSN	National Healthcare Safety Network
NIC	Nursing Intervention Classification
NLM	National Library of Medicine
NLP	natural language processing

NM	near miss
NNIS	National Nosocomial Infections Surveillance
NOC	Nursing Outcomes Classifications
NPSF	National Patient Safety Foundation
NPV	negative predictive value
NQF	National Quality Forum
NRC	National Research Council
NYPORTS	New York Patient Occurrence Reporting and Tracking System
OASIS	Outcome and Assessment Information Set for Home Care
PATH	Program for Appropriate Technology in Health
PCDS	Patient Care Data Set
PCP	primary care physician
PHA	proactive hazard analysis
PMRI	patient medical record information
PNDS	Perioperative Nursing Data Set
PPV	positive predictive value
PQI	prevention quality indicator
PRA	probabilistic risk assessment
PS	patient safety
PSDS	patient safety data standards
PSRS	patient safety reporting system
QIPS	quality indicators for patient safety
QuIC	Quality Interagency Coordination Task Force
RCA	root-cause analysis
R-Demo	reporting demonstration
RIM	Reference Information Model
RSNA	Radiological Society of North America
RxNORM	normalized notations for clinical drugs
SAC	Safety Assessment Code
SNAEMS	Special Nutritionals Adverse Event Monitoring System
SNOMED CT	Systemized Nomenclature for Human and Veterinary Medicine, Clinical Terms
SPARCS	Statewide Planning and Research Cooperative System

| **TPS** | Toyota Production System |
| **TQM** | total quality management |

UCSF	University of California, San Francisco
UHI	universal health identifier
UMDNS	Universal Medical Device Nomenclature System
UMLS	Unified Medical Language System
USP	United States Pharmacopeial Convention, Inc.

VAERS	Vaccine Adverse Event Reporting System
VHA	Veterans Health Administration
VSD	Vaccine Safety Datalink

| **WONCA** | World Organization of National Colleges, Academies, and Academic Associations of General Practitioners and Family Physicians |

| **XML** | extensible markup language |

REFERENCES

Cimino, James J. 1998. Desiderata for controlled medical vocabularies in the twenty-first century. *Methods Inf Med* 37(4–5):394–403.

First Consulting Group. 2003. *Computerized Physician Order Entry: Costs, Benefits, and Challenges, A Case Study Approach.* Online. Available: http://www.leapfroggroup. org/CPOE/AHA%20FAH%20CPOE%20Report%20FINAL.pdf [accessed February 2, 2004].

Hammond, W. E. 2002. *Patient Safety Data Standards: View from a Standards Perspective.* PowerPoint Presentation to IOM Committee on Data Standards for Patient Safety on May 6, 2002. Online. Available: http://www.iom.edu/file.asp?id=9915 [accessed December 16, 2003].

Joint Commission on Accreditation of Healthcare Organziations. 2003. *2003 Hospital Accreditation Standards.* Oakbrook Terrace, Illinois: Joint Commission Resources.

National Committee on Vital and Health Statistics. 2000. *Uniform Data Standards for Patient Medical Record Information.* Online. Available at http://ncvhs.hhs.gov/ hipaa000706.pdf [accessed April 15, 2002].

National Committee on Vital and Health Statistics. 2001. *Information for Health: A Strategy for Building the National Health Information Infrastructure.* Online. Available at http://ncvhs.hhs.gov/nhiilayo.pdf [accessed April 18, 2002].

National Research Council. 1995. *Standards, Conformity Assessment, and Trade: Into the 21st Century.* Washington, DC: National Academy Press.

Newton, H. 2001. *Newton's Telecom Dictionary: The Official Dictionary of Telecommunications, Networking and the Internet.* 17th edition. New York, NY: CMP Books.

Shortliffe, E. H., L. E. Perreault, G. Wiederhold, and L. M. Fagan. 2001. *Medical Informatics: Computer Applications in Healthcare and Biomedicine.* New York: Springer-Verlag.

Spackman, K. A., K. E. Campbell, and R. A. Cotz. 1997. *SNOMED RT: A Reference Terminology for Health Care.* Northfield, Illinois: College of American Pathologists.

Sujansky, W. 2003. *Summary and Analysis of Terminology Questionnaires Submitted by Developers of Candidate Terminologies for PMRI Standards: A Draft Report to the National Committee on Vital and Health Statistics Subcommittee on Standards and Security.* National Committee on Vital and Health Statistics Meeting 5.

van Bemmel, J. H., and M. A. Musen. 1997. *Handbook of Medical Informatics.* Heidelberg: Springer-Verlag.

Van Hentenryck, K. 2001. *HL7: The Art of Playing Together.* Online. Available: www.medicalcomputingtoday.com [accessed September 25, 2001].

C

Examples of Federal, State, and Private-Sector Reporting Systems

The *To Err Is Human* report (Institute of Medicine, 2000) boosted existing patient safety initiatives and stimulated new ones. In the United States, many types of patient safety reporting systems are now in operation or under development at the federal, state, and private-sector levels. The Institute of Medicine Committee on Data Standards for Patient Safety reviewed a large number of these systems during the study. This appendix summarizes a sample of reporting systems. For each sector the following areas are described:

- Type of system—reporting or surveillance
- History of reporting/surveillance system
- Voluntary or mandatory
- Reportable events
- Classification system and severity index
- Reporting time frame
- Data collected—format and summary
- Method of reporting
- Who reports
- Root-cause analysis trigger
- Follow-up, including root cause
- Other information collected
- Confidentiality issues
- Relationship with other reporting systems
- Relationship with JCAHO

I. FEDERAL REPORTING SYSTEMS

Overview

Within the federal government, eight major patient safety reporting and surveillance systems (see Tables C–1a, C–1b, and C–1c for details) were examined. Most of these systems were initiated by the federal agencies that manage them; however, one was mandated in legislation—the Vaccine Adverse Event Reporting System (VAERS). These federal agencies include the Centers for Disease Control and Prevention (CDC), the Food and Drug Administration (FDA), and the Centers for Medicare and Medicaid Services (CMS), which are all part of the Department of Health and Human Services (DHHS); the Department of Defense (DOD); and the Department of Veterans Affairs (VA).

The CDC manages two of the eight systems: the National Nosocomial Infections Surveillance (NNIS) System and the Dialysis Surveillance Network (DSN). The NNIS system has two components—nosocomial infections and antimicrobial use and resistance. The CDC also works jointly with the FDA to manage VAERS.

The FDA manages MedWatch, which handles reporting of medical device, biologic and blood product, drug product, and special nutritionals events. CMS is developing and will manage the Medicare Patient Safety Monitoring Program (MPSMS), and the DOD manages the Military Health System Patient Safety Program (MHS PSP).

The VA manages the National Center for Patient Safety (NCPS) and is working with the National Aeronautics and Space Administration (NASA) to develop a complementary system called the Patient Safety Reporting System (PSRS).

The longest operating of these systems is NNIS, which was initiated by CDC in 1970. The rest began operating after 1990, including several in the past few years. The newest systems are the MPSMS, MHS PSP, and PSRS.

Surveillance or Reporting Systems

Two types of systems are used: surveillance and reporting. In general, surveillance systems abstract data from patient and other records and/or health care personnel to determine if an adverse event has occurred and/or to analyze the data in order to monitor trends. Reporting systems are designed for individuals to report specific events and, in some cases, conduct root-cause analyses (RCAs) to determine the causal factors for these events.

Like surveillance systems, reporting can be used to monitor trends. The two CDC-managed systems and the CMS MPSMS are considered surveillance systems; the other five are for event reporting. Most of these systems are essentially voluntary, with the exception of VAERS and MedWatch, which mandate reporting by certain parties (health professionals, manufacturers, and/or user facilities). In the cases where reporting is mandatory, specific time frames are established within which reports must be received; these time frames vary according to the seriousness of the event.

Reportable Events

In terms of the events reported and monitored by the federal systems, they vary a great deal from one to the next (see "Reportable events/events monitored" and "Classification system and/or severity index" rows of the tables). Some systems include reporting for close calls (i.e., near misses), while others focus solely on adverse events.[1] However, a few general statements can be made about them. The CDC- and FDA-managed systems tend to focus on specific types of adverse events, based on patient outcome or what caused the event—nosocomial infections; infections resulting from hemodialysis; vaccine events; and medical device, biologic and blood product, drug product, and special nutritionals events. Although these systems are quite specific in terms of events reported/monitored, they can be used across numerous health systems. The focus of the other four systems—MPSMS, MHS PSP, NCPS, and PSRS—is essentially the opposite of the first four. They are designed for use within the health systems that serve their members: Medicare, the MHS, and the Veterans Health Administration (VHA). The types of events reported to and monitored by these systems are more general and, in some cases, are not categorized at all. Adverse/serious events are included in all of these systems; however, four of them—MHS PSP, NCPS, PSRS, and MedWatch (for device problems only via MedSun)—also include close calls and/or near misses. Additionally, the MHS PSP includes nonpatient specific events such as a fire or system failure in the facility. Often, an organization will classify an event or determine whether an RCA is needed based on a risk assessment scale. For example, the NCPS reporting system classifies events and close calls using the Safety Assessment Code (SAC) matrix and requires an RCA if a close call or adverse event has a high SAC score or at the discretion of the patient safety manager.

---

[1] Adverse/serious events and close calls/near misses are defined differently by each system (see tables).

Format for Reporting

Each system requires different data to be abstracted or reported, and most of them have a standard format for collecting those data (see "Data collected: Format and summary" row in the tables). The MHS PSP and NCPS do not use a standardized format for initially collecting data—they allow facilities to use locally accepted methods for reporting—but then report the data to their central agencies in a standardized manner. Most of the systems include patient-specific data in their reports; however, patient (and health care worker) identifiers are removed when the data are shared across the system or with an outside party. All of the data in these systems are protected from discovery by law or regulation.

Method of Reporting

Five of the systems allow for electronic transmission (via disk, e-mail, or the Internet) of reports to the central office; the rest require submission of hardcopy reports, which are then entered into databases by agency personnel. In terms of who can report to these systems and who abstracts the data, most are open to all personnel at participating facilities. The NNIS, however, uses trained personnel at participating hospitals to compile the data. The MHS PSP and NCPS allow reporting according to their facilities' locally accepted methods, but specific personnel are responsible for compiling and transmitting the data to the central offices. Only two of these systems currently allow consumers (patients and their families) to report events—VAERS and MedWatch. The MHS PSP also welcomes reports from patients and families but has not yet developed the mechanisms to facilitate this avenue of reporting.

Analysis of More Serious Events

All of the systems have in place some means for following up on events, although the type and amount of follow-up vary a great deal across the systems. The primary means of follow-up used by the surveillance systems is data analysis and trend monitoring. Most of the systems allow facilities to do this on a local level. Overall analyses and comparisons are usually conducted by the central agency. In such cases, these analyses are often shared with the individual facilities. VAERS and MedWatch both involve reviews of the most serious events by the FDA. These reviews may result in several actions from alerts and label/packaging changes to recalls of vaccine batches or products.

MHS PSP and NCPS both involve extensive RCAs and action plans, which must be monitored for effectiveness. NCPS and MHS PSP also require prompt feedback to the reporter, and patients are informed when they have been involved in an adverse event. PSRS involves the least follow-up—it was built as a complement to the NCPS and is used primarily for learning purposes; however, reporters do receive a confirmation by mail that their report has been received.

Tabular Information

All of this information is broken out in more detail in the tables. Table C–1a includes the two CDC-managed systems and the joint FDA- and CDC-managed VAERS. Table C–1b includes the FDA-managed MedWatch system, CMS's MPSMS, and the MHS PSP. Table C–1c includes the two VA-managed systems.

TABLE C–1a Selected Examples of Federal Patient Safety/Health Care Reporting
and Surveillance Systems

Federal Agency	CDC
Name of System	National Nosocomial Infections Surveillance System[a]
Type of System	Surveillance.
History of reporting/ surveillance system	The NNIS system is a cooperative effort that began in 1970 between CDC and participating hospitals. The system is used to describe the epidemiology of nosocomial infections and antimicrobial resistance trends.
Voluntary or mandatory	Voluntary.
Reportable events/events monitored	The NNIS system has two components: (1) nosocomial infections and (2) antimicrobial use and resistance (AUR). In two situations, an infection is considered nosocomial: (1) infection that is acquired in the hospital but does not become evident until after hospital discharge and (2) infection in a neonate that results from passing through the birth canal. There are two special situations when an infection is NOT considered nosocomial: (1) infection associated with a complication or extension of infection already present on admission, unless a change in pathogen or symptoms strongly suggests the acquisition of a new infection, and (2) in an infant an infection known or proved to have been acquired transplacentally and evident 48 hours or less after birth.

[a]Information on the NNIS system has been obtained from the following sources: Gaynes (1998), Gaynes and Horan (1999), Gaynes and Solomon (1996), Horan and Emori (1998), Richards et al. (2001), Centers for Disease Control and Prevention (2002).

CDC	Joint FDA/CDC
Dialysis Surveillance Network[b]	Vaccine Adverse Event Report System[c]
Surveillance.	Reporting.
DSN is a national surveillance system for monitoring bloodstream and vascular infections. It was initiated by CDC in August 1999.	The National Childhood Vaccine Injury Act (NCVIA) of 1986 mandated the reporting of certain adverse events following vaccination to help ensure the safety of vaccines distributed in the United States. This act led to the establishment of VAERS in November 1990 by the U.S. Department of Health and Human Services.
Voluntary.	Mandatory for health professionals and manufacturers to report events listed in the Reportable Events Table. Voluntary for health professionals and consumers to report reactions to other vaccines not listed in the Reportable Events Table.
Only chronic hemodialysis patients are included. Reportable events are significant bacterial infections resulting from hemodialysis. These events are identified because they include either a hospitalization or in-unit intravenous (IV) antimicrobial start.	The NCVIA requires reporting of: • Any event set forth in the Reportable Events Table that occurs within a specified time period (these are summarized below). • Any event listed in the manufacturer's package insert as a contraindication to subsequent doses. *Vaccine/toxoid = Tetanus in any combination* • Anaphylaxis or anaphylactic shock • Brachial neuritis

Continued

___

[b]Information on DSN has been obtained from the following sources: Centers for Disease Control and Prevention (1999), Centers for Disease Control and Prevention: Hospital Infections Program (2000).

[c]Information on VAERS has been obtained from the following sources: Food and Drug Administration (1999, 2001b).

TABLE C–1a *Continued*

Federal Agency	CDC
Name of System	National Nosocomial Infections Surveillance System[a]

The two conditions that are NOT infections include: (1) colonization or the presence of microorganisms that are not causing adverse clinical signs or symptoms, and (2) inflammation that results from tissue response to injury or stimulation by noninfectious agents, such as chemicals.

The AUR surveillance system requires, for a range of pathogens, the reporting of antimicrobial resistance. Each pathogen requires data for different antimicrobial agents.

The pathogens are *Staphylococcus aureus*, coagulase-negative *staphylococci, Enterococcus species, Streptococcus pneumoniae, Escherichia coli, Klebsiella pneumoniae, Enterobacter species,* and *Pseudomonas aeruginosa.*

CDC	Joint FDA/CDC
Dialysis Surveillance Network[b]	Vaccine Adverse Event Report System[c]

| | • Any sequela (including death) of above events
• Events described in manufacturer's package insert as contraindications to additional doses of vaccine
Vaccine/toxoid = Pertussis in any combination
• Anaphylaxis or anaphylactic shock
• Encephalopathy (or encephalitis)
• Any sequela (including death) of above events
• Events described in manufacturer's package insert as contraindications to additional doses of vaccine
Vaccine/toxoid = Measles, mumps, and rubella in any combination
Same events as pertussis in any combination
Vaccine/toxoid = Rubella in any combination
• Chronic arthritis
• Any sequela (including death) of above events
• Events described in manufacturer's package insert as contraindications to additional doses of vaccine
Vaccine/toxoid = Inactivated Polio (IPV)
• Anaphylaxis or anaphylactic shock
• Any sequela (including death) of above events
• Events described in manufacturer's package insert as contraindications to additional doses of vaccine
Vaccine/toxoid = Hepatitis B
Same events as IPV |

Continued

TABLE C–1a *Continued*

Federal Agency	CDC

Name of System	National Nosocomial Infections Surveillance System[a]

Classification system and/or severity index	All infections are categorized into major and specific infection sites, using standard CDC definitions that include laboratory and clinical criteria. Surgical site infection roles are stratified by a risk index based on wound classification, duration of operation, and the American Society of Anesthiologists severity assessment score.

Reporting time frame	Not applicable—surveillance is ongoing.

CDC	Joint FDA/CDC
Dialysis Surveillance Network[b]	Vaccine Adverse Event Report System[c]

	Vaccine/toxoid = Hemophilus influenzae type b (polysaccharide) • Early-onset Hib disease • Any sequela (including death) of above events • Events described in manufacturer's package insert as contraindications to additional doses of vaccine *Vaccine/toxoid = Hemophilus influenzae type b (conjugate)* • Events described in manufacturer's package insert as contraindications to additional doses of vaccine *Vaccine/toxoid = Varicella* • Same events as Hemophilus influenzae type b (conjugate) *Vaccine/toxoid = Rotavirus* • Same events as Hemophilus influenzae type b (conjugate) *Vaccine/toxoid = Pneumococcal conjugate* • Same events as Hemophilus influenzae type b (conjugate)
Events are classified initially according to outcome: hospitalization or in-unit IV antimicrobial start. They are further classified according to the vascular accesses that the patient has, the problems that led to hospitalization or in-unit IV antimicrobial start, and the results of blood cultures done in the hospital or dialysis unit. No severity index.	Reported adverse events that are listed on the Reportable Events Table are categorized by type of vaccine, to the extent possible. No severity index, but outcomes are recorded.
Not applicable—surveillance is ongoing.	For consumers: No restriction on the time lapse between the vaccination and the start of the event or between the event and the time the report is made.

Continued

TABLE C–1a *Continued*

Federal Agency	CDC

Name of System	National Nosocomial Infections Surveillance System[a]

Data collected: Format and summary	Standard format—data are collected using four standardized protocols called surveillance components: adult and pediatric intensive care unit, high-risk nursery, surgical patient, and antimicrobial use and resistance.
	Essential data collected for infections include patient name, age, and sex; hospital identification number; service; ward/intensive care unit (ICU); admission date; infection onset date and site of infection; and laboratory data, including pathogen(s) and antibiogram.
	AUR surveillance system: Prescribing practices—each hospital must identify its antimicrobial agent prescribing practices. For each antimicrobial agent, identify whether it is in the formulary. If it is, whether an automatic stop order exists, whether approval for use is needed outside the ICU(s), and whether approval for use is needed inside the ICU(s).
	Microbiology lab data: For the purposes of data collection, a hospital unit is defined to be an individual ICU or the total non-ICU inpatient care area or the total outpatient care area. Each unit must report: (1) the total number of clinical cultures processed for the particular month; (2) for each pathogen the total number of bacterial isolates classified as susceptible, intermediate, and resistant to at least one of the relevant antimicrobial agents; and (3) for each pathogen the total number of isolates processed in the laboratory that month.
	Pharmacy data: Each inpatient unit must report the total number of grams or millions of units of each parental antimicrobial agent received and the total number of grams of each oral antimicrobial agent received in the particular month.
Method of reporting	Entered into CDC-provided software and transmitted routinely to CDC via dedicated phone line and modem. Reports are provided on a monthly basis.
Who reports	Trained infection control personnel at the participating 300 hospitals. To participate, a hospital must have 100 or more "set up and staffed" acute care beds to meet minimum requirements for infection control staffing.

CDC	Joint FDA/CDC
Dialysis Surveillance Network[b]	Vaccine Adverse Event Report System[c]
	For health professionals: Time frame between administration of the vaccine and onset of an adverse event varies according to type of vaccine and event. The onset interval is listed in the Reportable Events Table.
Standard format—information collected *for hospitalizations*: that patients have been hospitalized; the problem or diagnoses prompting hospital admission, especially whether the patient had signs and symptoms of access infection; and the results of blood cultures done in the hospital soon after admission. Information collected *for in-unit IV antimicrobial starts*: that patients were started on an IV antimicrobial in-unit; the problem or diagnosis prompting use of the IV antimicrobial, especially whether patients had signs and symptoms of access infection; and the results of blood cultures done in the unit.	Standard format: Data collected include: description of adverse event; relevant diagnostic tests and/or laboratory data; information about the vaccines administered (e.g., type, manufacturer, lot number, date administered); and patient information, including relevant history.
Paper forms that are mailed to CDC or via an Internet-based system.	Form available online or by calling VAERS. It must be printed and mailed back to VAERS.
Dialysis center personnel.	Consumers, health professionals, and manufacturers.

Continued

TABLE C–1a *Continued*

Federal Agency	CDC
Name of System	National Nosocomial Infections Surveillance System[a]
RCA trigger	None. However, a hospital compares its data to the aggregate and makes decisions about whether to intervene based on its own prevention targets.
Follow-up (including RCA)	Hospitals may use the data collected to compare its infection rates with similar patient populations within the hospital or with external benchmark rates or by comparing changes in rates over time in their own hospital.
Other information collected through the system	Information describing important risk factors for infection can be collected if it will be analyzed and used by the hospital. Corresponding denominator data are collected so that risk-adjusted infection rates can be calculated. Information on adverse outcomes of nosocomial infection is also collected (death, secondary bloodstream infection).
Confidentiality issues	The CDC Division of Healthcare Quality Improvement (formerly Division of Hospital Infections) obtained authorization to collect these data under the protection of Section 308(d) of the Public Health Service Act. The legislation stipulates that no information in a project protected by 308(d) can be used for any purpose other than the purpose for which it was supplied, nor be published or released in an identifiable format unless the establishment or person supplying the information or described in it has consented to such release.

CDC	Joint FDA/CDC
Dialysis Surveillance Network[b]	Vaccine Adverse Event Report System[c]
None.	None.
No direct follow-up on events. However, centers using the Internet-based system can generate and print data analysis reports whenever desired.	The FDA reviews reports of individual serious events (including hospitalizations, life-threatening events, and deaths) weekly. The FDA also analyzes patterns of reporting associated with vaccine lots, looking for more death reports than would be expected on the basis of factors such as time in use and chance variation and for any unusual patterns in other serious reports within a lot. If evaluation of reports signaling a safety risk confirms that risk, the batch of vaccine can be recalled.
None.	Health professionals and consumers may report any clinically significant adverse event occurring after the administration of any vaccine licensed in the United States.
The CDC Division of Healthcare Quality Improvement (formerly Division of Hospital Infections) obtained authorization to collect these data under the protection of Section 308(d) of the Public Health Service Act. The legislation stipulates that no information in a project protected by 308(d) can be used for any purpose other than the purpose for which it was supplied, nor be published or released in an identifiable format unless the establishment or person supplying the information or described in it has consented to such release.	The National Childhood Vaccine Injury Act of 1986 provides liability protection through the Vaccine Injury Compensation Program. Therefore, practitioner liability is unaffected by the VAERS reporting requirement. VAERS data are made available to the public only after removal of patient identification information.

Continued

TABLE C–1a *Continued*

Federal Agency	CDC
Name of System	National Nosocomial Infections Surveillance System[a]
Relationship with other reporting systems	None. However, NNIS data are used with hospital discharge data for projections of how many patients had an infection at discharge.
Relationships with Joint Commission on Accreditation of Healthcare Organizations (JCAHO)/ Medicare certification	NNIS central line–associated bloodstream infection rate and device utilization measures are being pilot tested as JCAHO core measures.

CDC	Joint FDA/CDC
Dialysis Surveillance Network[b]	Vaccine Adverse Event Report System[c]
None.	None.
None.	None.

TABLE C–1b Selected Examples of Federal Patient Safety/Health Care Reporting and Surveillance Systems

Federal Agency	FDA

Name of System	MedWatch[a]

Type of system	Reporting.
History of reporting/ surveillance system	The FDA has had a postmarketing surveillance program in place since 1961. The FDA's system evolved into five separate reporting forms for different products. Then, in 1993, the FDA developed MedWatch to consolidate the forms and eliminate confusion. Three FDA centers are currently responsible for handling reports: The Center for Devices and Radiological Health (CDRH) handles medical device events, the Center for Biologics Evaluation and Research (CBER) handles biologic and blood product events, and the Center for Drug Evaluation and Research (CDER) handles drug product events. In addition to these centers, the Office of Special Nutritionals handles reports of events or product problems associated with special nutritionals, such as dietary supplements, infant formulas, and medical foods. Most recently, in 2002, the CDRH launched a pilot program called MedSun (Medical Product Surveillance Network), which provides a secure, Internet-based data entry system that automates the MedWatch form for reporting medical device problems. MedSun is managed by CODA, a professional research organization.

[a]Information on MedWatch has been obtained from the following sources: Henkel (1998), Food and Drug Administration (1996, 2001a, 2002).

[b]Information on MPSMS has been obtained from the following sources: personal communication, S. Jencks and S. Kellie, 2002; personal communication, S. Kellie, March 27, 2002.

CMS	DOD
Medicare Patient Safety Monitoring System[b]	Military Health System Patient Safety Program[c]
Surveillance.	Reporting.

MPSMS is being built under the auspices of DHHS's Patient Safety Task Force, announced by Secretary Thompson in April 2001. Four federal agencies (AHRQ, CDC, FDA, VHA), which make up the Federal Agency Work Group, are working with CMS to build MPSMS. In addition, CMS has selected Qualidigm, the Connecticut QIO (Quality Improvement Organization), to provide administrative and technical support for the development and maintenance of the MPSMS. The CMS Clinical Data Abstraction Centers will provide data collection support. The MPSMS is being developed to measure and track over time adverse events and their associated patient risk factors among the Medicare population. The goal is to have the system producing national estimates for the initial groups of adverse events by the end of 2002 and to have them included in the National Quality Report in 2003.

Following the release of the IOM report, *To Err Is Human* (1999), and President Clinton's Executive Memorandum of December 7, 1999, DOD convened the Patient Safety Working Group, an interdisciplinary group of individuals from the Armed Services, the Uniformed Services University, the Armed Forces Institute of Pathology (AFIP), and the Office of the Assistant Secretary of Defense to review patient safety in the MHS. This group consulted with the VA and implemented a pilot patient safety reporting system from October 2000 to April 2001; in August 2001, DOD Instruction Number 6025.17 "Military Health System Patient Safety Program" was signed. The instruction established a system for identifying and reporting actual and potential problems in medical systems and processes and implementing actions to improve patient safety and health care quality throughout the MHS. The instruction directed that the MHS reporting system would emulate, to the extent that is practical, the reporting system established by the VA. In June 2003, the DOD Working

Continued

---

[c]Information on MHS PSP has been obtained from the following sources: personal communications, F. Stewart, February 20 and April 12, 2002; Armed Forces. Confidentiality of Medical Quality Assurance Records: Qualified Immunity for Participants. 10 U.S.C. SS Number 1102 (1986); U.S. Department of Defense 1986; Department of Defense (2001a, b, c).

TABLE C–1b *Continued*

Federal Agency	FDA

Name of System	MedWatch[a]

Voluntary or mandatory	Voluntary for consumers and health professionals; mandatory for user facilities, such as hospitals and nursing homes. In addition, MedSun allows for voluntary reporting by user facilities of "close calls" related to medical devices.
Reportable events/events monitored	*Serious* adverse events and product problems are reported to the FDA directly or via the manufacturer. These include: • Death: Report if patient's death is suspected as being a direct outcome of the adverse event. • Life threatening: Report if patient was at substantial risk of dying at the time of the adverse event or it is suspected that the use or continued use of the product would result in the patient's death. • Hospitalization (initial or prolonged): Report if admission to the hospital or prolongation of a hospital stay results because of the adverse event. • Disability: Report if the adverse event resulted in a significant, persistent, or permanent damage or disruption in the patient's body function/structure, physical activities, or quality of life. • Congenital anomaly: Report if there are suspicions that exposure to a medical product prior to conception or during pregnancy resulted in an adverse outcome in the child.

CMS	DOD
Medicare Patient Safety Monitoring System[b]	Military Health System Patient Safety Program[c]
	Group (now the Patient Safety Planning and Coordination Committee) established requirements on a Web-based Patient Safety Reporting System that will be implemented throughout the MHS. Anticipated deployment is 18 to 24 months. The system will enable voluntary reporting from point of care to the Patient Safety Center located at the AFIP, where deidentified data will be collected, analyzed, and reported. The DOD PSP has also been working with the Agency for Healthcare Research and Quality to integrate with the National Patient Safety Database currently under construction.
Voluntary.	Voluntary.
Adverse events are defined as unintended, measurable harms made more likely by the processes of health care delivery. The Federal Agency Work Group developed five criteria to select adverse event categories for inclusion in the MPSMS: • The adverse event category represents a significant burden to the Medicare population as reflected in the frequency of its occurrence, associated severity of patient harm, morbidity, and/or mortality. • The adverse event category falls within the participating agencies' missions and priorities. • The adverse event categories representing outcomes of interest across participating agencies are of higher priority.	Close calls: Defined by DOD Instruction Number 6025.17 as events or situations that may have resulted in harm to a patient but did not, either by chance or through timely intervention; such events also have been referred to as "near-miss" incidents. This definition has since been clarified further to state that near misses are events that did not reach the patient. Adverse events: Defined by DOD Instruction Number 6025.17 as occurrences or conditions associated with care or services provided that cause unexpected harm to a patient during such care or services. These may be due to acts of commission or omission. Adverse events

Continued

TABLE C–1b *Continued*

Federal Agency	FDA

Name of System	MedWatch[a]

      • Requires intervention to prevent permanent impairment or damage: Report if it is suspected that the use of a medical product may result in a condition that required medical or surgical intervention to preclude permanent impairment or damage to a patient.

In addition, MedSun allows for reporting by user facilities of close calls or the rejection of a device over safety concerns.

Classification system and/or severity index	Adverse events or product problems are classified according to whether they are attributed to medical device, biologic and/or blood product, drug product, or special nutritional product. No severity index—only serious adverse events or product problems are required to be reported.

CMS	DOD
Medicare Patient Safety Monitoring System[b]	Military Health System Patient Safety Program[c]

- The adverse event category has been demonstrated to be associated with commonly occurring exposures or hazards.
- The adverse event category measures may include adverse events themselves, surrogates for adverse events, or modifiable risk factors.

Using these five criteria, the following adverse event categories are currently under development and scheduled for inclusion in the initial version of MPSMS:

- Adverse events associated with use of central vascular catheters
- Postoperative pneumonia, urinary tract infection, deep vein thrombosis, and pulmonary embolus.
- Adverse events associated with joint replacements—specifically hip and knee replacements—and including prosthetic device complications.
- Bloodstream infections and sepsis syndrome.
- Adverse drug events.

For each adverse event, three primary elements are precisely defined:

1. An explicit exposure case definition.
2. An explicit event case definition, including associated symptoms, physical findings, laboratory values, and treatments particular to that event.
3. An explicitly defined set of risk factors associated with the event; these risk factors help identify factors contributing to the occurrence of the events. Methodologically, these risk factors may be either confounding or effect-modifying variables.

do not include intentional unsafe acts.
Sentinel events: Defined by DOD Instruction Number 6025.17 as unexpected occurrences involving death or serious physical or psychological injury or risk thereof (as defined by JCAHO).

Events are categorized according to the following types:
Patient suicides/attempts
Wrong site/person/procedure or surgery
Death/injury in restraints
Transfusion errors
Patient falls
Medication errors
Patient elopement
Delay in diagnosis/treatment
Perinatal death
Maternal death
Death associated with transfer
Infant abduction/wrong family

Continued

TABLE C–1b *Continued*

Federal Agency	FDA

Name of System	MedWatch[a]

Reporting time frame	Mandatory reporting regarding **pharmaceuticals**: For each serious or unexpected adverse event, report must be submitted within 15 working days; all non-15-day reports must be reported quarterly for the first 3 years after drug approval, then annually; the frequency of reports of (1) serious and unexpected adverse events and (2) therapeutic failures must be periodically monitored, and any significant increase must be reported within 15 days. Mandatory reporting regarding **devices** (as outlined by the Safe Medical Devices Act of 1990): *User facility:* Deaths within 10 working days to the FDA and manufacturer; serious injuries/illnesses within 10 working days to manufacturer or the FDA if manufacturer is unknown; semiannual reports to the FDA and/or manufacturer. *Manufacturer:* Deaths, serious injuries, malfunctions to the FDA within 30 calendar days of becoming aware of event; within 5 working days if (1) event necessitates remedial action to prevent an unreasonable risk of substantial harm to the public health or (2) event is one the FDA has requested be reported within 5 days.

CMS	DOD
Medicare Patient Safety Monitoring System[b]	Military Health System Patient Safety Program[c]
No severity index.	Ventilator death or injury Anesthesia-related event Medical equipment event Fire Perioperative complication Other less frequent types All close calls and adverse events are also classified according to the Safety Assessment Code. The SAC matrix takes into account (1) the actual severity of the event and (2) the probability of occurrence according to specific definitions. The matrix scores are 3 = highest risk, 2 = intermediate risk, and 1 = lowest risk. Events with scores of SAC 3 are put into one of two groups: adverse event or sentinel event. Events with scores of SAC 1 are also put into two groups: no harm and harm.
Not applicable.	Time frame from occurrence of event/close call to filing a report at an individual facility is determined by that facility's locally accepted method. Facilities submit a monthly summary of all close calls and events to the Patient Safety Center. If an event requires an RCA, the facility has 45 days from the date the facility's patient safety manager becomes aware of the event to submit the RCA.

Continued

TABLE C–1b *Continued*

Federal Agency	FDA

Name of System	MedWatch[a]

Distributor: Deaths, serious injuries/illnesses, and malfunctions to the FDA and manufacturer within 10 working days.

Mandatory reporting regarding biologics/blood products: All events must be reported as soon as possible but no later than 45 calendar days from the date of discovery that a reportable event has occurred.

Data collected: Format and summary	Standard format: Data collected include description of event or problem, relevant tests and/or patient history, suspect product information, and reporter name and contact information.

CMS	DOD
Medicare Patient Safety Monitoring System[b]	Military Health System Patient Safety Program[c]

The MPSMS will secure data from administrative records and medical records that are already being submitted to the CMS Clinical Data Abstraction Centers for the Medicare Payment Error Prevention Program.

The proportion of hospitalized Medicare beneficiaries with central venous catheters (CVCs), for example, who have evidence of an infection can be calculated using the following numerator and denominator:

Numerator: Number of Medicare beneficiaries who have at least one CVC inserted during index hospitalization, who have an infection and (1) who are continuously entitled to Part A of Medicare for 12 months prior to index admission, (2) who are not enrolled in a managed care organization, (3) who are of any age, (4) whose index hospitalization occurs in an acute care hospital, and (5) whose hospital dates of discharge occur during specified time period.

Denominator: Number of Medicare beneficiaries who have at least one CVC inserted during index hospitalization and (1) who are continuously entitled to Part A of Medicare for 12 months prior to index admission, (2) who are not enrolled in a managed care organization, (3) who are of any age, (4) whose index

Data collected remain in an Excel spreadsheet with all the reportable events mentioned in the classification system. Medication errors have been collected by a medication error reporting system (MedMARx) since June 1, 2003. MedMARx data are centrally collected in the Patient Safety Center.

Data collected by the Patient Safety Center at the AFIP are in two forms: (1) a monthly summary report on a standard form, including number of events in each category broken down according to whether it was a near miss, adverse event (SAC 1–3), or sentinel event (SAC 3), and (2) a copy of every RCA on a standard form.

Continued

TABLE C–1b *Continued*

Federal Agency	FDA

Name of System	MedWatch[a]

Method of reporting	Online (MedWatch directly or via MedSun for device problems) or by phone, mail, or fax (MedWatch only).

Who reports	Consumers, health professionals, and user facilities.

CMS	DOD
Medicare Patient Safety Monitoring System[b]	Military Health System Patient Safety Program[c]

hospitalization occurs in an acute care hospital, and (5) whose hospital dates of discharge occur during specified time period.

Explicit exposure and event case definitions embedded in an electronic medical record abstraction tool are used to identify exposures and any associated adverse events. Analysis of these data is then conducted to determine whether the patient did, in fact, suffer an adverse event.

In addition, to increase the efficiency of identifying medical records likely to include relevant exposures and associated adverse events, claims-based algorithms are used to target medical records for abstraction.

As a component of the beta test, cognitive interviews are being conducted with an interdisciplinary group of professionals, including clinicians and hospital epidemiologists, to validate the exposure and event case definitions as well as the associations between the exposures and adverse events.

MHS personnel can use a facility's locally accepted method of reporting an adverse event or close call.

Each medical facility's patient safety manager submits monthly summary reports (as Excel spreadsheets) and RCAs (including the action plans) to the Patient Safety Center at the AFIP.

Trained medical record abstractors.

Any MHS personnel can report. Patients and families are also welcome to report, but mechanisms to facilitate this reporting have not yet been developed. Names of reporting individuals are deleted from all reports. Prompt feedback to reporting individuals is required.

Continued

TABLE C–1b *Continued*

Federal Agency	FDA

Name of System	MedWatch[a]

RCA trigger	None. However, all reports from health professionals and specific reports from manufacturers are reviewed individually by an FDA health professional safety evaluator, with attention to all serious events that are not due to labeling in the case of pharmaceuticals.

Follow-up (including RCA)	MedWatch: No direct follow-up with reporter.
	Based on review of incidents, the FDA can follow up with these actions: a "Dear Health Professional" letter or Safety Alert; labeling, name, or packaging changes; further epidemiologic investigations; requests for manufacturer-sponsored postmarketing studies; inspections of manufacturers' facilities or records; or work with a manufacturer regarding possible withdrawal of a medical product from the market.
	MedSun allows for additional follow-up, including a monthly newsletter reviewing all reports; alerts, advisories, and recall notices; access to special analyses of the MedSun and MAUDE[d] databases; and an annual conference.

Other information collected through the system	Health professionals may report any adverse event that they judge to be clinically significant, whether it is considered serious by the FDA definition or not.

---

[d]MAUDE is the Manufacturer and User Data Experience database, which serves as the reporting system for events involving medical devices.

CMS	DOD
Medicare Patient Safety Monitoring System[b]	Military Health System Patient Safety Program[c]
None. However, the presence of risk factors is noted during the medical record abstraction process.	All events with an actual SAC score of 3 require a full RCA. Facilities are also encouraged to do an RCA on any event or near miss when they believe it would be helpful. If an event has an SAC score of 3 AND it is a fall or medication error, more data are collected and aggregated for an analysis done every quarter.
None at this time.	If an event/close call warrants an individual RCA, a team is formed to conduct the RCA. The team facilitator is the performance improvement subject matter expert and the team leader is the content expert. Three to five other members are selected for the team. This team can use several tools: (1) a computer-aided software tool (TapRoot) that leads them through the steps of an RCA and (2) a list of "triage" or "memory jogger" questions. The team then completes an RCA form (a set of Microsoft Word templates that include the RCA and the proposed action plan) for submission to the medical treatment facility, JCAHO if needed, and the Patient Safety Center.
None.	None.

Continued

TABLE C–1b *Continued*

Federal Agency	FDA

Name of System	MedWatch[a]

Confidentiality issues	Identities of both reporters and patients are protected by FDA regulations. In 1995, an additional regulation went into effect extending this protection against disclosure by preempting state discovery laws regarding voluntary reports held by pharmaceutical, biological, and medical device manufacturers.
Relationship with other reporting systems	Receives medication error reports from the U.S. Pharmacopeia's (USP's) Medication Errors Reporting (MER) Program and USP's MedMARx system. Receives reports of transfusion errors from the Medical Event Reporting System for Transfusion Medicine (MERS-TM).
Relationships with JCAHO/ Medicare certification	Adverse event monitoring is linked to JCAHO standards. To be accredited, JCAHO requires each hospital to monitor for adverse events involving pharmaceuticals and devices.

CMS	DOD
Medicare Patient Safety Monitoring System[b]	Military Health System Patient Safety Program[c]

CMS	DOD
The MPSMS is a QIO quality study, and information collected is protected by federal law against disclosure in a form that identifies individuals or providers, as well as against discovery or subpoena in civil actions.	All records and information of the MHS PSP are considered medical quality assurance records and are confidential under 10 U.S.C. 1102 and DOD Directive 6040.37 (references (d) and (e)). Aggregate statistical information at the DOD-wide or service-wide levels may be provided consistent with references (d) and (e). Except as specifically authorized (e.g., JCAHO sentinel events reporting), MHS PSP records or information are not to be disclosed unless authorized by references (d) and (e) and also by other applicable authority or authorized by the Assistant Secretary of Defense for Health Affairs. No patient or health care provider identifiers are included in the reports, RCAs, action plans, or aggregate reviews.
None.	No direct relationships.
	All sentinel events meeting the JCAHO definition of reviewable sentinel event are to be reported to JCAHO. The completed RCA and action plan also should be made available to JCAHO consistent with JCAHO's policy and time limits.

TABLE C–1c Federal Patient Safety/Health Care Reporting and Surveillance
Systems

Federal Agency	VHA	VHA/NASA
Name of System	National Center for Patient Safety Reporting System[a]	Patient Safety Reporting System[b]
Type of system	Reporting.	Reporting.
History of reporting/ surveillance system	In 1997, the VA implemented the Patient Safety Improvement (PSI) initiative after identifying patient safety as a high priority within its health care system. The PSI included a Sentinel Event Reporting System, whose purpose was to prevent adverse events through an understanding of systems-level causes and then following up with corrective actions. This system was in place until late 1998 when, based on the recommendations of the External Panel on Patient Safety System Design, the VA established the dedicated National Center for Patient Safety to redesign the PSI in order to increase reporting and enhance the utility of reports. Then, after conducting two pilot studies, full-scale national rollout of the reporting system took place between April and August 2000.	In May 2000, the VHA formalized an agreement with NASA to develop PSRS, which is designed to be a complementary external system to the internal NCPS Reporting System. For the VA, the NCPS is a "safety valve" for incidents that otherwise may go unreported to the internal NCPS system. Pilot testing of PSRS began in March 2001 at a few selected VA medical centers, and the system became available to all VA medical centers in FY 2002. The VA pays NASA to independently operate PSRS according to the Memorandum of Understanding between the two agencies. PSRS builds on more than 25 years of NASA experience in running the Aviation Safety Reporting System for the Federal Aviation Administration.

[a]Information on the NCPS Reporting System has been obtained from the following sources: Agency for Healthcare Research and Quality (2002); Overhage (2003), U.S. Code (1980), Department of Veterans Affairs (2001, 2002).

[b]Information on the PSRS has been obtained from the following sources: Agency for Healthcare Research and Quality (2002), U.S. Code (1980), Department of Veterans Affairs (2001), Department of Veterans Affairs and National Aeronautics and Space Administration (2000).

TABLE C–1c *Continued*

Federal Agency	VHA	VHA/NASA
Name of System	National Center for Patient Safety Reporting System[a]	Patient Safety Reporting System[b]
Voluntary or mandatory	Participation in the program is mandatory. Performing RCAs on adverse events that score high on the NCPS Safety Assessment Code is mandatory. Those incidents that are reported locally must be transmitted to the NCPS.	Voluntary.
Reportable events/events monitored	Close calls: Defined as events or situations that could have resulted in an accident, injury, or illness but did not, either by chance or through timely intervention. Adverse events: Defined as untoward incidents, therapeutic misadventures, iatrogenic injuries, or other adverse occurrences directly associated with care or services provided within the jurisdiction of a medical center, outpatient clinic, or other facility. Adverse events may result from acts of commission or omission. An event that is believed by a potential reporter to be a result of an "intentionally unsafe act" is NOT to be reported to the NCPS system but should be reported to the facility director or other authorities. An "intentionally unsafe act" is defined as a criminal act, a purposefully unsafe act, an act related to alcohol or substance abuse by an impaired provider and/or staff, or events involving alleged or suspected patient abuse of any kind.	Adverse events and close calls (as defined by NCPS) and lessons learned or safety ideas. Intentionally unsafe acts (as defined by NCPS) are NOT to be reported to PSRS.

Continued

TABLE C–1c *Continued*

Federal Agency	VHA	VHA/NASA
Name of System	National Center for Patient Safety Reporting System[a]	Patient Safety Reporting System[b]
Classification system and/or severity index	All close calls and adverse events are classified to establish their priority for analysis according to the Safety Assessment Code. The SAC matrix takes into account (1) the actual or potential severity of the event and (2) the probability of occurrence according to specific definitions. The matrix scores are 3 = highest risk, 2 = intermediate risk, and 1 = lowest risk. When developing root-cause/contributing factor (RC/CF) statements, the team uses a paper tool called "NCPS Triage Cards" that include several prompting questions. The applicable questions are documented with the RC/CF statements. Additionally, four types of events —falls, medication errors, missing patients, and parasuicidal behavior—are categorized for aggregate RCA review. Additional categorization of reports began in late 2002 using an NCPS-developed Primary Analysis and Categorization (PAC) methodology, which includes key attributes of the event such as the location of occurrence within the VA Medical Center, the activity or process under way at the time, and other aspects of the adverse events or close calls.	The reporter enters data that can aid in categorization or sorting of reports, such as staff position, where the event occurred, the time of occurrence, environmental factors that may have contributed, and other factors such as medical devices or medical records that may have been involved.

TABLE C–1c *Continued*

Federal Agency	VHA	VHA/NASA
Name of System	National Center for Patient Safety Reporting System[a]	Patient Safety Reporting System[b]
Reporting time frame	Time frame from occurrence of event/close call to filing a report at an individual facility is determined by that facility's locally accepted method. Once an event/close call is entered into the Patient Safety Information System AND if an RCA is required, the facility has 45 days to complete the RCA.	None.
Data collected: Format and summary	Initial report is not in a standard format; each VA facility has its own locally accepted method of reporting an adverse event or close call to the local VAMC patient safety manager. The Patient Safety Information System is a computer-aided software tool (SPOT) that is used to record a standard set of data to be used to manage and analyze the adverse event or close call reported. Data collected in the Patient Safety Information System include date of event/close call; actual and potential SAC score; description of event/close call; type of event (if it falls into one of the four categories of falls, medication errors, missing patients, and parasuicidal behavior); flowcharts indicating the initial and final understanding of the event; references, resources, and personnel consulted in the investigation; root-cause contributing factors, lessons	Standard paper form that is mailed to NASA directly by the individual reporting the incident. Data collected include background information about the reporter's position and experience, general event characteristics, and a narrative description of the event.

Continued

TABLE C–1c *Continued*

Federal Agency	VHA	VHA/NASA
Name of System	National Center for Patient Safety Reporting System[a]	Patient Safety Reporting System[b]
	learned, and corrective actions to be taken; and the outcome measures for each action, concurrence, and dialogue with leadership and time, money, and resources expended for RCAs.	
Method of reporting	VA personnel can use a facility's locally accepted method of reporting an adverse event or close call; a facility's Patient Safety Manager (PSM) then uses a computer-aided software tool to triage and manage the event. Safety reports and RCAs are sent in a secure electronic fashion to the NCPS database when completed.	Forms can be obtained in paper format from a VA medical facility or by requesting them from NASA or in electronic (PDF) format from the PSRS Internet homepage. Forms then must be filled out by hand and mailed to NASA.
Who reports	Any VA personnel can report to each facility's PSM.	Any VA personnel.
RCA trigger	• All events with an actual SAC score of 3 receive a full RCA. • If a close call is a potential SAC score of 3 and it is one of the four categories indicated earlier, more data are collected and aggregated for an analysis done every quarter. • Any other close calls with a potential SAC score of 3 receive a full RCA. • At the discretion of the PSM and the facility director, any event or close call can undergo an RCA.	None (reports are not subject to RCA).

TABLE C–1c *Continued*

Federal Agency	VHA	VHA/NASA
Name of System	National Center for Patient Safety Reporting System[a]	Patient Safety Reporting System[b]
Follow-up (including RCA)	If an event/close call warrants an individual RCA, a team of frontline VA personnel not involved in the event under consideration performs the RCA. This team uses two tools: (1) a computer-aided software tool (SPOT) that leads them through the steps of an RCA and (2) a cognitive aid called "Triage Questions for Root-Cause Analysis." Then, based on the results of the RCA for an event/close call, corrective actions are proposed by the RCA team. The facility director can choose to "concur" or "nonconcur" with these proposed actions. If the director issues a "nonconcur" statement, he or she must furnish a written rationale for this decision; then the RCA team proposes an alternative correction action. The RCA team also outlines the parties responsible for enacting the corrective actions, including a due date and how the effectiveness of these actions will be evaluated to verify that they had the intended effect. Aggregate RCA review of the four most common events can be done quarterly. Additionally, VA personnel who submit reports that result in an RCA receive prompt feedback on actions being taken as a result of their report.	NASA will return a portion of the reporting form, called the Reporter Return Receipt, to the reporter as proof that the report has been received. Although NASA does not retain any of the information on the return receipt prior to being returned, that information on the receipt may be used to contact the reporter for clarifications if necessary. PSRS is designed to identify vulnerabilities but does not provide detailed solutions, except as proposed by the reporter.

Continued

TABLE C–1c *Continued*

Federal Agency	VHA	VHA/NASA
Name of System	National Center for Patient Safety Reporting System[a]	Patient Safety Reporting System[b]
	Informing patients: The VHA requires disclosure to patients who have been injured by adverse events. This is not associated with the RCA process and the results of RCAs are kept confidential, for use only in efforts to improve the quality and safety of care provided.	
Other information collected through the system	None.	None.
Confidentiality issues	RCAs of adverse events and close calls are protected from disclosure under 38 U.S.C. 5705, as part of a medical quality assurance program. Although there is a requirement to disclose adverse events to patients and families, legal restrictions limit disclosures that violate patient privacy. Specifically, the Privacy Act limits disclosures to families, and 38 U.S.C. 7332 limits disclosures related to a patient's treatment for substance abuse, sickle cell anemia disease, and HIV status, even after a patient's death. No patient or VA personnel identifiers are included in the reports entered into the Patient Safety Information System, which contains RCA information.	PSRS reports are considered confidential and privileged quality assurance documents under the provisions of 38 U.S.C. 5705. PSRS removes all personal names, facility names and locations, and other potentially identifying information before entering reports into its database.

TABLE C–1c *Continued*

Federal Agency	VHA	VHA/NASA
Name of System	National Center for Patient Safety Reporting System[a]	Patient Safety Reporting System[b]
	VA has developed detailed guidance on disclosing adverse events that is available online at http://www.va.gov/publ/direc/health/infolet/10200301.pdf.	
Relationship with other reporting systems	No direct relationships.	No direct relationships. It is designed to be complementary to the VA's NCPS Reporting System.
Relationships with JCAHO/ Medicare certification	If an event is an actual adverse event meeting the JCAHO definition of reviewable sentinel event, the facility can make the determination if it will report the event to JCAHO. If an event is reported to JCAHO, then the results of the RCA are also reported to JCAHO. VHA policy requiring disclosure to patients who have been injured by adverse events is consistent with JCAHO requirements that hospitalized patients and their families be told of "unanticipated outcomes" of care.	None.

II. STATE REPORTING SYSTEMS

Overview

In April 2000, the National Academy for State Health Policy (NASHP) reported on a survey to determine the extent states had developed reporting systems for medical errors and adverse events (Rosenthal et al., 2000). All 50 states and the District of Columbia responded to the survey. The survey found that 15 states required mandatory reporting from acute and general hospitals of adverse events. Twenty-one states now require reporting (Rosenthal, 2003).

For illustrative purposes, this section of Appendix C gives an overview of the state-based reporting systems in place in New York and Florida (see Table C–2). These systems represent the broad differences in the types of reporting systems that have been developed to date. For a comprehensive review of the reporting systems for all 21 states, refer to the NASHP Web site at http://www.nashp.org.

Reportable Events

The NASHP reports (Rosenthal et al., 2000, 2001) confirmed the lack of a universal definition of the terms "adverse event" and "medical error." Some states do not have generic definitions and, instead, specify the types of events that must be reported.

New York State provides the following preamble: "For the purpose of the New York Patient Occurrence and Reporting System (NYPORTS) reporting, an occurrence is an unintended adverse and undesirable development in an individual patient's condition occurring in a hospital." New York State also provides a detailed list of events that must be reported (see Table C–2a).

Florida provides this preamble: "The term 'adverse incident' means an event over which health care personnel could exercise control and which is associated in whole or in part with medical intervention, rather than the condition for which such intervention occurred, and which results in one of the following injuries." Lists of events for annual report and code 15 report are provided in Table C–2e.

Format for Reporting

Most states have specified formats for reporting. The 2001 NASHP study examined the commonality of data requirements for eight states and discovered the following:

- All states collected information on the facility name, the date the incident occurred, and the type of incident.
- A majority of states collected information on patient identification, provider identification, description of the incident, person reporting the incident, action taken by facility, patient outcome, and notification to other parties (e.g., professional bodies).
- A minority of states collected information on the identity of witnesses.

In New York State, certain categories of occurrences (i.e., codes 201–854 in Table C–2a) only require the submission of a short form (the data collected are in Table C–2b). There is no specific time frame for reporting these occurrences. The idea is to aggregate the data for each category and carry out trend analyses to identify areas where a review of the process might yield improvements. A second set of codes (i.e., 901, 902, 914, 931–935, and 939 at the end of Table C–2a) represent more serious events or those that are statutorily required to be reported. These must reported within 24 hours or one business day from occurrence of the event. These also only require the submission of the short form (see Table C–2b). The final set of codes (i.e., 108–110, 911–913, 915–923, 938, 961–963 in Table C–2a) represent the most serious occurrences and require notification to the New York State Patient Safety Center within 24 hours or one business day from occurrence of the event using the short form (see Table C–2b) and an RCA carried out by the hospital (see Analysis of More Serious Events below).

Florida state law prescribes what data are to be collected. Some of the data elements are coded using existing health care data standards. All events in Table C–2e must be reported on annually, providing the data given in Table C–2f. More serious events must be reported on within 15 days (i.e., Code 15 reports—see Table C–2g for an overview of the data collected).

Method of Reporting

The most common method of delivery of information for state reporting systems is by fax. Regular or certified mail is also used (Rosenthal et al., 2001).

Of those included in the 2001 NASHP report, the New York State system has the most sophisticated delivery system—an Internet-based system with secure firewalls. The Florida system uses fax or certified mail.

Analysis of More Serious Events

Most states use the information collected to trigger on-site investigations and corrective action (Rosenthal et al., 2001), although RCAs are not always explicitly required.

As noted earlier, in New York State the most serious offenses (i.e., codes 108–110, 911–913, 915–923, 938, and 961–963 in Table C–2a) require notification to the New York State Patient Safety Center within 24 hours or one business day from occurrence of the event and an RCA carried out by the hospital. The RCA must be completed within 30 days and reported electronically to NYPORTS (an overview of the data required for the RCA is in Table C–2c). Medication errors (i.e., codes 108–110) are recognized as a special category and therefore require the collection of additional data (see Table C–2d).

The Florida reporting system does not explicitly require the carrying out of formal RCAs for any group of reportable events. However, code 15 reports require an extensive data collection exercise and descriptions of the causes of the incident and corrective or proactive actions taken (see Table C–2f).

Tabular Information

- Table C–2: General information on the New York State and Florida reporting systems.
- Table C–2a: New York State reportable events.
- Table C–2b: Data collected for all New York State reportable events.
- Table C–2c: Overview of the data required for all New York State reportable events needing an RCA.
- Table C–2d: Extra data for all New York State reportable medication errors.
- Table C–2e: Florida State reportable events.
- Table C–2f: Data collected annually for all Florida State reportable events.
- Table C–2g: Data collected with 15 days for all serious Florida State reportable events.

TABLE C–2 Selected Examples: The New York and Florida Reporting Systems

State	New York
Name of System	New York Patient Occurrence Reporting and Tracking System[b]
Type of system	Reporting.
History of reporting/ surveillance system	Initial regulations requiring incident reporting were promulgated in 1985. Shortly after, a medical malpractice crisis during the mid-1980s led to the enactment of a statutory reporting requirement—New York State Public Health Law Section 2805-1, Incident Reporting, which created the NYPORTS reporting system. The system covers all hospitals (inpatient and outpatient) and extension clinics listed on its Article 28 operating certificate. Freestanding diagnostic and treatment centers, including ambulatory surgery centers, report a limited list of incidents to the New York State Department of Health (NYSDOH) by regulation, such as patient deaths or transfers to hospitals. It does not cover long-term care (e.g., nursing homes, hospices), private medical practices, retail pharmacies, and home care.
Voluntary or mandatory	Mandatory.
Reportable events/ events monitored	For the purpose of NYPORTS reporting, an occurrence is an unintended adverse and undesirable development in an individual patient's condition occurring in a hospital.

---

[a]Information on the Florida State reporting system has been obtained from Florida Health and Human Services, Agency for Health Care Administration (2003); personal communication, A. Polk, Florida Agency for Health Care Administration, 2002; Rosenthal et al. (2001).

[b]Information on the New York Patient Occurrence Reporting and Tracking System has been obtained from the following sources: New York Patient Occurrence Reporting and Tracking System (2001) and Rosenthal et al. (2001).

Florida[a]

Reporting.

The medical malpractice crisis during the mid-1980s led to the promulgation of the Comprehensive Medical Malpractice Act of 1985, with provisions mandating reporting of adverse or untoward incidents to the Agency for Health Care Administration (AHCA), Bureau of Health Facility Regulation. Legislation modified the reporting requirements in 1998, adding a 24-hour reporting provision and narrowing the scope of reportable incidents.

Mandatory.

For purposes of reporting, the term "adverse incident" means an event over which health care personnel could exercise control and which is associated in whole or in part with medical intervention, rather than the condition for which such intervention occurred, and which:
1. Results in one of the following injuries:

a. Death;
b. Brain or spinal damage;
c. Permanent disfigurement;
d. Fracture or dislocation of bones or joints;
e. A resulting limitation of neurological, physical, or sensory function that continues after discharge from the facility;
f. Any condition that required specialized medical attention or surgical intervention resulting from nonemergency medical intervention, other than an emergency medical condition, to which the patient has not given informed consent; or
g. Any condition that required the transfer of the patient, within or outside the facility, to a unit providing a more acute level of care due to the adverse incident, rather than the patient's condition prior to the adverse incident;

Continued

TABLE C–2 *Continued*

State	New York

Name of System	New York Patient Occurrence Reporting and Tracking System[b]

Classification system and/or severity index	Serious occurrences (codes 108–110, 911–913, 915–923, 938, 961–963, below): patient deaths unrelated to the natural course of illness, disease, or proper treatment in accordance with generally accepted medical standards; injuries and impairments of bodily functions in circumstances other than those related to the natural course of illness, disease, or proper treatment in accordance with generally accepted medical standards; equipment malfunction resulting in death or serious injury. Less serious occurrences (codes 201–854): adverse events with less serious patient outcomes, such as complications of surgery, burns, and falls. Other occurrences (codes 901, 902, 914, 931–935, and 939), fires or external disasters, strikes, and unscheduled termination of services vital to the continued safe operation of the facility or safety of its patients and personnel. See Table C–2a for a detailed list of NYPORTS codes.
Reporting time frame	• Serious occurrences: 24 hours/one business day. • Other occurrences: 24 hours/one business day. • Less serious occurrences: Within 30 days.
Data collected: Format and summary	• Serious occurrences: Short form (see Table C–2b) plus RCA. Extra data collected for medication errors (see Table C–2d). • Other occurrences: Short form (see Table C–2b) only. • Less serious occurrences: Short form (see Table C–2b) only.

Florida[a]

2. Was the performance of a surgical procedure on the wrong patient, a wrong surgical procedure, a wrong-site surgical procedure, or a surgical procedure otherwise unrelated to the patient's diagnosis or medical condition;
3. Required the surgical repair of damage resulting to a patient from a planned surgical procedure, where the damage was not a recognized specific risk, as disclosed to the patient and documented through the informed-consent process; or
4. Was a procedure to remove unplanned foreign objects remaining from a surgical procedure.

(1) Events that need to be reported within 15 days (code 15 reports—see Table C–2e).
(2) Events that must be reported on an annual basis (annual reports—see Table C–2e).

As identified above, events need to be reported:
- Within 15 days, or
- On an annual basis.

Notification to patient: An appropriately trained person designated by each licensed facility shall inform each patient, or the individual identified as the patient's health care surrogate, in person about adverse incidents that result in serious harm to the patient. Such notice shall be given as soon as possible to allow the patient an opportunity to minimize damage or injury.

Code 15 report.
Annual report.
See Tables C–2f, C–2g, and C–2h for details.

Continued

TABLE C–2 *Continued*

State	New York
Name of System	New York Patient Occurrence Reporting and Tracking System[b]
Method of reporting	Internet based with secure fire walls.
Who reports	Identified contact within facility; usually risk managers or quality divisions.
RCA trigger	All serious occurrences require an RCA or are performed at the request of the DOH.
Follow-up (including RCA)	The RCA must be completed within 30 days and reported electronically to NYPORTS (see Table C–2c for more information on the RCA form).
Other information collected through the system	None.
Confidentiality issues	Statutory provisions make reports that are submitted in compliance with the reporting requirement confidential and protect individuals making reports from civil lawsuits and monetary damages (Public Health Law 2805–m). The confidentiality provisions have been challenged under the state's Freedom of Information law. In a 1997 decision, the court ruled that under this law, incident reports are protected by the confidentiality statute. However, the court ruled that hospital-specific aggregate (annual) data can be released.
Relationship with other reporting systems	Within hospitals/freestanding clinics, there are other relevant New York State reporting systems—cardiac adverse events, perinatal adverse events, and hemolytic transfusion reactions and other types of blood- and tissue-related adverse events. These four systems collect and analyze statistics—RCA is not mandated, but in-depth assessment similar to RCA is undertaken for the hemolytic and radiologic events by their respective systems. None of the reporting systems are managed by the New York State Patient Safety Center.

Florida[a]

Fax or certified mail.

Each facility has a risk manager who collects the adverse event information.

The term "root-cause analysis" is not used in the statute; however, the statute does require the facility to investigate and analyze adverse incidents and to develop appropriate measures and other innovative approaches to minimize the risk of adverse incidents to patients. The Code 15 report requires an analysis of the cause of the incident and a list of the corrective or proactive actions taken.

As indicated above, a Code 15 report includes some description of the cause of the event and corrective or proactive actions taken. AHCA may require further documentation from the facility about the incident and its corrective action plan (or RCA), and/or can initiate a survey to assess risk management functions related to the adverse incident (patient safety) and patient quality of care.

Biennial risk management survey required of all licensed hospitals and ambulatory surgical centers. AHCA is collecting data on the citation for nonreporting of adverse incidents.

Statutory provision makes reports of an adviser and untoward incidents confidential and not subject to discovery or admission Into evidence in civil lawsuits. There has been no challenge to this provision to date.
Notification to patient of outcomes of care that result in harm to the patient under the section on patient notification shall not constitute an acknowledgment or admission of liability, nor can it be introduced as evidence.

Information is shared with professional boards. The Commission for Excellence in Health Care is exploring the coordination of data sources. Although AHCA is not responsible for the intake of complaints, the agency does investigate them and store information in a common database with incident reports.

Continued

TABLE C–2 *Continued*

State	New York
Name of System	New York Patient Occurrence Reporting and Tracking System[b]
	Although there is some degree of overlap among these systems and NYPORTS, efforts were made to reduce duplicative reporting as much as possible. In addition to the above three systems and NYPORTS, there is a voluntary "complaints" system covering all aspects of health care in the state. Complaints are processed on a case-by-case basis. Some effort is being made to integrate the complaints system and NYPORTS.
Relationships with JCAHO/Medicare certification	The New York State Department of Health does not deem JCAHO accreditation. However, it has a contract with JCAHO to share surveillance information. The contract is based on information sharing of the overall process, which includes complaint and incident investigations and a range of other surveillance activities. Additionally, there is direct overlap between the JCAHO sentinel events and NYPORTS serious events, with the exception of hemolytic transfusion reactions, which are captured in another unit within DOH.

Florida[a]

The Florida Agency for Health Care Administration deems JCAHO accreditation as meeting its biennial licensure requirements. The agency performs validation surveys on approximately 5 percent of JCAHO-accredited facilities each year as directed by CMS.

TABLE C–2a NYPORTS Reportable Events

Broad Category	Codes
Medication errors	108. A medication error occurred that resulted in permanent patient harm (harm that is enduring and cannot be rectified by treatment). 109. A medication error occurred that resulted in a near-death event (e.g., cardiac or respiratory arrest requiring Basic Life Support (BLS) or Advanced Cardiac Life Support (ACLS). 110. A medication error occurred that resulted in a patient death.
Aspiration	201. Aspiration pneumonitis/pneumonia in a nonintubated patient related to conscious sedation.
Intravascular catheter related	301. Necrosis or infection requiring repair (incision and drainage, debridgement, or other surgical intervention), regardless of the location of the repair. 302. Volume overload leading to pulmonary edema. 303. Pneumothorax, regardless of size or treatment.
Embolic and related disorders	401. New, acute pulmonary embolism, confirmed, or suspected and treated. 402. New documented deep-vein thrombosis.
Laparoscopic	501. All unplanned conversions to an open procedure because of an injury and/or bleeding during the laparoscopic procedure.
Perioperative/ periprocedural related	601. Any new central neurological deficit (e.g., stroke, hypoxic/anoxic encephalopathy). 602. Any new peripheral neurological deficit (e.g., palsy, paresis) with motor weakness. 603. Cardiac arrest with successful resuscitation. 604. Acute myocardial infarction—unrelated to a cardiac procedure. 605. Death occurring after procedure (specific to list of 10 procedures).
Burns, falls	701. Second- and/or third-degree burns. 751. Falls resulting in x-ray-proven fractures, subdural or epidural hematoma, cerebral contusion, traumatic subarachnoid hemorrhage, and/or internal trauma.
Procedure related	801. Procedure-related injury requiring repair, removal of an organ, or other procedural intervention. 803. Hemorrhage or hematoma requiring drainage, evacuation, or other procedural intervention. 804. Anastomatic leakage requiring repair.

TABLE C–2a *Continued*

Broad Category	Codes

	805. Wound dehiscence requiring repair.
	806. Displacement, migration, or breakage of an implant, device, graft, or drain, whether repaired, intentionally left in place, or removed.
	807. Thrombosed distal bypass graft requiring repair.
	808. Post-op wound infection following clean or clean/contaminated case, requiring drainage during the hospital stay or inpatient admission within 30 days. ASA class required.
	819. Any unplanned operation or reoperation related to the primary procedure, regardless of setting of primary procedure.
	851. Postpartum hysterectomy.
	852. Inverted uterus.
	853. Ruptured uterus.
	854. Circumcision requiring repair.
RCA required	911. Wrong patient, wrong site—surgical procedure.
	912. Incorrect procedure or treatment—invasive.
	913. Unintentionally retained foreign body due to inaccurate surgical count or break in procedural technique.
RCA required: Any unexpected adverse occurrence not directly related to the natural course of the patient's illness or underlying condition resulting in:	915. Death (e.g., brain death).
	916. Cardiac and/or respiratory arrest requiring BLS/ALCS intervention.
	917. Loss of limb or organ.
	918. Impairment of limb and Impairment present at discharge or for at least 2 weeks after occurrence if patient is not discharged.
	919. Loss or impairment of bodily function and present at discharge or for at least 2 weeks after occurrence if patient is not discharged.
	920. Errors of omission/delay resulting in death or serious injury related to the patient's underlying condition.
	921. Crime resulting in death or serious injury, as defined in 915–919.
	922. Suicides and attempted suicides with serious injury, as defined in 915–919.
	923. Elopement from the hospital resulting in death or serious injury, as defined in 915–919.
	938. Malfunction of equipment during treatment or diagnosis or a defective product that resulted in death or serious injury, as defined in 915–919.
	961. Infant abduction.
	962. Infant discharged to wrong family.
	963. Rape by another patient or staff (including alleged rape with clinical confirmation).

Continued

TABLE C–2a *Continued*

Broad Category	Codes
RCA NOT required	901. Serious occurrence warranting DOH notification, not covered by 911–963. 902. Patient transferred to the hospital from the diagnostic and treatment center. 914. Misadministration of radioactive material (as defined by the Bureau of Environmental Radioactive Protection, section 16.25, 10NYCRR). 931. Strike by hospital staff. 932. External disaster outside the control of the hospital that affects facility operations. 933. Termination of services vital to the continued safe operation of the hospital or to the health and safety of its patients or personnel (e.g., electricity, laundry services). 934. Poisonings occurring within the hospital (water, air, food). 935. Hospital fire disrupting patient care or causing harm to patients or staff. 937. Malfunction of equipment during treatment or diagnosis or a defective product that has a potential for adversely affecting patient or hospital personnel or resulting in a retained foreign body.

TABLE C–2b NYPORTS Short Form

The short form collects a limited amount of data items, including the following:

- Occurrence date
- Occurrence code (three-digit code above)
- ICD–9–CM code corresponding to the diagnosis for which patient was admitted
- ICD–9 procedure code most closely associated with occurrence
- Hospital medical record number
- Location in hospital where incident occurred
- SPARCS number—the Statewide Planning and Research Cooperative System is a comprehensive patient data system
- The service for which the patient was originally admitted
- Date of birth
- Sex
- Admission date
- Readmission date
- Do you believe that this occurrence will likely lead to (check all that apply) no action, change in policy, formal education/reeducation, discipline taken, process improvement, don't know yet?
- Brief summary of occurrence
- Description of any process improvement that others could learn from
- Any lesson learned that could be globally beneficial to others
- Report date and reporter—automatically filled in
- Hospital name
- Incident ID number

TABLE C–2c NYPORTS Root-Cause Analysis Form

The root-cause analysis form requires a description of the occurrence, answers to several yes/no questions about why the occurrence happened, and the details of a corrective action plan. The "why it happened" section consists of about 30 questions under several headings:

- Policy or process (system) in which the event occurred
- Human resource factors and issues
- Environment of care, including equipment and other related factors
- Information management and communication issues
- Standard of care
- Leadership: Corporate culture

An example question is, "Staff are properly qualified, yes/no?" If the answer to a question is "no," the respondent must elaborate on the root cause, develop a plan for improvement, and develop measures to assess effectiveness of risk reduction strategies.

Other elements required in the RCA form are:

- Literature search
- Executive summary
- List of participant titles

TABLE C–2d NYPORTS Medication Supplement

For codes 108–110 the following extra information is collected:

- Type of occurrence (e.g., wrong patient, wrong drug, wrong dose, wrong route, wrong frequency, wrong time, omission, administration after order discontinued/expired, wrong diluent/concentration/dosage form, monitoring error, other)
- Where in the process (e.g., prescribing, transcription, dispensing, administration, documentation on medical administration record)
- Medication given
- Medication intended to be given
- Categories of staff involved
- Discovery date/time
- How the occurrence was discovered

TABLE C–2e Florida State Reportable Events

Events that need to be reported within 15 days (Code 15 reports):

All the above, plus the following:
- The death of a patient
- Brain or spinal damage to a patient
- The performance of a surgical procedure on the wrong patient
- The performance of a wrong site surgical procedure
- The performance of a wrong surgical procedure
- Surgical procedure that is unnecessary or otherwise unrelated to the patient's diagnosis or medical condition
- The surgical repair of damage resulting to a patient from a planned surgical procedure, where the damage is not a recognized specific risk, as disclosed to the patient and documented through the informed-consent process
- The performance of procedures to remove unplanned foreign objects remaining from a surgical procedure

Events that must be reported on an annual basis (annual reports):

All the above, plus the following:
- Permanent disfigurement
- Fracture or dislocation of bones or joints
- A resulting limitation of neurological, physical, or sensory function that continues after discharge from the facility
- Any condition that requires specialized medical attention or surgical intervention resulting from nonemergency medical intervention, other than an emergency medical condition, to which the patient has not given informed consent
- Any condition that required the transfer of the patient, within or outside the facility, to a unit providing a more acute level of care due to the adverse incident, rather than the patient's condition prior to the adverse incident

TABLE C–2f Florida State Annual Report

- Facility information
- Total number of reportable incidents; total number of surgical incidents; total number of diagnostic incidents; total number of other actions causing injury
- Surgical, diagnostic, or treatment procedure being performed at time of incident (using ICD–9 Codes 01–99.9)
- Other actions causing medical injuries (using ICD–9 E Codes and Codes 800–999.9)
- Accident, event, circumstances, or specific agent that caused the injury or event (using ICD–9 E Codes)
- Resulting injury (using ICD–9 Codes 800–999.9)
- License numbers of personnel (or social security numbers of unlicensed personnel) directly involved in incident and relationship to facility
- A description of all malpractice claims filed against the facility, including the nature of the incident, license numbers of persons involved in the claim, and the status or disposition of each claim
- Total number of new claims
- Total number of claims pending
- Total number of claims closed during the reporting year
- Copy of the facility's policies and procedures to reduce risk of patient injuries and adverse incidents
- Copy of each regular summary to the facility governing board from the risk manager for the calendar year

TABLE C–2g Florida State Code 15 Report

- Facility information
- Patient information (i.e., name, identification number, address, age, sex, Medicaid/ Medicare, date of admission, admitting diagnosis, ICD–9 code for admit diagnosis)
- Incident information (date/time/location)
- Notification of medical examiner (yes/no/name/contact number)
- Autopsy performed (yes/no)
- Description of incident
- Surgical, diagnostic, or treatment procedure being performed at time of incident (using ICD–9 Codes 01–99.9)
- Accident, event, circumstances, or specific agent that caused the injury or event (using ICD–9 E Codes)
- Resulting injury (using ICD–9 Codes 800–999.9)
- List any equipment directly involved in incident
- Outcome (e.g., death, fetal death, brain damage, spinal damage, surgical procedure performed on the wrong patient, surgical procedure performed on the wrong site, wrong surgical procedure performed, surgical procedure unrelated to patient's diagnosis, surgical procedure to remove foreign objects remaining from a surgical procedure, surgical repair of injuries from a planned surgical procedure)
- License numbers of personnel and capacity or social security numbers of unlicensed personnel directly involved in incident
- License numbers of witnesses or docial decurity numbers of unlicensed witnesses)
- Analysis of cause of incident (description)
- Corrective or proactive actions taken (description)

III. PRIVATE-SECTOR REPORTING SYSTEMS

Overview

In the private sector, a number of initiatives are working to develop patient safety and/or health care reporting and surveillance systems. Some of these systems are being developed by universities and companies for use in multiple health care organizations and settings, whereas others are being developed by hospital systems for their own internal use or by groups with an interest in specific nonhospital-based practice settings (e.g., family practices). This section addresses the first of these system types.

As noted earlier, it is not the intention of this appendix to be comprehensive but instead to review a representative sample of the patient safety reporting and surveillance systems that are being developed in the private sector. The four private-sector systems summarized in the attached tables were all established for reporting purposes. These systems are:

• **The Medical Event Reporting System for Transfusion Medicine (MERS-TM)**, which is primarily based and managed at Columbia University and is funded under a grant from the National Heart, Lung, and Blood Institute of the National Institutes of Health.
• **The Medication Errors Reporting (MER) Program**, which is operated by the United States Pharmacopeia (USP) in cooperation with the Institute for Safe Medication Practices (ISMP).
• **MedMARx**, which is owned and managed by USP.
• **The Joint Commission on Accreditation of Healthcare Organizations (JCAHO) Sentinel Event Policy**

All of these systems were initiated in the 1990s. The longest operating of the four is the USP MER Program, which was begun in 1991 through a USP partnership with the ISMP. USP then purchased the MER Program from ISMP in 1994, but the two organizations continue to operate the system jointly.

In addition, all of these are essentially voluntary nonpunitive systems, with the possible exception of the JCAHO Sentinel Event Policy. JCAHO-accredited organizations are "encouraged, but not required" to report events meeting its criteria for reviewable sentinel events (see the "Reportable events" row of Table C–3b for more detail). However, if the Joint Commission becomes aware of a reviewable sentinel event that occurred at an accredited organization and was not reported, then that organization must prepare and submit an RCA and action plan to JCAHO. If an acceptable RCA and action plan are not submitted to the Joint Commission within a designated time frame, then the organization can be placed on Accreditation Watch and risk its accreditation status being changed to Preliminary Non-Accreditation or Not Accredited.

Reportable Events

Because these four systems were developed by private organizations and are essentially voluntary, they tend to be more limited in their scope than the federal patient safety/health care reporting systems. MERS-TM, the MER Program, and MedMARx systems focus on specific types of events based on what is believed to have caused the event—blood components/transfusion services and medication errors. MERS-TM and MedMARx also collect reports of near-miss events. Of these three systems, MERS-TM and the MER Program are the most applicable across multiple health care practice settings, whereas MedMARx is currently limited to hospital reporting of medication errors. In fact, MERS-TM is in the process of expanding the current transfusion medicine-based near-miss system to a hospital-wide application by investing in information technology for handling large amounts of incident data coming from many locations. The input forms feed directly into the database, which can compare incoming reports with those already in the database. However, all three of these systems are employed only by organizations that choose to participate, and therefore the three systems do not collect data on a nationwide level, as do several of the federal reporting and surveillance systems.

The Joint Commission's Sentinel Event Policy is more general than the other three—the types of events reported to JCAHO are not limited by causality. Any type of event meeting JCAHO's Sentinel Event definition (which may be interpreted slightly differently by each accredited organization) can be reported to JCAHO; however, the only events that must be reported are those meeting JCAHO's list of reviewable sentinel events (see the "Reportable events" row of Table C–3b for more detail). This system covers all organizations that are JCAHO accredited or seeking accreditation; approximately 80 percent of U.S. hospitals are currently involved in the JCAHO accreditation process (Joint Commission on Accreditation of Healthcare Organizations, 2002c).

Format for Reporting

Each system requires slightly different data to be reported, and most of them use a standard format for collecting these data (see "Data collected: Format and summary" row in Tables C–3a and C–3b). The only system that does not use a standard format is JCAHO. The Joint Commission does make a form available for organizations to use in self-reporting sentinel events but does not require use of the form. In addition, JCAHO allows RCAs and action plans to be conducted according to each organization's locally accepted method; however, these RCAs and action plans are required to be *thorough* and *credible* before they will be accepted by JCAHO. Most of these systems include patient information and information about the staff that were involved in, discovered, and in some cases reported an event, but no specific identifiers of individuals are used. In terms of classifying and/or coding the data collected, the MERS-TM and MedMARx systems have the most involved data models (see "Classification system and/or severity index" row in the tables).

Method of Reporting

Both the MER Program and MedMARx allow for online reporting of data, while the other two systems rely on paper forms transmitted via mail. The only one of the four that currently allows for reporting by patients and their families is JCAHO.

Analysis of More Serious Events

All of these systems have some means for following up on reported events. Three of the four have trigger mechanisms in place to indicate when an RCA should be conducted. Those three systems also provide guidelines for how to conduct the RCAs as well as for how to develop subsequent action plans. The exception in this area is the MER Program. Although the MER Program does not include RCAs event reports submitted to the program are forwarded to the FDA MedWatch system and to the product manufacturer where applicable. The FDA and the manufacturer can then follow up on these events as appropriate. In addition, events reported to MedMARx are also forwarded to the FDA.

The managers of the systems discussed in this section, with the exception of the MER Program, maintain a database of their reports. These databases then allow for data analysis, such as monitoring event trends so that alerts can be issued when necessary.

Tabular Information

All of this information is broken out in more detail in the following tables. Table C–3a includes MERS-TM, the MER Program, and MedMARx. Table C–3b includes JCAHO's Sentinel Event Policy.

TABLE C–3a Selected Examples of Private Patient Safety/Health Care Reporting and Surveillance Systems

Name of System	Medical Event Reporting System for Transfusion Medicine[a]
System owner or manager	Primarily based at **Columbia University** (under a grant from the **National Heart, Lung, and Blood Institute** of the National Institutes of Health).
Type of system	Reporting.
History of reporting/ surveillance system	In 1995, the University of Texas (UT) Southwestern Medical Center at Dallas received a grant from the National Heart, Lung, and Blood Institute to design, develop, and implement an event-reporting system in transfusion medicine. UT Southwestern researchers brought together an interdisciplinary team of experts to design a prototype medical event-reporting system for transfusion medicine. The FDA, American Association of Blood Banks, America's Blood Centers, American Blood Resources Association, American Red Cross, and Blood Systems, Inc., all participated in the early design of MERS-TM. Initial implementation in hospital Transfusion Services and Blood Centers began in 1997. Management of the system moved to Columbia University in 1998, when the principal investigator relocated. MERS-TM has since grown from a PC-based to a Web-based system and is now in use in 27 transfusion services and one blood center. It is being piloted as the national system for Canada and Ireland (as a near-miss system).
Voluntary or mandatory	Voluntary.

[a]Information on MERS-TM has been obtained from the following sources: Battles et al. (1998), Callum et al. (2001), Columbia University (2001), Kaplan et al. (1998), and Westat (2001).

[b]Information on the MER Program has been obtained from the following sources: U.S. Pharmacopeia (1997, 2001).

[c]Information on MedMARx has been obtained from the following sources: Cousins (2001) and National Coordinating Council for Medication Error Reporting and Prevention (1998).

Medication Errors Reporting Program[b]	MedMARx[c]
United States Pharmacopeia	**United States Pharmacopeia**
Reporting.	Reporting.
In 1991, USP began coordinating the MER Program with the Institute for Safe Medication Practices; in 1994, USP purchased the MER Program from ISMP. The USP MER Program is presented in cooperation with ISMP.	In 1998, USP spearheaded the formation of the National Coordinating Council for Medication Error Reporting and Prevention (NCC MERP). NCC MERP established a standardized definition of medication error and an Index for Categorizing Medication Errors. The council has issued recommendations on the error-prone aspects of prescription writing, drug dispensing and administering, and on labeling and packaging of drug products. In early 1997, USP began receiving requests for guidance from risk managers, quality assurance staff, pharmacists, and nurses on medication error analysis and reporting. In response to these questions, USP developed MedMARx— an Internet-accessible medication errors database for hospitals to anonymously report to a centralized system that resides at USP.
Voluntary.	Voluntary.

Continued

TABLE C–3a *Continued*

Name of System	Medical Event Reporting System for Transfusion Medicine[a]
System owner or manager	Primarily based at **Columbia University** (under a grant from the **National Heart, Lung, and Blood Institute** of the National Institutes of Health).
Reportable events/ events monitored	The system monitors all events (error, incident, deviation, variance, discovery, occurrence, or adverse or sentinel event) related to blood components and transfusion services. An event is defined as an occurrence with a potentially negative outcome that most often results from both latent conditions and human/active error. This includes: Near-miss event: Event in which unwanted consequences were prevented because of recovery by identification and correction of the failure. Such a recovery could be by a planned barrier or critical control point or unplanned. No-harm event: Event that has actually occurred (no recovery action was taken), but no actual harm has come to the patient or the organization. Except for "luck" (or in health care, the robust nature of human physiology), these accidents would have become misadventures. Misadventure: Event in which there was no recovery and in which the patient has been harmed or the mission of the organization has been harmed or compromised.
Classification system and/or severity (risk assessment) index	At the local level, events are coded according to where/when in the work process the event was discovered and where/when the event occurred. Events are assigned causal codes, which are based on the Eindhoven Classification Model—Medical Version (ECM). MERS-TM has 20 codes for describing causes of both active and latent errors. These codes are divided among three groups of causes: technical factors, organizational factors, and human factors. Risk is measured as severity (or potential severity) multiplied by the probability of recurrence. Severity is termed the Quantified Estimate of Severity (QES) and the probability of recurrence is called Quantified Estimate of Probability (QEP). QES and QEP have numerical values assigned to them, and these numbers are multiplied to calculate the Risk Assessment Index (RAI) for an event. The RAI is then adjusted based on whether or not a product was issued and the type of recovery, if any.

Medication Errors Reporting Program[b]	MedMARx[c]
United States Pharmacopeia	**United States Pharmacopeia**
Medication errors (both actual and potential).	Medication errors: Defined by the NCC MERP as any preventable event that may cause or lead to inappropriate medication use or patient harm while the medication is in the control of the health care professional, patient, or consumer. Such events may be related to professional practice, health care products, procedures, and systems, including prescribing; order communications; product labeling, packaging, and nomenclature; compounding; dispensing; distribution; administration; education; monitoring; and use.

Events are categorized according to the categorization index developed by the NCC MERP. This index consists of nine categories (A through I):

No error

A. Circumstances or events that have the capacity to cause error.

Error, no harm

B. An error occurred, but the medication did not reach the patient.

C. An error occurred that reached the patient but did not cause patient harm.

D. An error occurred that reached the patient and required monitoring to confirm that it resulted in no harm to the patient and/or required intervention to preclude harm.

Events are categorized according to the categorization index developed by the NCC MERP. This index consists of nine categories (A through I):

No error

A. Circumstances or events that have the capacity to cause error.

Error, no harm

B. An error occurred, but the medication did not reach the patient.

C. An error occurred that reached the patient but did not cause patient harm.

D. An error occurred that reached the patient and required monitoring to confirm that it resulted in no harm to the patient and/or required intervention to preclude harm.

Continued

TABLE C–3a *Continued*

Name of System	Medical Event Reporting System for Transfusion Medicine[a]
System owner or manager	Primarily based at **Columbia University** (under a grant from the **National Heart, Lung, and Blood Institute** of the National Institutes of Health).

Reporting time frame	Not applicable.

Data collected: Format and summary	**Event Discovery Report** (standard format): *Section A:* Data collected include date and time of discovery, where the event was discovered, information about who

[a]Harm is defined as impairment of the physical, emotional, or psychological function or structure of the body and/or resulting pain.

Medication Errors Reporting Program[b]	MedMARx[c]
United States Pharmacopeia	**United States Pharmacopeia**

Error, harm

E. An error occurred that may have contributed to or resulted in temporary harm to the patient and required intervention.

F. An error occurred that may have contributed to or resulted in temporary harm to the patient and required initial or prolonged care.

G. An error occurred that may have contributed to or resulted in permanent patient harm.

H. An error occurred that required intervention necessary to sustain life.

Error, death

I. An error occurred that may have contributed to or resulted in the patient's death.

Not applicable.

Standard format: Data collected include description of event (actual or potential), type of staff or health care practitioner

Error, harm[d]

E. An error occurred that may have contributed to or resulted in temporary harm to the patient and required intervention.

F. An error occurred that may have contributed to or resulted in temporary harm to the patient and required initial or prolonged care.

G. An error occurred that may have contributed to or resulted in permanent patient harm.

H. An error occurred that required intervention necessary to sustain life.

Error, death

I. An error occurred that may have contributed to or resulted in the patient's death.

The NCC MERP also developed a standard taxonomy for use in classifying and coding all of the data elements in the reports.

Not applicable. However, a hospital may hold a report aside in the database for 45 days in order to ensure that it has collected all of the necessary information and performed necessary follow-up and that the information in the database is as complete and accurate as possible. During this time, other hospitals cannot view that report.

Standard format: Amount of data collected is related to the category of error; therefore, category A error reports

Continued

TABLE C–3a *Continued*

Name of System	Medical Event Reporting System for Transfusion Medicine[a]
System owner or manager	Primarily based at **Columbia University** (under a grant from the **National Heart, Lung, and Blood Institute** of the National Institutes of Health).

discovered the event, a description of what was discovered and how it was discovered, when in the work sequence the event was discovered, and the action taken with regard to the product or record.

Section B: Data collected include date and time of occurrence, job classification and name of person involved in the event, where in the process the event first occurred, location of the occurrence, and information about whether the product was issued and administered.

Quality Assurance Systems Operator (QA Sys Op)[e] Investigation Report (standard format):

First section: Data collected include the report accession number, event codes, an additional description of the event, risk information, follow-up action, preventive action to be taken, and type of investigation the event will receive.

Second section: Cause codes and other information for events undergoing routine investigation. Option to link to a similar event already in the database.

Third section: Used to record notes.

Causal Tree Worksheet (standard format, but boxes can be added or deleted as necessary): Data collected include the consequent event, antecedent events, root causes, and root-cause classification codes.

Root-Cause Analysis Report (standard format): Consequent event code and description, antecedent events codes and descriptions, and system action.

---

[e]Information on the Joint Commission on Accreditation of Healthcare Organizations (JCAHO) Sentinel Event Policy has been obtained from the following sources: Joint Commission on Accreditation of Healthcare Organizations (2002a, c), and Schyve (2002).

Medication Errors Reporting Program[b]	MedMARx[c]
United States Pharmacopeia	**United States Pharmacopeia**

who made the initial error, patient outcome, any intervention that prevented the medication from reaching the patient, who discovered the error, when and how the error was discovered, where the error occurred, if another practitioner was involved in the error, if patient counseling wasprovided, description of product involved, relevant patient information (no patient identifiers included), recommendations by reporter as to how to prevent this error in the future, reporter information, and whether or not the reporter chooses to have his/her information released to the manufacturer, the FDA, or other persons.

capture significantly less information than reports on category E errors, where the patient is harmed.

Data collected for category E errors and above are as follows: date and time of error, description of event, type of error, possible causes of error, contributing factors, node in the process at which initial error occurred (e.g., prescribing, dispensing), location at which error was made, level of staff who made the initial error, level of staff who were involved in the error, level of staff who discovered the error, actions taken to avoid similar errors of this type, and a summary of the RCA.

Once these elements are completed, if a product is involved, information can be entered about that product. These data include generic and brand names; therapeutic classification; dosage, route, and strength; manufacturer; repacker; compounded ingredients; and container.

Also, for error categories C through I, a patient profile section captures data that include age and gender, outcome, and other relevant information.

Standardized pick lists are used for nearly all of the data entries; however, reporters are not limited to these lists. These pick lists are constructed based on the NCC MERP Taxonomy of Medication Errors.

Continued

TABLE C–3a *Continued*

Name of System	Medical Event Reporting System for Transfusion Medicine[a]
System owner or manager	Primarily based at **Columbia University** (under a grant from the **National Heart, Lung, and Blood Institute** of the National Institutes of Health).
Method of reporting	MERS-TM is a Web-based system. Paper forms may be downloaded if desired for initial data collection, or information may be entered directly into the hospital's database. The server resides at Columbia University.
Who reports	Everyone in a participating organization is encouraged to report any and all events that have the potential for having an adverse effect on blood products or patient or donor safety.
RCA trigger	For events that are new or unique or that have an RAI of ≥0.5, the QA Sys Op performs/facilitates RCAs and constructs causal trees to further characterize the event. In addition, if an event has an RAI of less than 0.5, BUT it represents a significant risk to the organization (i.e., potential for financial loss or damaged reputation), the QA Sys Op may decide to perform an expanded investigation.
Follow-up (including RCA)	The data are collected and interpreted for three main purposes: modeling, monitoring, and mindfulness. Modeling the types of events and recovery steps that occur in the transfusion process allows for the identification of factors or system elements that have the potential to cause future errors. Monitoring the existing areas of concern to determine whether the incidence of near misses and accidents is changing and to evaluate the impact of corrective actions. Mindfulness increases alertness by disseminating information about potential risks and error-producing precursors. RAI value (<0.5 – monitor; ≥0.5 and ≤0.7 – monitor and consider change; >0.7 – propose change), and the potential for organizational risk. Two MERS-TM software tools allow for database searching and monitoring. "Query by Field" searches for events with exact matches to user-selected fields. "HAWK" is

Medication Errors Reporting Program[b]	MedMARx[c]
United States Pharmacopeia	**United States Pharmacopeia**
Online or by mail or fax.	Online.
Individuals in hospitals that do not participate in MEDMARx and health professionals who practice in other settings.	There is usually a "gatekeeper" or administrator at each hospital who is responsible for releasing records into the system—most often this person is the pharmacist. However, multiple users are permitted at each site and may be given read-only or read-and-write levels of access by the administrator.
None.	All errors that result in harm as defined by the NCC MERP—Category E to Category I errors—merit an RCA.
Reporters may be contacted with additional questions for clarification. Reports are forwarded to the FDA MedWatch system and to the manufacturer and those entities may conduct follow-up.	Hospitals should conduct RCAs on Category E to Category I errors. These RCAs can be conducted according to each hospital's locally accepted method. However, certain RCA data elements are collected for Category E to I errors in a standardized manner, using the NCC MERP taxonomy (see "Data collected" row above). In addition, the following options are available to participating hospitals: 1. They can track and analyze trends in medication errors through a standardized format that can be inculcated into the hospital's internal quality improvement

Continued

TABLE C–3a *Continued*

Name of System	Medical Event Reporting System for Transfusion Medicine[a]
System owner or manager	Primarily based at **Columbia University** (under a grant from the **National Heart, Lung, and Blood Institute** of the National Institutes of Health).
	based on the theories of case-based reasoning (CBR) and searches the database for similar cases based on weighted form fields. Users may analyze and interpret both their local data and the central aggregate database using preprogrammed online reports or by downloading their sites' data into Excel or Access. This allows for benchmarking. The local database is evaluated regularly to assess the effectiveness of the system and impact of corrective actions. After evaluation, regular feedback about the system to all staff and immediate feedback to incident reporters are strongly recommended. The central database is evaluated for trends and analyzed using data mining software.
Other information collected through the system	None.
Confidentiality issues	Event reporting is completely confidential and not linked to employee performance assessment.
Relationship with other reporting systems	Any events defined by the FDA as reportable are transmitted to the FDA's Blood Products Deviation (BPD) system.
Relationships with JCAHO/Medicare certification	For JCAHO-accredited organizations: All sentinel events meeting the JCAHO definition of a reviewable sentinel event can be reported to JCAHO (this is determined at the local level).

Medication Errors Reporting Program[b]	MedMARx[c]
United States Pharmacopeia	**United States Pharmacopeia**
	activities and pharmacy and therapeutics committee activities.
	2. They can do comparative analyses against similar institutions.
	3. Eventually, they will be able to use MedMARx for benchmarking.
None.	None.
Although reporters provide their contact information, they can require that their identities be kept anonymous when the reports are forwarded to ISMP, the FDA, the manufacturer, and other persons requesting a copy of their reports.	Reports are anonymous, but randomly assigned facility IDs (each facility only knows its own ID) are used to group the reports. These IDs are associated with facility profiles, which allow each facility to compare its information with similar facilities without knowing the actual identities of those facilities.
All information is forwarded to the FDA MedWatch system.	
	All sentinel events meeting the JCAHO definition of reviewable sentinel event can be downloaded into a JCAHO template located in MedMARx.

TABLE C–3b Selected Examples of Private Patient Safety/Health Care Reporting and Surveillance Systems

Name of System	Sentinel Event Policy[a]
System Owner or Manager	Joint Commission on Accreditation of Healthcare Organizations
Type of system	Reporting.
History of reporting/ surveillance system	JCAHO has been involved in patient safety reporting systems since 1995. In 1996, the Sentinel Event Policy was implemented. This was followed by the establishment of a Sentinel Event Database and the implementation of sentinel event standards. These standards were first included in the Joint Commission accreditation manual in 1999, and in July 2001 additional patient safety standards went into effect for hospitals.
Voluntary or mandatory	Voluntary; organizations are "encouraged, but not required" to report any sentinel event meeting the JCAHO criteria for reviewable sentinel events (see below). If the Joint Commission becomes aware of a reviewable sentinel event that occurred at an accredited organization, whether self-reported or not, that organization must prepare and submit an RCA and action plan to JCAHO or otherwise provide evidence of having completed a thorough and credible RCA and action plan (see "Method of reporting" below for available alternatives).
Reportable events/ events monitored	A sentinel event is defined as an unexpected occurrence involving death or serious physical or psychological injury, or the risk thereof. Serious injury specifically includes loss of limb or function. The phrase "or the risk thereof" includes any process variation for which a recurrence would carry a significant chance of a serious adverse outcome. Note that the definition does include "near misses." Such events are called "sentinel" because they signal the need for immediate investigation and response. The following events are defined as reviewable sentinel events and should be reported to JCAHO: 1. An event that has resulted in an unanticipated death or major permanent loss of function, not related to the natural course of the patient's illness or underlying condition or

[a]Information on the JCAHO Sentinel Event Policy has been obtained from the following sources: Joint Commission on Accreditation of Healthcare Organizations (2002a, b) and personal communication, P. Schyve, JCAHO, 2002.

TABLE C–3b *Continued*

Name of System	Sentinel Event Policy[a]
System Owner or Manager	Joint Commission on Accreditation of Healthcare Organizations

	2. An event that is one of the following (even if the outcome was not death or major permanent loss of function): (a) Suicide of a patient in a setting where the patient receives round-the-clock care (e.g., hospital, residential treatment center, crisis stabilization center), (b) Infant abduction or discharge to the wrong family, (c) Rape, (d) Hemolytic transfusion reaction involving administration of blood or blood products having major blood group incompatibilities, (e) Surgery on the wrong patient or wrong body part. Note: This subset of events excludes "near-miss" sentinel events.
Classification system and/or severity (risk assessment) index	No standard system. Leadership standard (LD.5.1) requires each accredited organization to define sentinel event for its own purposes in establishing mechanisms to identify, report, and manage these events. At a minimum, an organization's definition must include those events defined as reviewable sentinel events by JCAHO; however, they have latitude in setting more specific parameters to define "unexpected," "serious," and "the risk thereof."
Reporting time frame	If the Joint Commission becomes aware (through voluntary self-reporting or otherwise) of a reviewable sentinel event that occurred at an accredited organization, that organization must prepare and submit an RCA and action plan to JCAHO within 45 calendar days of the event or of becoming aware of the event. If an organization fails to submit or make available an acceptable RCA and action plan within 45 days, the Accreditation Committee can place the organization on Accreditation Watch.[b] An organization on Accreditation Watch has an additional 15 days to submit an acceptable RCA and action plan.
Data collected: Format and summary	There is a form that organizations may use when reporting the occurrence of a sentinel event. The information collected on this form includes name and address of organization, date of incident, textual summary of incident (which should not include

Continued

---

[b]Accreditation Watch status is considered information that can be publicly disclosed.

TABLE C–3b *Continued*

Name of System	Sentinel Event Policy[a]
System Owner or Manager	Joint Commission on Accreditation of Healthcare Organizations

	names of patients, caregivers, or other individuals involved in the event), method for sharing event-related information (via mail or one of the four alternatives—see "Method of reporting" below for more detail on these alternatives), and contact information for the event reporter. There are no standard formats for RCAs and action plans; they may be conducted according to each organization's locally accepted method. However, JCAHO does require that RCAs be *thorough* and *credible* before they will accept them (see "Follow-up" below for more detail on these requirements). In addition, JCAHO does provide a sample framework for an RCA and action plan, which may be used as an aid for organizing the steps in RCAs. The JCAHO Sentinel Event Database has certain required data elements that are abstracted from RCAs, action plans, and follow-up activities. The three major categories of data elements included are sentinel event data, root-cause data, and risk reduction data.
Method of reporting	The primary means of submitting RCAs and action plans to JCAHO is via the mail. JCAHO then acknowledges receipt of the information and, once it has been processed, will return the original RCA and destroy all remaining copies of the document. *Alternative 1:* The organization can schedule an appointment to personally bring the RCA and other sentinel event-related documents to the JCAHO headquarters building for review by JCAHO staff, then leave with all of these documents still in the organization's possession. *Alternative 2:* The organization can request an on-site review of the RCA and other sentinel event–related documents by a JCAHO surveyor. This surveyor can then review these documents and interview staff. No copy of the RCA will be retained by JCAHO. *Alternative 3:* The organization can request an on-site visit by a JCAHO surveyor to conduct interviews and review relevant documentation to obtain information about the process and findings of the RCA and action plan, without actually reviewing the RCA documents. No copy of the RCA will be requested or retained by JCAHO.

TABLE C–3b *Continued*

Name of System	Sentinel Event Policy[a]
System Owner or Manager	Joint Commission on Accreditation of Healthcare Organizations

	Alternative 4: The organization can request an on-site review of its process for responding to a sentinel event and the relevant policies and procedures preceding and following the organization's review of a specific event. This option is to be used in those instances where the organization meets specified criteria respecting the risk of waiving legal protections for RCA information shared with JCAHO.
Who reports	JCAHO-accredited organizations are self-reporting often through the quality improvement coordinator, sometimes the chief executive officer or another senior executive, or the risk manager. Also, JCAHO can be made aware of sentinel events through patients and their families, employees of the accredited organizations, or the media.
RCA trigger	All events defined by the accredited organization as sentinel events, which will, at a minimum, include JCAHO reviewable sentinel events, require an RCA.
Follow-up (including RCA)	Each organization can conduct RCAs and develop action plans according to its own locally accepted methods. JCAHO then determines if the RCA and action plan are acceptable. An RCA will be considered acceptable for accreditation purposes if it has the following characteristics: • The analysis focuses primarily on systems and processes, not individual performance. • The analysis progresses from special causes in clinical processes to common causes in organizational processes. • The analysis repeatedly digs deeper by asking "Why?" Then, when answered, "Why?" again, and so on. • The analysis identifies changes that could be made in systems and processes—either through redesign or development of new systems or processes—that would reduce the risk of such events occurring in the future. • The analysis is *thorough* and *credible*. To be *thorough*, the RCA must include: • A determination of the human and other factors most directly

Continued

TABLE C–3b *Continued*

Name of System	Sentinel Event Policy[a]
System Owner or Manager	Joint Commission on Accreditation of Healthcare Organizations

associated with the sentinel event and the process(es) and systems related to its occurrence;
- Analysis of the underlying systems and processes through a series of "Why?" questions to determine where redesign might reduce risk;
- Inquiry into all areas appropriate to the specific type of event as described in the current edition of *Minimum Scope of Review of Root Cause Analysis;*
- Identification of risk points and their potential contributions to this type of event; and
- A determination of potential improvement in processes or systems that would tend to decrease the likelihood of such events in the future or a determination, after analysis, that no such improvement opportunities exist.

To be *credible*, the RCA must:
- Include participation by the leadership of the organization and by the individuals most closely involved in the processes and systems under review;
- Be internally consistent;
- Provide an explanation for all findings of "not applicable" or "no problem"; and
- Include consideration of any relevant literature.

An action plan will be considered *acceptable* if it:
- Identifies changes that can be implemented to reduce risk or formulates a rationale for not undertaking such changes; and
- Where improvement actions are planned, identifies who is responsible for implementation, when the action will be implemented, and how the effectiveness of the actions will be evaluated.

After the RCA and action plan are accepted by JCAHO, an *Official Accreditation Decision Report* is issued. This report:
- Reflects JCAHO's determination to continue or modify the organization's current accreditation status and to terminate the Accreditation Watch, if previously assigned; and
- Assigns an appropriate follow-up activity, typically a written progress report or follow-up visit, to be conducted within 6 months.

TABLE C–3b *Continued*

Name of System	Sentinel Event Policy[a]
System Owner or Manager	Joint Commission on Accreditation of Healthcare Organizations
	Follow-up activities are conducted when the organization believes it can demonstrate effective implementation, but no later than 6 months following receipt of the *Official Accreditation Decision Report.*
Other information collected through the system	None.
Confidentiality issues	Handling of any submitted RCA and action plan is restricted to specially trained staff in accordance with procedures designed to protect the confidentiality of the documents. Upon completing the review of any submitted RCA and action plan and abstracting the required data elements for the Joint Commission's Sentinel Event Database: • The original RCA documents will be returned to the organization and any copies will be shredded. • The action plan resulting from the analysis of the sentinel event will be initially retained to serve as the basis for the follow-up activity. Once the action plan has been implemented to the satisfaction of the Joint Commission, as determined through follow-up activities, the Joint Commission will return the action plan to the organization.
Relationship with other reporting systems	No direct relationships, but organizations can use other reporting and surveillance systems to facilitate their reporting to JCAHO. However, aggregate data on event characteristics, root causes, and risk reduction strategies contribute to the evidence base for publication of *Sentinel Event Alert* and the Joint Commission's patient safety bulletin and for the annual JCAHO National Patient Safety Goals, which are utilized by other organizations.
Relationships with JCAHO/Medicare certification	Failure to comply with the JCAHO Sentinel Event Policy by accredited organizations can result in being placed on Accreditation Watch or having status changed to Preliminary Non-accreditation or nonaccredited.

REFERENCES

Agency for Healthcare Research and Quality. 2002. *Patient Safety Database: Request for Proposal No. AHRQ-02-0015.*

Battles, J.B., H. S. Kaplan, T. W. Van der Schaaf, and C. E. Shea. 1998. The attributes of medical event-reporting systems: Experience with a prototype medical event-reporting system for transfusion medicine. *Arch Pathol Lab Med* 122(3):231–238.

Callum, J. L., H. S. Kaplan, L. L. Merkley, P. H. Pinkerton, B. Rabin Fastman. R. A. Romans, A. S. Coovadia, and M. D. Reis. 2001. Reporting of near-miss events for transfusion medicine: Improving transfusion safety. *Transfusion (Paris)* 41(10): 1204–1211.

Centers for Disease Control and Prevention. 1999. *Dialysis Surveillance Network (DSN).* [Online]. Available: http://www.cdc.gov/ncidod/hip/Dialysis/dsn.htm [accessed April 10, 2002].

———. 2002. *NNIS—National Nosocomial Infections Surveillance System.* [Online]. Available: http://www.cdc.gov/ncidod/hip/SURVEILL/NNIS.HTM [accessed April 15, 2002].

———, Hospital Infections Program. 2000. *Surveillance for Bloodstream and Vascular Access Infections in Outpatient Hemodialysis Centers: Procedure Manual.* Atlanta: Public Health Service, Department of Health and Human Services.

Columbia University. 2001. *Medical Event Reporting System—Transfusion Medicine.* [Online]. Available: http://www.mers-tm.net/ [accessed March 20, 2002].

Cousins, D. D. 2001. *Medication Errors, MedMARx and Hospitals. MedMARx: The National Database to Reduce Hospital Medication Errors* (pamphlet). U.S. Pharmacopeia.

Department of Defense. 1986. *Department of Defense Directive Number 6040.37.*

———. 2001a. *Near Miss/Adverse Events/Sentinel Event Reporting Form* (unpublished).

———. 2001b. *Root Cause Analysis (RCA) Form.* Used with permission (as modified) from the VA National Center for Patient Safety (unpublished).

———, Aug. 16, 2001c. Department of Defense Instruction Number 6025.17.

Department of Veterans Affairs. 2001. Excerpt from VA Briefing Book on Major Quality Improvement and Evaluation Programs: The VA's National Center for Patient Safety (NCPS) (unpublished).

———. 2002. *Veterans Health Administration (VHA) National Patient Safety Improvement Handbook.* Washington, DC: U.S. Department of Veterans Affairs.

Department of Veterans Affairs and National Aeronautics and Space Administration. 2000. *The Patient Safety Reporting System (PSRS)* (pamphlet). Moffett Field, CA: National Aeronautics and Space Administration and U.S. Department of Veterans Affairs.

Florida Health and Human Services, Agency for Health Care Administration. 2003. *AHCA Risk Management.* [Online]. Available: http://www.fdhc.state.fl.us/MCHQ/Health_Facility_Regulation/Risk/index.shtml [accessed July 14, 2003].

Food and Drug Administration. 1996. *The Clinical Impact of Adverse Event Reporting: A MedWatch Continuing Education Article.* [Online]. Available: http://www.fda.gov/medwatch/articles/medcont/medcont.htm [accessed February 26, 2002].

————. 1999. *Vaccine Adverse Event Reporting System: Table of Reportable Events Following Vaccination.* [Online]. Available: http://www.fda.gov/cber/vaers/eventtab.htm [accessed March 13, 2002].

————. 2001a. *MedWatch: What Is a Serious Adverse Event?* [Online]. Available: http://www.fda.gov/medwatch/report/desk/advevnt.htm [accessed September 4, 2001].

————. 2001b. *Vaccine Adverse Event Reporting System.* [Online]. Available: http://www.fda.gov/cber/vaers/vaers.htm [accessed September 4, 2001].

Food and Drug Administration and CODA. 2002. *MedSun: Playing a Vital Role in Ensuring Medical Device Safety.* [Online]. Available: https://www.medsun.net/about.html [accessed August 12, 2003].

Gaynes, R. P. 1998. Surveillance of nosocomial infections. In: D. Abrutyn, D. A. Goldmann, and W. E. Scheckler, eds. *Saunders Infection Control Reference Service.* Philadelphia: W. B. Saunders.

Gaynes, R. P., and T. C. Horan. 1999. Surveillance of nosocomial infections. In: C. G. Mayhall, ed. *Hospital Epidemiology and Infection Control.* 2nd ed. Philadelphia: Lippincott, Williams and Wilkins. Pp. 1285–1318.

Gaynes, R. P., and S. Solomon. 1996. Improving hospital-acquired infection rates: The CDC Experience. *Jt Comm J Qual Improv* 22(7):457–467.

Henkel, J. 1998. MedWatch: FDA's "Heads Up" on Medical Product Safety. *FDA Consumer Magazine.*

Horan, T. C., T. G. Emori. 1998. Definitions of nosocomial infections. In: E. Abrutyn, D. A. Goldmann, and W. E. Scheckler, eds. *Saunders Infection Control Reference Service.* Philadelphia: W. B. Saunders. Pp. 308–316.

Institute of Medicine. 2000. *To Err Is Human: Building a Safer Health System.* L. T. Kohn, J. M. Corrigan, and M. S. Donaldson, eds. Washington, DC: National Academy Press.

Jencks, S., and S. Kellie. 2002. Personal communication: conference call on the Medicare Patient Safety Monitoring System.

Joint Commission on Accreditation of Healthcare Organizations. 2002a. *Sentinel Events Main Page.* [Online]. Available: http://www.jcaho.org/sentinel/sentevnt_main.html [accessed April 24, 2002].

————. 2002b. *Sentinel Event Policy and Procedures.* [Online]. Available: http://www.jcaho.org/sentinel/se_pp.html [accessed April 24, 2002].

————. 2002c. *Understanding the 2001 Hospital Performance Report.* [Online]. Available: http://www.jcaho.org/lwapps/perfrep/undrstd/hap/2001.htm [accessed May 3, 2002].

Kaplan, H. S., J. B. Battles, T. W. Van der Schaaf, C. E. Shea, and S. Q. Mercer. 1998. Identification and classification of the causes of events in transfusion medicine. *Transfusion (Paris)* 38(11–12):1071–1081.

Kellie, S. March 27, 2002. Personal communication to IOM Staff. E-mail regarding the Medicare Patient Safety Monitoring System: Overview, Technical Specifications, and Contact List.

National Coordinating Council for Medication Error Reporting and Prevention. 1998. *NCC MERP Taxonomy of Medical Errors.*

New York Patient Occurrence Reporting and Tracking System. 2001. *NYPORTS User's Manual.* Version 2.1.

Overhage, M. 2003. *Enhancing Public Health, Healthcare System, and Clinician Preparedness: Strategies to Promote Coordination and Communication.* The Indiana Network for Patient Care.

Polk, A. 2002. Personal communication to IOM Staff. Conference call regarding the Agency for Health Care Administration, Florida.

Richards, C., T. G. Emori, J. Edwards, S. Fridkin, J. Tolson, and R. Gaynes. 2001. Characteristics of hospitals and infection control professionals participating in the National Nosocomial Infections Surveillance System. 1999. *Am J Infect Control* 29(6):400–403.

Rosenthal, J. 2003. List of States with Mandatory Reporting Systems. Personal communication to Institute of Medicine's Committee on Data Standards for Patient Safety.

Rosenthal, J., T. Riley, and M. Booth. 2000. *State Reporting of Medical Errors and Adverse Events: Results of a 50-State Survey.* Portland, ME: National Academy for State Health Policy.

Rosenthal, J., M. Booth, L. Flowers, and T. Riley. 2001. *Current State Programs Addressing Medical Errors: An Analysis of Mandatory Reporting and Other Initiatives.* Portland, ME: National Academy for State Health Policy.

Schyve, P. 2002. Personal communication to IOM Staff. Joint Commission on Accreditation of Healthcare Organizations. Conference call regarding JCAHO Sentinel Event Policy.

Stewart, F. February 20, 2002a. Personal communication to IOM Staff. Conference call regarding the IOM study on Data Standards for Patient Safety.

———. April 12, 2002b. Personal communication to IOM Staff. MHS Patient Safety System. Conference call regarding the DoD patient safety reporting system in development.

The Kevric Company. 2003. *National Patient Safety Database Project: Coding & Classification Report.* Silver Spring: The Kevric Company, Inc.

U.S. Code. Oct. 7, 1980. Title 38—Veterans' Benefits. Sec. 5705—Confidentiality of Medical Quality-Assurance Records.

———. Nov. 14, 1986. Title 10—Armed Forces. Sec. 1102—Confidentiality of Medical Quality Assurance Records: Qualified Immunity for Participants.

U.S. Pharmacopeia. 1997. *USP Medication Errors Reporting Program (Reporting Form).* [Online]. Available: http://www.usp.org/reporting/medform.pdf [accessed January 30, 2002].

———. 2001. *Practitioner Reporting: Medication Errors Reporting (MER) Program.* [Online]. Available: http://www.usp.org/reporting/mer.htm [accessed October 12, 2001].

Westat. 2001. *MERS-TM: Medical Event Reporting System for Transfusion Medicine Reference Manual.* In support of Columbia University under a grant from the National Heart, Lung, and Blood Institute, National Institutes of Health (Grant RO1 HL53772, Harold S. Kaplan, M.D., Principal Investigator). Version 3.0. New York: Trustees of Columbia University.

D

Clinical Domains for Patient Safety

Consolidated Health Informatics Initiative Clinical Domain Areas	Additional Domains for Patient Safety
Demographics	

Diagnosis/problem lists for:
  Signs
  Symptoms
  Diseases
  Social problems
	Patient risk factors/precursors (e.g., designation of comorbid diagnosis)

Interventions/procedures including:
  Laboratory orders
  Laboratory results contents
	Complications associated with specific procedures

Encounters	Episodes
	Process-specific risk factors (e.g., managing coronary health failure) Departmental risk factors (e.g., delays in the emergency room) Clinical data measures for health conditions

Medications including:
  Clinical drugs
  Warnings
	Alternative medicines
	Nutritional supplements
	Vitamins

Consolidated Health Informatics Initiative Clinical Domain Areas	Additional Domains for Patient Safety
Allergic reactions Adverse drug events (ADE)	Over-the-counter medications Previous known adverse drug reactions Triggers Medication orders Drug interactions Patient-specific drug dosing Diagnosis-specific drug indications Diagnosis-specific drug contraindications
Text-based reports including: Clinical document architecture Clinical document naming	Clinical template
History and physical including: History Vital signs Anatomy Exam findings Functional status	Nutritional status Discharge or treatment plan Determinants for genetic testing/screening of family-related diseases
Immunizations	
	Provider information Training level, cultural factors, speaking language, health
Population health including: Nosocomial infections reporting Reportable infections reporting Other reportable conditions Hospital errors other than ADE Emergency room trauma reporting Other national health statistics	Near misses Patient complaints Readmission indicators Performance measurement Causal factors Malpractice claims Risk management reports Potential adverse events assessment through electronic surveillance
Genes and proteins	Pharmacogenomic markers for drug response or drug complication
Multimedia including but not limited to: Image Audio Waveforms	

Consolidated Health Informatics Initiative Clinical Domain Areas	Additional Domains for Patient Safety

Nursing including:
  Diagnoses
  Interventions
  Goals and outcomes
	Process-specific nursing factors
	Acuity levels for nurse staffing

Physiology	

	Knowledge bases (systematic reviews of):
	  Clinical guidelines
	  Medical literature
	  Health outcomes data
	  Disease registries

	Patient self-management
	  Data set and guidelines for self-care
	  Rx interaction program access

Functioning and disability	Rehabilitation therapies
	  Respiratory
	  Occupational
	  Speech, etc.

Supplies including:
  Ontology for the ordering physician
  Medical devices
	Medical device simulations and testing

	Organizational process factors
	  Organizational risk factors
	  Hazard analysis

Chemicals (Unified Medical Language System—UMLS)	
Billing (Health Insurance Portability and Accountability Act, Administrative Simplification, Transactions and Code Sets)	Data from claims attachment
Scientific/fundamental (UMLS)	
Units (UMLS)	

Continued

E

Key Capabilities of an Electronic Health Record System

Letter Report

Committee on Data Standards for Patient Safety
Board on Health Care Services

INSTITUTE OF MEDICINE
OF THE NATIONAL ACADEMIES

THE NATIONAL ACADEMIES PRESS
Washington, D.C.
www.nap.edu

THE NATIONAL ACADEMIES PRESS   500 Fifth Street, N.W.   Washington, DC 20001

NOTICE: The project that is the subject of this report was approved by the Governing Board of the National Research Council, whose members are drawn from the councils of the National Academy of Sciences, the National Academy of Engineering, and the Institute of Medicine. The members of the committee responsible for the report were chosen for their special competences and with regard for appropriate balance.

Support for this project was provided by the U.S. Department of Health and Human Services. The views presented in this report are those of the Institute of Medicine Committee on Data Standards for Patient Safety and are not necessarily those of the funding agencies.

Additional copies of this report are available in limited quantities from the Committee on Data Standards for Patient Safety through the Board on Health Care Services, 500 Fifth Street, N.W., Washington, DC 20001. This report is also available online at **www.nap.edu**.

For more information about the Institute of Medicine, visit the IOM home page at: **www.iom.edu**.

"Knowing is not enough; we must apply.
Willing is not enough; we must do."
—Goethe

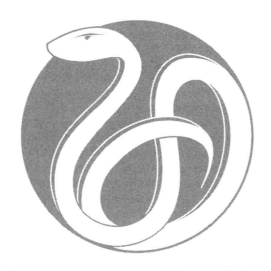

INSTITUTE OF MEDICINE
OF THE NATIONAL ACADEMIES

Shaping the Future for Health

THE NATIONAL ACADEMIES
Advisers to the Nation on Science, Engineering, and Medicine

The **National Academy of Sciences** is a private, nonprofit, self-perpetuating society of distinguished scholars engaged in scientific and engineering research, dedicated to the furtherance of science and technology and to their use for the general welfare. Upon the authority of the charter granted to it by the Congress in 1863, the Academy has a mandate that requires it to advise the federal government on scientific and technical matters. Dr. Bruce M. Alberts is president of the National Academy of Sciences.

The **National Academy of Engineering** was established in 1964, under the charter of the National Academy of Sciences, as a parallel organization of outstanding engineers. It is autonomous in its administration and in the selection of its members, sharing with the National Academy of Sciences the responsibility for advising the federal government. The National Academy of Engineering also sponsors engineering programs aimed at meeting national needs, encourages education and research, and recognizes the superior achievements of engineers. Dr. Wm. A. Wulf is president of the National Academy of Engineering.

The **Institute of Medicine** was established in 1970 by the National Academy of Sciences to secure the services of eminent members of appropriate professions in the examination of policy matters pertaining to the health of the public. The Institute acts under the responsibility given to the National Academy of Sciences by its congressional charter to be an adviser to the federal government and, upon its own initiative, to identify issues of medical care, research, and education. Dr. Harvey V. Fineberg is president of the Institute of Medicine.

The **National Research Council** was organized by the National Academy of Sciences in 1916 to associate the broad community of science and technology with the Academy's purposes of furthering knowledge and advising the federal government. Functioning in accordance with general policies determined by the Academy, the Council has become the principal operating agency of both the National Academy of Sciences and the National Academy of Engineering in providing services to the government, the public, and the scientific and engineering communities. The Council is administered jointly by both Academies and the Institute of Medicine. Dr. Bruce M. Alberts and Dr. Wm. A. Wulf are chair and vice chair, respectively, of the National Research Council.

www.national-academies.org

KEY CAPABILITIES OF AN
ELECTRONIC HEALTH RECORD SYSTEM

Letter Report

July 31, 2003

Dr. Carolyn Clancy
Director, Agency for Healthcare Research and Quality
John M. Eisenberg Building
540 Gaither Road
Rockville, MD 20850

Dear Dr. Clancy:

In May 2003, the Department of Health and Human Services (DHHS) asked the Institute of Medicine (IOM) to provide guidance on the key care delivery-related capabilities of an electronic health record (EHR) system. An EHR system includes (1) longitudinal collection of electronic health information for and about persons, where health information is defined as information pertaining to the health of an individual or health care provided to an individual; (2) immediate electronic access to person- and population-level information by authorized, and only authorized, users; (3) provision of knowledge and decision-support that enhance the quality, safety, and efficiency of patient care; and (4) support of efficient processes for health care delivery. Critical building blocks of an EHR system are the electronic health records (EHR) maintained by providers (e.g., hospitals, nursing homes, ambulatory settings) and by individuals (also called personal health records).

There is a great deal of interest within both the public and private sectors in encouraging all health care providers to migrate from paper-based health records to a system that stores health information electronically and employs computer-aided decision support systems. In part, this interest is due to a growing recognition that a stronger information technology (IT) infrastructure is integral to addressing such national concerns as the need to improve the safety and quality of health care, rising health care costs, and matters of homeland security related to the health sector. The efforts of all parties—purchasers, regulators, providers, and vendors—to advance the deployment of EHR systems would benefit from a common set of expectations about EHR capabilities.

The IOM was asked to respond very rapidly to this request from DHHS. Fortunately, a sizable project focused on patient safety data standards was already under way at the IOM, and this new task proved to be an appropriate expansion of that ongoing work. Thus the charge to the IOM Committee on Data Standards for Patient Safety (the IOM Committee) was expanded to address this additional task, and the committee devoted a portion of its previously scheduled meeting of June 9–10, 2003, to the development of this letter report. The IOM Committee's full report on data standards will be issued in fall 2003.

BACKGROUND

The development of an IT infrastructure has enormous potential to improve the safety, quality, and efficiency of health care in the United States (Institute of Medicine, 2001). Computer-assisted diagnosis and chronic care management programs can improve clinical decision making and adherence to clinical guidelines, and can provide focus on patients with those diseases (Durieux et al., 2000; Evans et al., 1998). Computer-based reminder systems for patients and clinicians can improve compliance with preventive service protocols (Balas et al., 2000). More immediate access to computer-based clinical information, such as laboratory and radiology results, can reduce redundancy and improve quality. Likewise, the availability of complete patient health information at the point of care delivery, together with clinical decision support systems such as those for medication order entry, can prevent many errors and adverse events (injuries caused by medical management rather than by the underlying disease or condition of the patient) from occurring (Bates et al., 1998, 1999; Evans et al., 1998). Via a secure IT infrastructure, patient health information can be shared amongst all authorized participants in the health care community (National Research Council, 2000).

An IT infrastructure also has great potential to contribute to achieving other important national objectives, such as enhanced homeland security and improved and informed public health services (Institute of Medicine, 2002b; National Committee on Vital and Health Statistics, 2001; Wagner et al., 2001). EHRs, combined with Internet-based communication, may enable early detection of and rapid response to bioterrorism attacks, including the organization and execution of large-scale inoculation campaigns and ongoing monitoring, detection, and treatment of complications arising from exposure to biochemical agents or immunizations (Tang, 2002; Teich et al., 2002). A more advanced health information infrastructure is also crucial for various forms of biomedical and health systems research, as well as educating patients, informal caregivers, and citizens about health (Detmer, 2003; National Committee on Vital and Health Statistics, 2001).

EHR system implementation and its continuing development is a critical element of the establishment of an IT infrastructure for health care. In 1991, the IOM issued a report calling for the elimination of paper-based patient records within 10 years, but progress has been slow, and this goal has not yet been met (Institute of Medicine, 1991; Overhage et al., 2002). It should be noted that the motivation is not to have a paperless record per se, but to make important patient information and data readily available and useable. In addition, computerizing patient data enables the use of various computer-aided decision supports.

There are some noteworthy examples of health care settings in both the private and public sectors in which EHRs have been deployed. A handful of communities and systems have established secure platforms for the exchange of data among providers; suppliers; patients; and other authorized users, such as the Veterans Health Administration, the New England Healthcare Electronic Data Interchange Network, the Indiana Network for Patient Care, the Santa Barbara County Care Data Exchange, the Patient Safety Institute's National Benefit Trust Network, and the Markle Foundation's Healthcare Collaborative Network (CareScience, 2003; Kolodner and Douglas, 1997; Markle Foundation, 2003b; New England Healthcare EDI Network, 2002; Overhage, 2003; Patient Safety Institute, 2002). But these examples are the exception, not the rule. In most of the nation's hospitals, orders for medications, laboratory tests, and other services are still written on paper, and many hospitals lack even the capability to deliver laboratory and other results in an automated fashion. The situation is no different in most small practice settings, where there has been little if any migration to electronic records.

In addition to the technical challenges, there are sizable policy, organizational, financial, and technological challenges that must be addressed to facilitate the adoption of EHR systems (Overhage et al., 2002). Some attempts to introduce order entry systems and other components of an EHR system have been unsuccessful (Auber and Hamel, 2001; Ornstein, 2003). Also, currently available personal health records, which allow patients to enter their own information, have demonstrated limited functionality to date (Kim and Johnson, 2002).

Government health care programs, along with various private-sector stakeholders, are considering options for encouraging the implementation of EHR systems by providers. To achieve widespread implementation, some external funding or incentive programs will be necessary (Institute of Medicine, 2001, 2002a). For example, the Centers for Medicare and Medicaid Services might provide some form of financial reward to providers participating in the Medicare program that have deployed EHR systems. On the private-sector side, various insurers, purchasers, and employer groups are instituting quality incentive programs for specific EHR system functionalities, such as computerized provider order entry for prescription drugs and electronic reporting of performance measures (National Health Care Purchasing Institute, 2003). In addition, a number of employers, health plans, and physicians have recently formed a coalition called Bridges to Excellence, which will provide financial bonuses to providers to encourage improved patient care management systems, including EHR systems (Bridges to Excellence, 2003). Another option is to provide grant funding or access to "low-cost" capital to enable providers, especially those with a safety net role, to invest in acquiring EHR systems (Health Technology Center and Manatt, Phelps and Phillips, LLP, 2003). Certain regulatory strategies might also be pursued, such as requiring providers to have an EHR system as a condition of participation in Medicare (Department of Health and Human Services, 2003).

To implement any of the above strategies, one must first clearly define a functional model of key capabilities for an EHR system. There have been many different views of what constitutes an EHR system. Some EHR systems include virtually all patient data, while others are limited to certain types of data, such as medications and ancillary results. Some EHR systems provide decision support (e.g., preventive service reminders, alerts concerning possible drug interactions, clinical guideline-driven prompts), while others do not. Most current EHR systems are enterprise-specific (e.g., operate within a specific health system or multi-hospital organization), and only a few provide strong support for communication and interconnectivity across the providers in a community. The functionality of EHR systems also varies across multiple settings—from the perspective of both what is available from vendors and what has actually been implemented. Some EHR systems have been developed locally and others by commercial vendors. In summary, EHR systems are actively under development and will remain so for many years.

A "functional model" of an EHR system will assist providers in acquiring and vendors in developing software. For most providers, the migration to an electronic environment will take place over a period of years. The development of a common set of requirements for the functional capabilities of various EHR system software components would allow providers to compare and contrast the systems that are available, and enable vendors to build systems more in line with providers' expectations. To be most useful, a functional model of an EHR system must also reflect a balance between what is desirable and what can feasibly be implemented immediately or within a short time frame. It will be important to update the functional model from time-to-time to reflect advancements in health care technology and care delivery.

PROJECT OVERVIEW

In response to the request from DHHS in May 2003, the charge to the IOM Committee on Data Standards for Patient Safety was expanded as follows:

> Provide guidance to DHHS on a set of "basic functionalities" that an electronic health record system should possess to promote patient safety. The IOM committee will consider functions, such as the types of data that should be available to providers when making clinical decisions (e.g., diagnoses, allergies, laboratory results); and the types of decision-support capabilities that should be present (e.g., the capability to alert providers to potential drug-drug interactions).

The IOM Committee was asked to focus on *care delivery functions*, and did not address infrastructure functions, such as database management and the use of health care data standards (e.g., terminology, messaging standards, network protocols). Although not within the scope of this project, the IOM Committee would like to emphasize the importance of two infrastructure functions—privacy and security (e.g., access control, encryption). It is absolutely critical that an EHR system be capable of safeguarding privacy and security.

DHHS requested a rapid response because of its desire to implement various programs in 2004 that would benefit from the availability of a functional model for an EHR system. Specifically, the Center for Medicare and Medicaid Services (CMS) is considering offering financial and other incentives to providers to encourage the deployment of EHR systems. The Agency for Healthcare Research and Quality is implementing an applied research program that will provide funding for the implementation and evaluation of innovative IT-related programs. The federal government is also working collaboratively with private sector stakeholders to facilitate the development of a national health information infrastructure (Department of Health and Human Services, 2003).

In addition, the IOM work is the first step of a two-step process. IOM is being asked to identify core care delivery–related functionalities of an EHR system. Health Level Seven (HL7), a leading standards-setting organization working on the development of an EHR functional model, will incorporate these core functionalities into the model, and further specify each functionality along three dimensions: (1) develop a functional statement or definition (what), (2) establish a rationale for the functionality (why included), and (3) establish a compliance metric or test (Dickinson et al., 2003).

Because of the quick turnaround required, the IOM Committee convened a small working group that met at the National Academies' Jonsson Conference Center in Woods Hole, Massachusetts, on June 7–8, 2003. The work of this group served as a starting point for discussions of the full IOM Committee at its June 9–10, 2003, meeting.

FRAMEWORK FOR IDENTIFYING CORE EHR FUNCTIONALITIES

In recent years, several IOM reports have recommended that the U.S. health care system make a commitment to the development of a health information infrastructure by the year 2010 (Institute of Medicine, 2001, 2002a, 2002c). This IOM Committee concurs with those recommendations.

It is recognized that the EHR system will be built incrementally utilizing clinical information systems and decision support tools as building blocks of the EHR, and the IOM Committee has strived to identify reasonable steps that can be taken by health care providers over the next 7 years to advance the accomplishment of this overall goal. It will be important for the Agency for Healthcare Research and Quality and others to pursue a robust research agenda if the EHR system is to reach full maturity in the years ahead.

Key EHR functionalities have been identified for four settings—hospital, ambulatory care, nursing home, and care in the community (i.e., the personal health record). Additional settings will need to be addressed in the future, such as home health agencies, pharmacies, and dental care.

In considering the core functionalities of EHR systems, it is important to recognize their many potential uses (see Box 1). EHR systems must support the delivery of personal health care services, including care delivery (e.g., care processes), care management, care support processes, and administrative processes (e.g., billing and reimbursement). As individuals engage more actively in management of their own health, they too become important users of electronic health information. There are also important secondary uses, including education, regulation (e.g., credentialing), clinical and health services research, public health and homeland security, and policy support. There are both individual users (e.g., patients, clinicians, manag-

---

BOX 1
Primary and Secondary Uses of an
Electronic Health Record System

Primary Uses
- Patient Care Delivery
- Patient Care Management
- Patient Care Support Processes
- Financial and Other Administrative Processes
- Patient Self-Management

Secondary Uses
- Education
- Regulation
- Research
- Public Health and Homeland Security
- Policy Support

SOURCE: Adapted from Institute of Medicine (1997).

---

ers) and institutional users (e.g., hospitals, public health departments, accreditation organizations, educators, and research entities).

To guide the process of identifying core EHR system functionalities, the IOM Committee formulated five criteria, which are listed below. Although each functionality independently may not fulfill all five criteria, when taken together as part of an EHR system, the core functionalities should address all criteria.

- *Improve patient safety.* Safety is the prevention of harm to patients. Each year in the United States, tens of thousands of people die as a result of preventable adverse events due to health care (Institute of Medicine, 2000).
- *Support the delivery of effective patient care.* Effectiveness is providing services based on scientific knowledge to those who could benefit and at the same time refraining from providing services to those not likely to benefit (Institute of Medicine, 2001). Only about one-half (55 percent) of Americans receive recommended medical care that is consistent with evidence-based practice guidelines (McGlynn et al., 2003).
- *Facilitate management of chronic conditions.* Chronic conditions are now the leading cause of illness, disability, and death in the United States (Hoffman et al., 1996). Persons with chronic conditions account for over 75 percent of all health care spending, and more than half of that spending is on behalf of people with multiple such conditions (Partnership for Solutions, 2002; U.S. Department of Health and Human Services, 2002). More than half of those with chronic conditions have three or more different providers and report that they often receive conflicting information from those

providers; moreover, many undergo duplicate tests and procedures, but still do not receive recommended care (Leatherman and McCarthy, 2002; Partnership for Solutions, 2002). Physicians also report difficulty in coordinating care for their patients with chronic conditions, and believe that this lack of coordination produces poor outcomes (Partnership for Solutions, 2002).

• *Improve efficiency.* Efficiency is the avoidance of waste, in particular, waste of equipment, supplies, ideas, and energy (Institute of Medicine, 2001). Methods must be found to enhance the efficiency of health care professionals and reduce the administrative and labor costs associated with health care delivery and financing. Staffing shortages have developed in multiple health care professions, placing added pressure on providers to continually improve care processes with current staffing levels (AHA Commission on Workforce for Hospitals and Health Systems, 2002). The cost of private health insurance is increasing at an annual rate of greater than 12 percent, while individuals are paying more out of pocket and receiving fewer benefits (Edwards et al., 2002; Kaiser Family Foundation and Health Research and Educational Trust, 2002). And rising health care costs will likely contribute to growing numbers of uninsured, who currently total over 41 million, or 1 in 7 Americans (U.S. Census Bureau, 2002). Addressing these issues represents a major challenge.

• *Feasibility of implementation.* The IOM Committee considered this criterion in determining the time frames within which it is reasonable to expect providers' EHR systems will be capable of demonstrating the key functionalities. The timing of this study did not allow for a thorough evaluation of feasibility, so the IOM Committee had to rely on its collective knowledge of the field. In assessing feasibility, the IOM Committee considered whether software is currently available or under development; the time period necessary for vendors to develop, produce, and market new software to achieve certain functionalities; and the willingness of users to purchase and implement such systems. It would be advisable to reassess periodically the feasibility of implementing certain EHR functionalities and modify expectations regarding timing, as appropriate.

CORE EHR FUNCTIONALITIES

The IOM Committee identified core functionalities falling into eight categories (see Box 2).

> **BOX 2**
> **Core Functionalities for an**
> **Electronic Health Record System**
>
> - Health information and data
> - Results management
> - Order entry/management
> - Decision support
> - Electronic communication and connectivity
>
> - Patient support
> - Administrative processes
> - Reporting & population health management

Health Information and Data

Although not truly a functionality attribute per se, in order to achieve the objectives set forth for an EHR system, it must contain certain data about patients. Physicians and other care providers require certain information to make sound clinical decisions; however, their information needs are often not met (Bates et al., 2003; Covell et al., 1985; McKnight et al., 2001; Tang et al., 1994). This lack of information can lead to lesser-quality and inefficient care.

As noted, for example, the capability to display previous laboratory test results can significantly reduce the number of redundant tests ordered, not only saving money, but also preventing the patient from undergoing unnecessary tests (Bates et al., 1999; Stair, 1998; Tierney et al., 1987). Also as noted earlier, information on patient allergies and other medications, in combination with alerts and reminders, can decrease the number of medication-related adverse events and improve the prescribing practices of physicians and nurse practitioners (Bates et al., 1999; Kuperman et al., 2001; McDonald, 1976; Teich et al., 2000). In addition, urgent matters, such as abnormal test results, can be addressed on a more timely basis if the physician has the information at the point of care (Bates et al., 2003). EHR systems with a defined dataset that includes such items as, medical and nursing diagnoses, a medication list, allergies, demographics, clinical narratives, and laboratory test results, can therefore ensure improved access to at least some types of information needed by care providers when they need it.

It is also important to note that too much information and data may overwhelm or distract the end user, so EHR systems must have well designed interfaces. The health information and data captured by an EHR system must also evolve over time, as new knowledge becomes available, both clinical knowledge and knowledge regarding the information needs of different users.

Results Management

Managing results of all types (e.g., laboratory test results, radiology procedure results reports) electronically has several distinct advantages over paper-based reporting in terms of improved quality of care. Computerized results can be accessed more easily by the provider at the time and place they are needed; the reduced lag time increases both efficiency and patient safety by allowing for quicker recognition and treatment of medical problems (Bates et al., 2003). Additionally, the automated display of previous test results makes it possible to reduce redundant and additional testing, thus not only improving efficiency of treatment, but also decreasing costs (Bates et al., 2003; Shea et al., 2002; Tierney et al., 1987). Having electronic results can allow for better interpretation and for easier detection of abnormalities, thereby ensuring appropriate follow-up (Bates et al., 2003; Overhage et al., 2001; Schiff et al., 2003). Finally, access to electronic consults and patient consents can establish critical linkages and improve care coordination among multiple providers, as well as between provider and patient (Bates et al., 2003).

Order Entry/Order Management

The benefits of computerized provider order entry (CPOE) have been well documented (Bates and Gawande, 2003; Bates et al., 1998, 1999; Butler and Bender, 1999; Kuperman and Gibson, 2003; Kuperman et al., 2001; Mekhjian et al., 2002; Schiff and Rucker, 1998; Sittig and Stead, 1994; Teich et al., 2000; Tierney et al., 1993). Even with little or no decision support capabilities, such systems can improve workflow processes by eliminating lost orders and ambiguities caused by illegible handwriting, generating related orders automatically, monitoring for duplicate orders, and reducing the time to fill orders (Lepage et al., 1992; Mekhjian et al., 2002; Sittig and Stead, 1994). The use of computerized order entry, in conjunction with an electronic health record, is also beginning to demonstrate a positive effect on clinician productivity (Overhage et al., In press).

The strongest evidence of the clinical effectiveness of CPOE is seen in medication order entry. Relatively simple systems have been shown to reduce the number of non-intercepted medication errors by up to 83 percent by using "forcing functions" for medication dose and frequency (Bates and

Gawande, 2003), displaying relevant laboratories, and checking for drug–allergy and drug–drug interactions. CPOE is expected to offer similar benefits for laboratory, microbiology, pathology, radiology, nursing, and supply orders, as well as for ancillary services and consults (Butler and Bender, 1999; Sanders and Miller, 2001; Schiff et al., 2003; Schuster et al., 2003; Teich et al., 1992; Wang et al., 2002). Financial benefits—such as reducing the amount of money spent on preprinted forms, assuring that prescribing practices are consistent with a facility's established formulary, and informing physicians and other providers about cost-saving options and duplicate test orders—have also been demonstrated (Butler and Bender, 1999; Mekhjian et al., 2002; Sittig and Stead, 1994).

Decision Support

Computerized decision support systems have demonstrated their effectiveness in enhancing clinical performance for many aspects of health care, including prevention, prescribing of drugs, diagnosis and management, and detection of adverse events and disease outbreaks (Bates and Gawande, 2003; Hunt et al., 1998; Johnston et al., 1994; Tang et al., 1999b). In two meta-analyses, computer reminders and prompts were shown to significantly improve preventive practices in such areas as vaccinations, breast cancer screening, colorectal screening, and cardiovascular risk reduction (Balas et al., 2000; Shea et al., 1996). Several studies have also been conducted on the use of computerized decision support to improve drug dosing, drug selection, and screening for drug interactions; these studies have shown overall positive effects on the quality of patient care (Abookire et al., 2000; Evans et al., 1998; Hunt et al., 1998; Schiff and Rucker, 1998). A study comparing clinical decisions made by physicians in the same practice using an EHR system and traditional paper records found that the former group made more appropriate clinical decisions as a result of all the tools available in an EHR system, including decision support (Tang et al., 1999a).

There is also a small but growing evidence base for the effectiveness of such systems in the area of computer-assisted diagnosis and disease treatment and management. In 1992, an expert diagnostic system demonstrated the ability to detect more serious quality problems arising from diagnostic errors than those detected by a state-based peer review organization, suggesting that computerized tools may help prevent such diagnostic misadventures (Lee and Warner, 1992). A 1999 study comparing the performance of clinicians with and without the aid of a diagnostic computerized decision support system found a significant improvement in the generation of correct diagnoses when the system was used (Friedman et al., 1999). Two additional recent studies have revealed that decision support tools could improve clinician compliance with established evidence-based guidelines and protocols (Morris, 2003; Starmer et al., 2000). Other studies on the use of decision support tools have not found improvements, however (Eccles et al., 2002; Rollman et al., 2002).

More sophisticated tools, such as artificial neural networks, have also demonstrated their effectiveness in detecting acute myocardial infarction, breast cancer, and cervical cancer (Bates and Gawande, 2003; Heden et al., 1997; Kok and Boon, 1996; Petrick et al., 2002). In addition, computerized tools can be used to identify and track the frequency of adverse events (Bates et al., 2001; Classen et al., 1991; Honigman et al., 2001) and hospital-acquired infections (Evans et al., 1986), as well as disease outbreaks and bioterrorism events (Pavlin, 2003; Tsui et al., 2003).

Electronic Communication and Connectivity

Effective communication—among health care team members and other care partners (e.g., laboratory, radiology, pharmacy) and with patients—is critical to the provision of quality health care. Its lack can contribute to the occurrence of adverse events (Bates and Gawande, 2003; Petersen et al., 1994; Schmidt and Svarstad, 2002; Wanlass et al., 1992). Improved communication among care partners, such as laboratory, pharmacy, and radiology, can enhance patient safety and quality of care (Schiff et al., 2003), and improve public health surveillance (Schiff and Rucker, 1998; Wagner et al., 2001). Electronic connectivity is essential in creating and populating EHR systems, especially for those patients with chronic conditions, who characteristically have multiple providers in multiple settings that must coordinate care plans (Wagner, 2000; Wagner et al., 1996). While communication interfaces are becoming well established for administrative data exchange, there are very few such interfaces for the exchange of clinical data.

Electronic communication tools, such as e-mail and web messaging, have been shown to be effective in facilitating communication both among providers and with patients, thus allowing for greater continuity of care (Balas et al., 1997; Liederman and Morefield, 2003; Worth and Patrick, 1997) and more timely interventions (Kuebler and Bruera, 2000). One recent study found that automatic alerts to providers regarding abnormal laboratory results reduced the time until an appropriate treatment was ordered (Kuperman et al., 1999). Another important communication tool is an integrated health record, both within a setting and across settings and institutions. Such a record allows for improved access to patient data at the point where clinical decisions are made (Institute of Medicine, 1997). In addition, telemedicine has demonstrated effectiveness in certain settings, including pulmonary clinics and intensive care units (Pacht et al., 1998; Rosenfeld et al., 2000; Shafazand et al., 2000); home telemonitoring has been shown to be successful as well (Finkelstein et al., 2000; Johnston et al., 2000; Rogers et al., 2001; Shea et al., 2002; Whitlock et al., 2000).

Patient Support

Patient education has demonstrated significant effectiveness in improving control of chronic illnesses (Weingarten et al., 2002). Computer-based patient education in particular has been found to be successful in primary care (Balas et al., 1996). In a 1997 study of 22 clinical trials, interactive educational interventions showed positive results for several major clinical applications, the most frequently targeted of these being diabetes (Krishna et al., 1997). Additionally, as noted earlier, several studies have demonstrated the feasibility of home monitoring by patients (Finkelstein et al., 2000; Johnston et al., 2000; Rogers et al., 2001; Whitlock et al., 2000). In a recent study, for instance, spirometry self-testing by asthma patients during home telemonitoring was found to provide valid results comparable to those of tests collected under the supervision of a clinician (Finkelstein et al., 2000). A multidimensional telehealth system has also demonstrated the ability to decrease stress for some caregivers of patients with Alzheimer's disease (Bass et al., 1998).

Administrative Processes

Electronic scheduling systems for hospital admissions, inpatient and outpatient procedures, and visits not only increase the efficiency of heath care organizations, but also provide better, more timely service to patients (Everett, 2002; Hancock and Walter, 1986; Woods, 2001). Use of communication and content standards is equally important in the billing and claims management area—close coupling of authorization and prior approvals can, in some cases, eliminate delays and confusion. Additionally, immediate validation of insurance eligibility should add value for both providers and patients through improved access to services, more timely payments and less paperwork.

Moreover, computerized decision support tools are being used in a variety of settings to identify eligible or potentially eligible patients for clinical trials (Breitfeld et al., 1999; Carlson et al., 1995; Ohno-Machado et al., 1999; Papaconstantinou et al., 1998). Other effective electronic administrative tools include reporting tools that support drug recalls (Schiff and Rucker, 1998) and artificial neural networks that can assist in identifying candidates for chronic disease management programs (Heden et al., 1997; Kok and Boon, 1996; Petrick et al., 2002).

Reporting and Population Health Management

Institutions currently have multiple public and private sector reporting requirements at the federal, state, and local levels for patient safety and quality, as well as for public health. In addition, the internal quality improvement efforts of many health care organizations include routine reporting of key quality indicators (sometimes referred to as clinical dashboards) to clinicians. Most of the data for these reports must be abstracted from claims data, paper records, and surveys, a process that is labor-intensive and time-consuming, and usually occurs retrospectively. Thus such reporting is often limited to entities that have sufficient administrative infrastructure to develop the necessary data (Institute of Medicine, 2002c). Additionally, chart abstraction has been shown to involve a number of significant errors (Green and Wintfeld, 1993). Having clinical data represented with a standardized terminology and in a machine-readable format would reduce the significant data collection burden at the provider level, as well as the associated costs, and would likely increase the accuracy of the data reported.

CORE FUNCTIONAL REQUIREMENTS

When identifying the core functional requirements for an EHR system, the IOM Committee was asked to consider both the *care setting* of each function and the *time frame* for its introduction. Table 1 at the end of this report lists the eight key EHR system capabilities described above, broken down at a more detailed level, according to these two dimensions. The committee was asked to provide guidance pertaining to four care settings: (1) hospitals; (2) ambulatory care settings, including small practice settings, community health centers, and group practices; (3) nursing homes; and (4) care in the community.

In addressing the fourth setting, care in the community, the IOM Committee focused on functional requirements for the personal health record (PHR), defined to include (1) a subset of data from the individual's EHR, and (2) information recorded by the individual, including health maintenance and monitoring data. A PHR may be used in a number of ways by the patient to support their care, disease management, and clinical communication. (Markle Foundation, 2003a). As computer-based PHRs become part of the EHR system, being able to access patients' own narratives of their illnesses will become a valuable source of information for improving care through comparisons with the clinicians' records.

Assuming that the migration from paper records to a comprehensive EHR system will take 7 or more years for most providers, the IOM Committee strived to identify functional requirements for three time periods:

• In the immediate future (2004–2005), it is assumed that providers (i.e., ambulatory care settings, hospitals, and nursing homes) will focus on (1) the capture of essential patient data already found frequently in electronic form, such as laboratory and radiology results; (2) the acquisition of limited decision support capabilities for which software is readily available in the marketplace (e.g., order entry, electronic prescribing); and (3) the generation of reports required by external organizations for quality and safety oversight and public health reporting.

• In the near term (2006–2007), providers' EHR systems should (1) allow for the capture of defined sets of health information, (2) incorporate a core set of decision support functions (e.g., clinical guideline support, care plan implementation), and (3) support the exchange of basic patient care data and communication (e.g., laboratory results, medication data, discharge summaries) among the care settings (e.g. pharmacies, hospitals, nursing homes, home health agencies, etc.) within a community.

• In the longer term (2008–2010), the committee believes that fully functional, comprehensive EHR systems will be available and implemented by some health systems and regions. It may take considerably longer, however, for all providers to be using a comprehensive EHR system that provides for the longitudinal collection of complete health information for an individual; immediate access to patient information by all authorized users within a secure environment; extensive use of knowledge support and decision support systems; and extensive support for applications that fall outside immediate patient care (e.g., homeland security, public health, clinical research).

In identifying core functionalities for specific provider settings, the IOM Committee also considered the current level of information technology capabilities within a sector. Specifically, the IOM Committee assumed that the migration pathway for hospitals would be more rapid than that for nursing homes, recognizing that many hospitals have some EHR system capabilities already in place while most nursing homes do not, and that hospitals generally have greater access to technical expertise. The migration can also be expected to take longer for physicians' offices than for hospitals, given the differences between the two in financial resources available for IT investments. The IOM Committee set these targets within the context of the current momentum it is observing in the public and private sectors. A loss of momentum would adversely affect these estimates. It is recognized that not every provider will meet the functional requirements by the times indicated. The functional requirements are intended to be challenging but achievable for a sizable proportion of the health care sector.

CONCLUSION

The IOM Committee is pleased to have had the opportunity to provide guidance on this important issue. The committee hopes its work will be useful to HL7 in its efforts to develop functional statements for an EHR system; to government programs and private purchasers in their efforts to encourage and assist health care providers in deploying EHR systems; to providers and vendors as they strive to acquire and build software products that form part of the foundation for a comprehensive health information infrastructure; and to patients as they seek to participate more fully in decisions regarding their own care.

Paul C. Tang, *Chair*
Committee on Data Standards for Patient Safety

Cc: Ann Marie Lynch, Acting Assistant Secretary for Planning and
            Evaluation (ASPE), Department of Health and Human Services
        Thomas A. Scully, Administrator, Centers for Medicare and
            Medicaid Services, Department of Health and Human Services
        Gary Christopherson, Senior Advisor for the Undersecretary for
            Health, Department of Veterans Affairs

TABLE 1 EHR System Capabilities by Time Frame and Site of Care

Core Functionality	Hospitals		
	2004–5	2006–7	2008–10

1. Health Information and Data

Key data (using standardized code sets where available)

	2004–5	2006–7	2008–10
– Problem list	X		
– Procedures	X		
– Diagnoses	X		
– Medication list	X		
– Allergies	X		
– Demographics	X		
– Diagnostic test results	X		
– Radiology results	X		
– Health maintenance	X		
– Advance directives	X		
– Disposition	X		
– Level of service		X	

Minimum dataset (MDS) for nursing homes

	2004–5	2006–7	2008–10
– Defined MDS for nursing homes	NA[a]		
– Expanded/refined MDS	NA		

Narrative (clinical and patient narrative)

	2004–5	2006–7	2008–10
– Free text	X		
– Template-based		X	
– Deriving structure from unstructured text			
- Natural Language Processing			X
– Structured and coded			
- Signs and Symptoms			X
- Diagnoses	X		
- Procedures	X		
- Level of service	X		
– Treatment plan			
- Single discipline	X		
- Interdisciplinary			X

Patient acuity/severity of illness/risk adjustment

	2004–5	2006–7	2008–10
– Nursing workload	X		
– Severity adjustment		X	

[a]NA = not applicable.

Ambulatory Care			Nursing Homes			Care in the Community (Personal Health Record)		
2004–5	2006–7	2008–10	2004–5	2006–7	2008–10	2004–5	2006–7	2008–10
X						X		
X						X		
X			See Minimum Dataset Below			X		
X						X		
X						X		
X						X		
X						X		
X						X		
X						X		
X						X		
X						X		
X							X	
NA			X			NA		
NA				X		NA		
X				X		X		
	X				X	X		
		X			X	NA		
		X			X			X
X			X			X		
X			X			X		
X			NA			NA		
	X				X			X
		X			X			X
NA				X		NA		
		X			X	NA		

Continued

TABLE 1 *Continued*

Core Functionality	Hospitals		
	2004–5	2006–7	2008–10
1. Health Information and Data *(continued)*			
Capture of identifiers			
– People and roles	X		
– Products/devices	X		
– Places (including directions)	X		
2. Results Management			
Results Reporting			
– Laboratory	X		
– Microbiology	X		
– Pathology	X		
– Radiology Reports	X		
– Consults		X	
Results Notification	X		
Multiple views of data/Presentation	X		
Multimedia support			
– Images			X
– Waveforms			X
– Scanned documents			
- Patient consents		X	
– Pictures			X
– Sounds			X
3. Order Entry/Management			
Computerized provider order entry			
– Electronic prescribing	X		
– Laboratory	X		
– Microbiology	X		
– Pathology	X		
– XR	X		
– Ancillary	X		
– Nursing	X		
– Supplies	X		
– Consults	X		

Ambulatory Care			Nursing Homes			Care in the Community (Personal Health Record)		
2004–5	2006–7	2008–10	2004–5	2006–7	2008–10	2004–5	2006–7	2008–10
X				X			X	
X				X			X	
X				X			X	
X			X			X		
X				X		X		
X				X		X		
X				X		X		
	X			X				X
X				X		X		
X				X			X	
		X			X			X
		X			X			X
	X				X			X
		X			X			X
		X			X			X
X			X			NA		
X				X		NA		
X					X	NA		
X					X	NA		
X					X	NA		
	X				X	NA		
	X				X	NA		
	X				X	NA		
	X			X		NA		

Continued

TABLE 1 *Continued*

Core Functionality	Hospitals		
	2004–5	2006–7	2008–10
4. Decision Support			
Access to knowledge sources			
– Domain knowledge	X		
– Patient education	X		
Drug alerts			
– Drug dose defaults	X		
– Drug dose checking		X	
– Allergy checking	X		
– Drug interaction checking	X		
– Drug–lab checking		X	
– Drug–condition checking		X	
– Drug–diet checking		X	
Other rule-based alerts			
(e.g., significant lab trends, lab test because of drug)		X	
Reminders			
– Preventive services	X		
Clinical guidelines and pathways			
– Passive	X		
– Context-sensitive passive		X	
– Integrated		X	
Chronic disease management	NA		
Clinician work list	X		
Incorporation of patient and/or family preferences		X	
Diagnostic decision support			X
Use of epidemiologic data			X
Automated real-time surveillance			
– Detect adverse events and near misses		X	
– Detect disease outbreaks		X	
– Detect bioterrorism		X	

Ambulatory Care			Nursing Homes			Care in the Community (Personal Health Record)		
2004–5	2006–7	2008–10	2004–5	2006–7	2008–10	2004–5	2006–7	2008–10
X				X		X		
X					X	X		
X			X			NA		
	X			X		NA		
X			X			NA		
X			X			NA		
	X				X	NA		
	X				X	NA		
	X				X	NA		
	X			X		NA		
X				X		X		
X				X		X		
	X				X			X
	X				X	NA		
	X				X			X
X				X		NA		
	X				X			X
		X			X	NA		
		X			X	NA		
	X			X		NA		
	X			X		NA		
	X		NA			NA		

Continued

TABLE 1 *Continued*

Core Functionality	Hospitals		
	2004–5	2006–7	2008–10
5. Electronic Communication & Connectivity			
Provider–provider	X		
Team coordination		X	
Patient–provider			
– E-mail	X		
– Secure web messaging	X		
Medical devices		X	
Trading partners (external)			
– Outside pharmacy		X	
– Insurer	X		
– Laboratory	X		
– Radiology		X	
Integrated medical record[b]			
– Within setting	X		
– Cross-setting			
- Inpatient–outpatient	X		
- Other cross-setting		X	
– Cross-organizational			X
6. Patient Support			
Patient education			
– Access to patient education materials	X		
– Custom patient education		X	
– Tracking		X	
Family and informal caregiver education		X	
Data entered by patient, family, and/or informal caregiver			
– Home monitoring		NA	
– Questionnaires		X	

[b]Defined as the extent to which a single record integrates data from different settings, providers, and organizations (e.g., Primary Care Physician, specialist, hospital).

Ambulatory Care			Nursing Homes			Care in the Community (Personal Health Record)		
2004–5	2006–7	2008–10	2004–5	2006–7	2008–10	2004–5	2006–7	2008–10
X			X			NA		
		X			X	NA		
X			NA			X		
X			NA			X		
		X		X				X
	X			X		X		
X				X		X		
X				X		NA		
	X				X	NA		
X				X		NA		
X				X			X	
	X			X			X	
		X		X				X
X				X		X		
	X			X			X	
	X				X		X	
	X			X			X	
	X			NA			X	
	X			NA		X		

Continued

TABLE 1 *Continued*

Core Functionality	Hospitals		
	2004–5	2006–7	2008–10
7. Administrative Processes			
Scheduling management			
– Appointments	X		
– Admissions	X		
– Surgery/procedure schedule	X		
Eligibility determination			
– Insurance eligibility	X		
– Clinical trial recruitment	X		
– Drug recall	X		
– Chronic disease management	X		
8. Reporting and Population Health Management			
Patient safety and quality reporting			
– Clinical dashboards	X		
– External accountability reporting	X		
– Ad hoc reporting	X		
Public health reporting			
– Reportable diseases	X		
– Immunization	X		
Deidentifying data		X	
Disease registries	X		

Ambulatory Care			Nursing Homes			Care in the Community (Personal Health Record)		
2004–5	2006–7	2008–10	2004–5	2006–7	2008–10	2004–5	2006–7	2008–10
X					X	X		
NA					X	NA		
X			NA			NA		
X			X			X		
X			NA				X	
X			NA			NA		
X				X		NA		
X			X			NA		
X			X			NA		
X			X			NA		
X			X			NA		
X				X		NA		
	X			X		NA		
X			X				X	

REFERENCES

Abookire, S. A., J. M. Teich, H. Sandige, M. D. Paterno, M. T. Martin, G. J. Kuperman, and D. W. Bates. 2000. Improving Allergy Alerting in a Computerized Physician Order Entry System. *Proc AMIA Symp* 2-6.

AHA Commission on Workforce for Hospitals and Health Systems. 2002. *In Our Hands: How Hospital Leaders Can Build a Thriving Workforce.* Washington, D.C.: American Hospital Association.

Auber, B. A., and G. Hamel. 2001. Adoption of Smart Cards in the Medical Sector: the Canadian Experience. *Soc Sci Med* 53 (7):879-94.

Balas, E. A., S. M. Austin, J. A. Mitchell, B. G. Ewigman, K. D. Bopp, and G. D. Brown. 1996. The Clinical Value of Computerized Information Services. A Review of 98 Randomized Clinical Trials. *Arch Fam Med* 5 (5):271-8.

Balas, E. A., F. Jaffrey, G. J. Kuperman, S. A. Boren, G. D. Brown, F. Pinciroli, and J. A. Mitchell. 1997. Electronic Communication With Patients. Evaluation of Distance Medicine Technology. *JAMA* 278 (2):152-9.

Balas, E. A., S. Weingarten, C. T. Garb, D. Blumenthal, S. A. Boren, and G. D. Brown. 2000. Improving Preventive Care by Prompting Physicians. *Arch Intern Med* 160 (3):301-8.

Bass, D. M., M. J. McClendon, P. F. Brennan, and C. McCarthy. 1998. The Buffering Effect of a Computer Support Network on Caregiver Strain. *J Aging Health* 10 (1):20-43.

Bates, D. W., M. Cohen, L. L. Leape, J. M. Overhage, M. M. Shabot, and T. Sheridan. 2001. Reducing the Frequency of Errors in Medicine Using Information Technology. *J Am Med Inform Assoc* 8 (4):299-308.

Bates, D. W., M. Ebell, E. Gotlieb, J. Zapp, and H. C. Mullins. 2003. A Proposal for Electronic Medical Records in U.S. Primary Care. *J Am Med Inform Assoc* 10 (1):1-10.

Bates, D. W., and A. A. Gawande. 2003. Improving Safety With Information Technology. *N Engl J Med* 348 (25):2526-34.

Bates, D. W., G. J. Kuperman, E. Rittenberg, J. M. Teich, J. Fiskio, N. Ma'luf, A. Onderdonk, D. Wybenga, J. Winkelman, T. A. Brennan, A. L. Komaroff, and M. Tanasijevic. 1999. A Randomized Trial of a Computer-Based Intervention to Reduce Utilization of Redundant Laboratory Tests. *Am J Med* 106 (2):144-50.

Bates, D. W., L. L. Leape, D. J. Cullen, N. Laird, L. A. Petersen, J. M. Teich, E. Burdick, M. Hickey, S. Kleefield, B. Shea, M. Vander Vliet, and D. L. Seger. 1998. Effect of Computerized Physician Order Entry and a Team Intervention on Prevention of Serious Medication Errors. *JAMA* 280 (15):1311-6.

Bates, D. W., J. M. Teich, J. Lee, D. Seger, G. J. Kuperman, N. Ma'Luf, D. Boyle, and L. Leape. 1999. The Impact of Computerized Physician Order Entry on Medication Error Prevention. *J Am Med Inform Assoc* 6 (4):313-21.

Bellazzi, R., A. Riva, S. Montani, C. Larizza, G. d'Annunzio, R. Lorini, A. Monteforte, and M. Stefanelli. 1998. A Web-Based System for Diabetes Management: the Technical and Clinical Infrastructure. *Proc AMIA Symp* 972.

Breitfeld, P. P., M. Weisburd, J. M. Overhage, G. Sledge Jr, and W. M. Tierney. 1999. Pilot Study of a Point-of-Use Decision Support Tool for Cancer Clinical Trials Eligibility. *J Am Med Inform Assoc* 6 (6):466-77.

Bridges to Excellence. 2003. "Bridges to Excellence: Rewarding Quality Across the

Healthcare System." Online. Available at http://www.bridgestoexcellence.org [accessed July 1, 2003].

Butler, M. A., and A. D. Bender. 1999. Intensive Care Unit Bedside Documentation Systems. Realizing Cost Savings and Quality Improvements. *Comput Nurs* 17 (1):32-8; quiz 39-40.

CareScience. 2003. "Santa Barbara County Care Data Exchange." Online. Available at http://www.carescience.com/healthcare_providers/cde/care_data_exchange_santabarbara_cde.shtml [accessed July 10, 2003].

Carlson, R. W., S. W. Tu, N. M. Lane, T. L. Lai, C. A. Kemper, M. A. Musen, and E. H. Shortliffe. 1995. Computer-Based Screening of Patients With HIV/AIDS for Clinical-Trial Eligibility. *Online J Curr Clin Trials* Doc No 179:[3347 words; 32 paragraphs].

Classen, D. C., S. L. Pestotnik, R. S. Evans, and J. P. Burke. 1991. Computerized Surveillance of Adverse Drug Events in Hospital Patients. *JAMA* 266 (20):2847-51.

Covell, D. G., G. C. Uman, and P. R. Manning. 1985. Information Needs in Office Practice: Are They Being Met? *Ann Intern Med* 103 (4):596-9.

Detmer, Don E. 2003. Building the National Health Information Infrastructure for Personal Health, Health Care Services, Public Health,a Nd Research. *BioMed Central* 3(1)

Dickinson, Gary, Linda Fischetti, and Sam Heard. 2003. *EHR Functional Model and Standard.* (PowerPoint Presentation): Health Level Seven (HL7) EHR SIG.

Durieux, Pierre, Remy Nizard, Philippe Ravaud, et al. 2000. A Clinical Decision Support System for Prevention of Venous Thromboembolism. *JAMA* 283 (21):2816-21.

Eccles, M., E. McColl, N. Steen, N. Rousseau, J. Grimshaw, D. Parkin, and I. Purves. 2002. Effect of Computerised Evidence Based Guidelines on Management of Asthma and Angina in Adults in Primary Care: Cluster Randomised Controlled Trial. *BMJ* 325 (7370):941.

Edwards, J. N., M. M. Doty, and C. Schoen. 2002. *The Erosion of Employer-Based Health Coverage and the Threat to Workers' Health Care: Findings From the Commonwealth Fund 2002 Workplace Health Insurance Survey.* New York, NY: The Commonwealth Fund.

Evans, R. S., R. A. Larsen, J. P. Burke, R. M. Gardner, F. A. Meier, J. A. Jacobson, M. T. Conti, J. T. Jacobson, and R. K. Hulse. 1986. Computer Surveillance of Hospital-Acquired Infections and Antibiotic Use. *JAMA* 256 (8):1007-11.

Evans, R. S., S. L. Pestotnik, D. C. Classen, T. P. Clemmer, L. K. Weaver, J. F. Orme Jr, J. F. Lloyd, and J. P. Burke. 1998. A Computer-Assisted Management Program for Antibiotics and Other Antiinfective Agents. *N Engl J Med* 338 (4):232-8.

Everett, J. E. 2002. A Decision Support Simulation Model for the Management of an Elective Surgery Waiting System. *Health Care Manag Sci* 5 (2):89-95.

Finkelstein, J., M. R. Cabrera, and G. Hripcsak. 2000. Internet-Based Home Asthma Telemonitoring: Can Patients Handle the Technology? *Chest* 117 (1):148-55.

Friedman, C. P., A. S. Elstein, F. M. Wolf, G. C. Murphy, T. M. Franz, P. S. Heckerling, P. L. Fine, T. M. Miller, and V. Abraham. 1999. Enhancement of Clinicians' Diagnostic Reasoning by Computer-Based Consultation: a Multisite Study of 2 Systems. *JAMA* 282 (19):1851-6.

Green, J., and N. Wintfeld. 1993. How Accurate Are Hospital Discharge Data for Evaluating Effectiveness of Care? *Med Care* 31 (8):719-31.

Hancock, W. M., and P. F. Walter. 1986. Reduce Hospital Costs With Admissions and Operating Room Scheduling Systems. *Softw Healthc* 4 (1):42-6.

Health Technology Center and Manatt, Phelps and Phillips, LLP. 2003. *Spending Our Money Wisely: Improving America's Healthcare System By Investing in Healthcare Information Technology.* New York, NY: Manatt, Phelps and Phillips, LLP.

Heden, B., H. Ohlin, R. Rittner, and L. Edenbrandt. 1997. Acute Myocardial Infarction Detected in the 12-Lead ECG by Artificial Neural Networks. *Circulation* 96 (6):1798-802.

Hoffman, C., D. Rice, and H. Y. Sung. 1996. Persons With Chronic Conditions. Their Prevalence and Costs. *JAMA* 276 (18):1473-9.

Honigman, B., J. Lee, J. Rothschild, P. Light, R. M. Pulling, T. Yu, and D. W. Bates. 2001. Using Computerized Data to Identify Adverse Drug Events in Outpatients. *J Am Med Inform Assoc* 8 (3):254-66.

Hunt, D. L., R. B. Haynes, S. E. Hanna, and K. Smith. 1998. Effects of Computer-Based Clinical Decision Support Systems on Physician Performance and Patient Outcomes: a Systematic Review. *JAMA* 280 (15):1339-46.

Institute of Medicine. 1991. *The Computer-Based Patient Record: An Essential Technology for Health Care.* eds. R. S. Dick and E. B. Steen. Washington, D.C: National Academy Press.

————. 1997. *The Computer-Based Patient Record: An Essential Technology for Health Care (Revised Edition).* eds. R. S. Dick, E. B. Steen, and D. E. Detmer. Washington, D.C: National Academy Press.

————. 2000. *To Err Is Human: Building a Safer Health System.* Linda T. Kohn, Janet M. Corrigan, and Molla S. Donaldson, eds. Washington, D.C: National Academy Press.

————. 2001. *Crossing the Quality Chasm: A New Health System for the 21st Century.* Washington, D.C.: National Academy Press.

————. 2002a. *Fostering Rapid Advances in Health Care: Learning From System Demonstrations.* J. M. Corrigan, A. Greiner, and S. M. Erickson, eds. Washington, D.C.: The National Academies Press.

————. 2002b. *The Future of the Public's Health in the 21st Century.* Washington, D.C.: The National Academies Press.

————. 2002c. *Leadership by Example: Coordinating Government Roles in Improving Health Care Quality.* eds. J. M. Corrigan, J. Eden, and B. M. Smith. Washingon, D.C.: The National Academies Press.

Johnston, B., L. Wheeler, J. Deuser, and K. H. Sousa. 2000. Outcomes of the Kaiser Permanente Tele-Home Health Research Project. *Arch Fam Med* 9 (1):40-5.

Johnston, M. E., K. B. Langton, R. B. Haynes, and A. Mathieu. 1994. Effects of Computer-Based Clinical Decision Support Systems on Clinician Performance and Patient Outcome. A Critical Appraisal of Research. *Ann Intern Med* 120 (2):135-42.

Kaiser Family Foundation and Health Research and Educational Trust. 2002. "2002 Employer Health Benefits Survey." Online. Available at http://www.kff.org/content/2002/20020905a/ [accessed Sept. 13, 2002].

Kim, M. I., and K. B. Johnson. 2002. Personal Health Records: Evaluation of Functionality and Utility. *J Am Med Inform Assoc* 9 (2):171-80.

Kok, M. R., and M. E. Boon. 1996. Consequences of Neural Network Technology for Cervical Screening: Increase in Diagnostic Consistency and Positive Scores. *Cancer* 78 (1):112-7.

Kolodner, R. M. and J. V. Douglas, eds. 1997. *Computerized Large Integrated Health Networks: The VA Success.* New York, NY: Springer-Verlag.

Krishna, S., E. A. Balas, D. C. Spencer, J. Z. Griffin, and S. A. Boren. 1997. Clinical Trials of Interactive Computerized Patient Education: Implications for Family Practice. *J Fam Pract* 45 (1):25-33.

Kuebler, K. K., and E. Bruera. 2000. Interactive Collaborative Consultation Model in End-of-Life Care. *J Pain Symptom Manage* 20 (3):202-9.

Kuperman, G. J., and R. F. Gibson. 2003. Computer Physician Order Entry: Benefits, Costs, and Issues. *Ann Intern Med* 139 (1):31-9.

Kuperman, G. J., J. M. Teich, T. K. Gandhi, and D. W. Bates. 2001. Patient Safety and Computerized Medication Ordering at Brigham and Women's Hospital. *Jt Comm J Qual Improv* 27 (10):509-21.

Kuperman, G. J., J. M. Teich, M. J. Tanasijevic, N. Ma'Luf, E. Rittenberg, A. Jha, J. Fiskio, J. Winkelman, and D. W. Bates. 1999. Improving Response to Critical Laboratory Results With Automation: Results of a Randomized Controlled Trial. *J Am Med Inform Assoc* 6 (6):512-22.

Leatherman, S. and D. McCarthy. 2002. *Quality of Health Care in the United States: A Chartbook.* New York, NY: The Commonwealth Fund.

Lee, M. L., and H. R. Warner. 1992. Performance of a Diagnostic System (Iliad) As Tool for Quality Assurance. *Comput Biomed Res* 25 (4):314-23.

Lepage, E. F., R. M. Gardner, R. M. Laub, and O. K. Golubjatnikov. 1992. Improving Blood Transfusion Practice: Role of a Computerized Hospital Information System. *Transfusion (Paris)* 32 (3):253-9.

Liederman, E. M., and C. S. Morefield. 2003. Web Messaging: a New Tool for Patient-Physician Communication. *J Am Med Inform Assoc* 10 (3):260-70.

Markle Foundation. 2003a. "Connecting for Health - A Public-Private Collaboration: The Personal Health Working Group, Executive Summary." Online. Available at http://www.connectingforhealth.org/resources/PHWG_Report.pdf [accessed July 16, 2003a].

———. 2003b. "Connecting for Health Unites Over 100 Organizations To Bring American Healthcare System into Information Age." Online. Available at http://www.markle.org/news/_news_pressrelease_060503.stm [accessed July 10, 2003b].

McDonald, C. J. 1976. Protocol-Based Computer Reminders, the Quality of Care and the Non-Perfectability of Man. *N Engl J Med* 295 (24):1351-5.

McGlynn, E. A., S. M. Asch, J. Adams, J. Keesey, J. Hicks, A. DeCristofaro, and E. A. Kerr. 2003. The Quality of Health Care Delivered to Adults in the United States. *N Engl J Med* 348 (26):2635-45.

McKnight, L., P. D. Stetson, S. Bakken, C. Curran, and J. J. Cimino. 2001. Perceived Information Needs and Communication Difficulties of Inpatient Physicians and Nurses. *Proc AMIA Symp* 453-7.

Mekhjian, H. S., R. R. Kumar, L. Kuehn, T. D. Bentley, P. Teater, A. Thomas, B. Payne, and A. Ahmad. 2002. Immediate Benefits Realized Following Implementation of Physician Order Entry at an Academic Medical Center. *J Am Med Inform Assoc* 9 (5):529-39.

Morris, A. H. 2003. Treatment Algorithms and Protocolized Care. *Curr Opin Crit Care* 9 (3):236-40.

National Committee on Vital and Health Statistics. 2001. "Information for Health: A Strategy for Building the National Health Information Infrastructure." Online. Available at http://ncvhs.hhs.gov/nhiilayo.pdf [accessed Apr. 18, 2002].

National Health Care Purchasing Institute. 2003. "Profiles of Organizations Using Quality Incentives." Online. Available at http://nhcpi.net/profiles.cfm [accessed July 10, 2003].

National Research Council. 2000. *Networking Health: Prescriptions for the Internet.* Washington, D.C.: National Academy Press.

New England Healthcare EDI Network. 2002. "NEHEN About Us." Online. Available at http://www.nehen.net/ [accessed July 10, 2003].

Ohno-Machado, L., S. J. Wang, P. Mar, and A. A. Boxwala. 1999. Decision Support for Clinical Trial Eligibility Determination in Breast Cancer. *Proc AMIA Symp* 340-4.

Ornstein, C. Jan. 22, 2003. California; Hospital Needs Doctors, Suspends Use of Software; Cedars-Sinai Physicians Entered Prescriptions and Other Orders In It, But Called It Unsafe. *Los Angeles Times.* Sect. B-1

Overhage, J. M. 2003. Enhancing Public Health, Health Care System, and Clinician Preparedness: Strategies to Promote Coordination and Communication—The Indiana Network for Patient Care [PowerPoint Presentation].

Overhage, J. M., B. Middleton, R. A. Miller, R. D. Zielstorff, and Hersh W. R. 2002. Does National Regulatory Mandate of Provider Order Entry Portend Greater Benefit Than Risk for Health Care Delivery? The 2001 ACMI Debate. *J Am Med Inform Assoc* 9 (3):199-208.

Overhage, J. M., S. Perkins, and C. J. McDonald. In press. The Impact of Direct Physician Time Utilization on a University Affiliated, Ambulatory Primary Care Internal Medicine Practice. *J Am Med Inform Assoc*

Overhage, J. M., J. Suico, and C. J. McDonald. 2001. Electronic Laboratory Reporting: Barriers, Solutions and Findings. *J Public Health Manag Pract* 7 (6):60-6.

Pacht, E. R., J. W. Turner, M. Gailiun, L. A. Violi, D. Ralston, H. S. Mekhjian, and R. C. St John. 1998. Effectiveness of Telemedicine in the Outpatient Pulmonary Clinic. *Telemed J* 4 (4):287-92.

Papaconstantinou, C., G. Theocharous, and S. Mahadevan. 1998. An Expert System for Assigning Patients into Clinical Trials Based on Bayesian Networks. *J Med Syst* 22 (3):189-202.

Partnership for Solutions, Johns Hopkins University, Prepared for The Robert Wood Johnson Foundation. 2002. *Chronic Conditions: Making the Case for Ongoing Care.* Baltimore, MD: Johns Hopkins University.

Patient Safety Institute. 2002. "Patient Safety Institute: Presentation to the Fifth National HIPAA Summit—Beyond HIPAA: Clinical Data Standards and the Creation of an Interconnected Electronic Health Information Infrastructure." Online. Available at http://www.ehcca.com/presentations/HIPAA5/walker.pdf [accessed July 10, 2003].

Pavlin, J. A. 2003. Investigation of Disease Outbreaks Detected by "Syndromic" Surveillance Systems. *J Urban Health* 80 (Suppl 1):I107-14.

Petersen, L. A., T. A. Brennan, A. C. O'Neil, E. F. Cook, and T. H. Lee. 1994. Does Housestaff Discontinuity of Care Increase the Risk for Preventable Adverse Events? *Ann Intern Med* 121 (11):866-72.

Petrick, N., B. Sahiner, H. P. Chan, M. A. Helvie, S. Paquerault, and L. M. Hadjiiski. 2002. Breast Cancer Detection: Evaluation of a Mass-Detection Algorithm for

Computer-Aided Diagnosis — Experience in 263 Patients. *Radiology* 224 (1):217-24.

Rogers, M. A., D. Small, D. A. Buchan, C. A. Butch, C. M. Stewart, B. E. Krenzer, and H. L. Husovsky. 2001. Home Monitoring Service Improves Mean Arterial Pressure in Patients With Essential Hypertension. A Randomized, Controlled Trial. *Ann Intern Med* 134 (11):1024-32.

Rollman, B. L., B. H. Hanusa, H. J. Lowe, T. Gilbert, W. N. Kapoor, and H. C. Schulberg. 2002. A Randomized Trial Using Computerized Decision Support to Improve Treatment of Major Depression in Primary Care. *J Gen Intern Med* 17 (7):493-503.

Rosenfeld, B. A., T. Dorman, M. J. Breslow, P. Pronovost, M. Jenckes, N. Zhang, G. Anderson, and H. Rubin. 2000. Intensive Care Unit Telemedicine: Alternate Paradigm for Providing Continuous Intensivist Care. *Crit Care Med* 28 (12):3925-31.

Sanders, D. L., and R. A. Miller. 2001. The Effects on Clinician Ordering Patterns of a Computerized Decision Support System for Neuroradiology Imaging Studies. *Proc AMIA Symp* 583-7.

Schiff, G. D., D. Klass, J. Peterson, G. Shah, and D. W. Bates. 2003. Linking Laboratory and Pharmacy: Opportunities for Reducing Errors and Improving Care. *Arch Intern Med* 163 (8):893-900.

Schiff, G. D., and T. D. Rucker. 1998. Computerized Prescribing: Building the Electronic Infrastructure for Better Medication Usage. *JAMA* 279 (13):1024-9.

Schmidt, I. K., and B. L. Svarstad. 2002. Nurse-Physician Communication and Quality of Drug Use in Swedish Nursing Homes. *Soc Sci Med* 54 (12):1767-77.

Schuster, D. M., S. E. Hall, C. B. Couse, D. S. Swayngim, and K. Y. Kohatsu. 2003. Involving Users in the Implementation of an Imaging Order Entry System. *J Am Med Inform Assoc* 10(4):315-21.

Shafazand, S., H. Shigemitsu, and A. B. Weinacker. 2000. A Brave New World: Remote Intensive Care Unit for the 21st Century. *Crit Care Med* 28 (12):3945-6.

Shea, S., W. DuMouchel, and L. Bahamonde. 1996. A Meta-Analysis of 16 Randomized Controlled Trials to Evaluate Computer- Based Clinical Reminder Systems for Preventive Care in the Ambulatory Setting. *J Am Med Inform Assoc* 3 (6): 399-409.

Shea, S., J. Starren, R. S. Weinstock, P. E. Knudson, J. Teresi, D. Holmes, W. Palmas, L. Field, R. Goland, C. Tuck, G. Hripcsak, L. Capps, and D. Liss. 2002. Columbia University's Informatics for Diabetes Education and Telemedicine (IDEATel) Project: Rationale and Design. *J Am Med Inform Assoc* 9 (1):49-62.

Sittig, D. F., and W. W. Stead. 1994. Computer-Based Physician Order Entry: the State of the Art. *J Am Med Inform Assoc* 1 (2):108-23.

Stair, T. O. 1998. Reduction of Redundant Laboratory Orders by Access to Computerized Patient Records. *J Emerg Med* 16 (6):895-7.

Starmer, J. M., D. A. Talbert, and R. A. Miller. 2000. Experience Using a Programmable Rules Engine to Implement a Complex Medical Protocol During Order Entry. *Proc AMIA Symp* 829-32.

Tang, P. C. 2002. AMIA Advocates National Health Information System in Fight Against National Health Threats. *J Am Med Inform Assoc* 9 (2):123-4.

Tang, P. C., D. Fafchamps, and E. H. Shortliffe. 1994. Traditional Medical Records As a Source of Clinical Data in the Outpatient Setting. *Proc Annu Symp Comput Appl Med Care* 575-9.

Tang, P. C., M. P. LaRosa, and S. M. Gorden. 1999a. Use of Computer-Based Records, Completeness of Documentation, and Appropriateness of Documented Clinical Decisions. *J Am Med Inform Assoc* 6 (3):245-51.

Tang, P. C., M. P. LaRosa, C. Newcomb, and S. M. Gorden. 1999b. Measuring the Effects of Reminders for Outpatient Influenza Immunizations at the Point of Clinical Opportunity. *J Am Med Inform Assoc* 6 (2):115-21.

Teich, J. M., J. F. Hurley, R. F. Beckley, and M. Aranow. 1992. Design of an Easy-to-Use Physician Order Entry System With Support for Nursing and Ancillary Departments. *Proc Annu Symp Comput Appl Med Care* 99-103.

Teich, J. M., P. R. Merchia, J. L. Schmiz, G. J. Kuperman, C. D. Spurr, and D. W. Bates. 2000. Effects of Computerized Physician Order Entry on Prescribing Practices. *Arch Intern Med* 160 (18):2741-7.

Teich, J. M., M. M. Wagner, C. F. Mackenzie, and K. O. Schafer. 2002. The Informatics Response in Disaster, Terrorism, and War. *J Am Med Inform Assoc* 9 (2):97-104.

Tierney, W. M., C. J. McDonald, D. K. Martin, and M. P. Rogers. 1987. Computerized Display of Past Test Results. Effect on Outpatient Testing. *Ann Intern Med* 107 (4):569-74.

Tierney, W. M., M. E. Miller, J. M. Overhage, and C. J. McDonald. 1993. Physician Inpatient Order Writing on Microcomputer Workstations. Effects on Resource Utilization. *JAMA* 269 (3):379-83.

Tsui, F. C., J. U. Espino, V. M. Dato, P. H. Gesteland, J. Hutman, and M. M. Wagner. 2003. Technical Description of RODS: A Real-Time Public Health Surveillance System. *J Am Med Inform Assoc* [Epub ahead of print]

U.S. Census Bureau. 2002. "Health Insurance Coverage: 2001." Online. Available at http://www.census.gov/prod/2002pubs/p60-220.pdf [accessed Sept. 30, 2002].

U.S. Department of Health and Human Services, Centers for Disease Control and Prevention. 2002. *The Burden of Chronic Diseases and Their Risk Factors: National and State Perspectives.* Atlanta, GA: Centers for Disease Control and Prevention.

Wagner, E. H. 2000. The Role of Patient Care Teams in Chronic Disease Management. *BMJ* 320 (7234):569-72.

Wagner, E. H., B. T. Austin, and M. Von Korff. 1996. Organizing Care for Patients With Chronic Illness. *Milbank Q* 74 (4):511-44.

Wagner, M. M., F. C. Tsui, J. U. Espino, V. M. Dato, D. F. Sittig, R. A. Caruana, L. F. McGinnis, D. W. Deerfield, M. J. Druzdzel, and D. B. Fridsma. 2001. The Emerging Science of Very Early Detection of Disease Outbreaks. *J Public Health Manag Pract* 7 (6):51-9.

Wang, S. J., B. H. Blumenfeld, S. E. Roche, J. A. Greim, K. E. Burk, T. K. Gandhi, D. W. Bates, and G. J. Kuperman. 2002. End of Visit: Design Considerations for an Ambulatory Order Entry Module. *Proc AMIA Symp* 864-8.

Wanlass, R. L., S. L. Reutter, and A. E. Kline. 1992. Communication Among Rehabilitation Staff: "Mild," "Moderate," or "Severe" Deficits? *Arch Phys Med Rehabil* 73 (5):477-81.

Weingarten, S. R., J. M. Henning, E. Badamgarav, K. Knight, V. Hasselblad, A. Gano Jr, and J. J. Ofman. 2002. Interventions Used in Disease Management Programmes for Patients With Chronic Illness-Which Ones Work? Meta-Analysis of Published Reports. *BMJ* 325 (7370):925.

Whitlock, W. L., A. Brown, K. Moore, H. Pavliscsak, A. Dingbaum, D. Lacefield, K.

Buker, and S. Xenakis. 2000. Telemedicine Improved Diabetic Management. *Mil Med* 165 (8):579-84.

Woods, L. 2001. What Works: Scheduling. Picture Perfect Solution. The Right Technology and an ASP Solution Bring Scheduling Efficiency and Added Revenue to a Community Hospital's Radiology Department. *Health Manag Technol* 22 (8):48-50.

Worth, E. R., and T. B. Patrick. 1997. Do Electronic Mail Discussion Lists Act As Virtual Colleagues? *Proc AMIA Annu Fall Symp* 325-9.

Appendix A
Committee and Staff

COMMITTEE ON DATA STANDARDS FOR PATIENT SAFETY

PAUL C. TANG (*Chair*), Chief Medical Information Officer, Palo Alto
  Medical Foundation
MOLLY JOEL COYE (*Vice Chair*), Chief Executive Officer, Health
  Technology Center
SUZANNE BAKKEN, Alumni Professor of Nursing and Professor of
  Biomedical Informatics, Columbia University
E. ANDREW BALAS, Dean, School of Public Health, Saint Louis
  University
DAVID W. BATES, Chief, Division of General Medicine, Brigham and
  Women's Hospital
JOHN R. CLARKE, Professor of Surgery, Drexel University
DAVID C. CLASSEN, Associate Professor of Medicine, Vice President,
  University of Utah, First Consulting Group
SIMON P. COHN, National Director of Health Information Policy,
  Kaiser Permanente
CAROL CRONIN, Consultant
JONATHAN S. EINBINDER, Assistant Professor, Harvard Medical
  School and Corporate Manager, Partners Health Care Information
  Systems
LARRY D. GRANDIA, Chief Technology Officer, Executive Vice
  President, Premier, Inc.
W. ED HAMMOND, Professor, Division of Medical Informatics, Duke
  University
BRENT C. JAMES, Executive Director, Intermountain Health Care
  Institute for Health Care Delivery Research, and Vice President for
  Medical Research, Intermountain Health Care
KEVIN JOHNSON, Associate Professor and Vice Chair, Department of
  Biomedical Informatics and Associate Professor, Department of
  Pediatrics, Vanderbilt University
JILL ROSENTHAL, Program Manager, National Academy for State
  Health Policy
TJERK W. van der SCHAAF, Associate Professor of Human Factors in
  Risk Control, Eindhoven University of Technology, Eindhoven Safety
  Management Group, Department of Technology Management

Special Consultant

J. MARC OVERHAGE, Associate Professor of Medicine and
Investigator, Regenstrief Institute for Health Care, Indiana University
School of Medicine

Study Staff

JANET M. CORRIGAN, Director, Board on Health Care Services
PHILIP ASPDEN, Study Director
JULIE WOLCOTT, Program Officer
SHARI ERICKSON, Research Associate
REBECCA LOEFFLER, Senior Project Assistant
ANTHONY BURTON, Administrative Assistant

The committee wishes to thank the co-chairs of the Health Level Seven (HL7) Special Interest Group (SIG), **Linda Fischetti** (U.S. Department of Veterans Affairs), **Gary L. Dickinson** (Misys Healthcare), and **Sam Herd** (Ocean Informatics, Australia), for the briefing and background materials they provided to the committee at its June 2003 meeting. The committee would also like to thank **Gary Christopherson** of the U.S. Department of Veterans Affairs, **William C. Rollow** of the Centers for Medicare and Medicaid Services, and **Scott Young** of the Agency for Healthcare Research and Quality for their helpful contributions to the report.

Appendix B
Reviewers

This report has been reviewed in draft form by individuals chosen for their diverse perspectives and technical expertise, in accordance with procedures approved by the NRC's Report Review Committee. The purpose of this independent review is to provide candid and critical comments that will assist the institution in making its published report as sound as possible and to ensure that the report meets institutional standards for objectivity, evidence, and responsiveness to the study charge. The review comments and draft manuscript remain confidential to protect the integrity of the deliberative process. We wish to thank the following individuals for their review of this report:

REED M. GARDNER, Professor, Medical Informatics, University of
  Utah
BLACKFORD MIDDLETON, Director of Clinical Informatics Research
  and Development, Partners Healthcare System, Inc., Brigham and
  Women's Hospital
DAVID N. MOHR, Professor of Medicine, Area Medicine, Mayo Clinic
JUDITH J. WARREN, Associate Professor, School of Nursing,
  University of Kansas

Although the reviewers listed above have provided many constructive comments and suggestions, they did not see the final draft of the report before its release. The review of this report was overseen by **Don E. Detmer**, Dennis Gillings Professor of Health Management, The Judge Institute of Management Studies, University of Cambridge, and Professor Emeritus, Professor of Medical Education, University of Virginia. Appointed by the National Research Council and Institute of Medicine, he was responsible for making certain that an independent examination of this report was carried out in accordance with institutional procedures and that all review comments were carefully considered. Responsibility for the final content of this report rests entirely with the authoring committee and the institution.

F

Quality Improvement and Proactive Hazard Analysis Models: Deciphering a New Tower of Babel

Commissioned Paper by
John E. McDonough, Milbank Memorial Fund
Ronni Solomon and Luke Petosa, ECRI

ABSTRACT

Health care leaders seeking to improve quality and prevent harm to patients have an array of tools to help them in this task. We propose dividing these tools into two categories: (1) quality improvement tools—including Continuous Quality Improvement, Six Sigma, and Toyota Production System—can be applied to many organizational challenges, including but not limited to safety concerns; and (2) proactive hazard analysis tools—including Health Care Failure Mode and Effect Analysis, Hazard Analysis and Critical Control Point, Hazard and Operability Studies, Proactive Risk Analysis—are designed specifically to identify hazards and to prevent harm. Each tool has common ancestry in the application of the scientific method to process analysis pioneered by Shewhart and Deming; each has unique attributes and advantages. This report explains each model in the context of patient safety. We recommend establishment of a clearinghouse to enable physicians and other practitioners to learn from experimentation with these models and to establish a common analytic framework. We also recommend use of models for personal health information as a methodology for medical specialties to address patient safety concerns.

471

I. INTRODUCTION

Two Institute of Medicine (IOM) reports, *To Err Is Human* (1999) and *Crossing the Quality Chasm* (2001), moved public and health care industry concerns about quality, patient safety, and hazard analysis to greater visibility. As patient safety and hazard analysis concerns rise, health industry leaders have sought tools to address these challenges more effectively. Many tools exist; the quality improvement and hazard analysis models that offer methodologies to make medicine safer include Six Sigma, Hazard Analysis and Critical Control Points (HACCP), Failure Mode and Effect Analysis/ Healthcare Failure Mode and Effect Analysis (FMEA/HFMEA™), Toyota Production System (TPS), Hazard and Operability Studies (HAZOP), Total Quality Management/Continuous Quality Improvement (TQM/CQI), Root Cause Analysis (RCA), and Probabilistic Risk Assessment (PRA).

Each approach has champions, supported by consultants ready to train managers and frontline workers in the rollout of each. Competing terms, acronyms, symbols, and techniques suggest a Tower of Babel—health leaders speaking different languages and using tools that do not resemble each other. As demands for improvements in patient safety escalate, the IOM's Patient Safety Data Standards Committee seeks a framework to understand these approaches to identify principles necessary for any quality improvement (QI) or proactive hazard analysis (PHA) methodology to succeed.

This paper provides an overview of key features of prominent methodologies, offers a framework to understand each, and shows how each relates to others. We outline principles to create effective hazard analysis in health care organizations, and we identify conceptual and methodological considerations in design and evaluation of risk/hazard identification. We relate hazard analysis to adverse event prevention and discuss strategies to apply this approach to health care. Finally, we discuss data requirements and measurement tools to support this approach.

As a caveat, we recall the words of Avedis Donabedian, who devised our modern framework for understanding quality in health care: "If we are truly committed to quality, almost any mechanism will work. If we are not, the most elegantly constructed of mechanisms will fail." While today's quality leaders dispute the first sentence, all affirm the validity of the second. While QI and PHA tools can assist any health care organization's commitment to making health care safer, none will succeed in the absence of deep and sustained leadership commitment.

II. OVERVIEW OF EXISTING QUALITY IMPROVEMENT/ HAZARD PREVENTION MODELS

Essential Features of Health Care Quality

The *Chasm* report identifies six attributes for a quality health care system: (1) safe, (2) effective, (3) patient centered, (4) timely, (5) efficient, and (6) equitable.[1] Safety is a preeminent feature of health care quality, first on the list, though not the only one. Health care quality may be thought of as a circle, with each of the six essential features forming smaller overlapping circles within the larger whole.

Over the past 60 years, many models have been developed to help organizations improve quality and enhance safety. Among the methodologies discussed here, we distinguish between tools that address all six aspects of quality versus tools with an explicit focus on safety and hazard analysis. General QI tools can be used to improve timeliness, efficiency, and other goals in addition to safety. PHA tools are more prescriptive and require more steps, including documentation; in cases where a tool is applied to an ongoing service operation (i.e., HACCP), it becomes a part of a firm's daily functioning.[2] This distinction provides the framework for discussion in this paper of the various methodologies:

Quality Improvement Tools (QI)	Proactive Hazard Analysis Tools (PHA)
Total Quality Management—TQM	Failure Mode and Effect Analysis—FMEA
Continuous Quality Improvement—CQI	Healthcare Failure Mode and Effect Analysis—HFMEA™
Toyota Production System	Hazard Analysis and Critical Control Points—HACCP
Six Sigma	Hazard and Operability Studies—HAZOP
	Probabilistic Risk Assessment—PRA

For comparative purposes, we also include discussion of Root Cause Analysis under PHA tools. Following is a brief outline of each approach, describing purpose and features, a thumbnail history, and key applications. Tables D–1 and D–2 summarize key points.

1. Quality Improvement Tools: TQM/CQI, Toyota Production System, Six Sigma

The three approaches we will describe can be used to improve all aspects of quality and are not targeted specifically at hazard prevention. Still,

TABLE D-1 Quality Improvement Approaches

Continuous Quality Improvement (Total Quality Management)	
Origin	TQM: Japanese and U.S. manufacturing, 1950s/1980s CQI: Berwick and Bataldan, 1980s
Purpose	Continuously improve quality by relentless focus on customer satisfaction
Core methodology	1. Plan a process improvement. 2. Do the intervention. 3. Study the results from the intervention. 4. Act on the results—if favorable by institutionalizing; if unfavorable by testing another intervention.
Key example	Ford Motor Company
Health care example	Institute for Healthcare Improvement; JCAHO accreditation requirement
Strength	Most widely dispersed and recognized improvement methodology

Toyota—Lean Production	Six Sigma
Toyota	Motorola in 1984
Lean production; endlessly reduce costs and lead time through elimination of waste	Achieve near zero defects (3.4 per million opportunities)
Rule 1. All work highly specified as to content, sequence, timing, and outcome. Rule 2. Every customer-supplier connection is direct, with unambiguous yes-or-no way to send requests and receive responses. Rule 3. The pathway for every product and service must be simple and direct. Rule 4. Improvement must be made in accord with scientific method, under guidance of a teacher, at the lowest possible level in organization.	1. Define: Identify problems, clarify scope, define goals 2. Measure performance to requirements, gather data, refine goals 3. Analyze: Develop hypotheses, identify root causes, analyze best practices 4. Improve: Conduct experiments to remove root cause, test solution, measure results, standardize solutions, implement new process 5. Control: Establish standard measures to maintain performance and correct problems as needed
Toyota, Alcoa	General Electric
Pittsburgh Regional Healthcare Initiative	University of Virginia Health System; Virtua Health, New Jersey
Focus on elimination of waste, empowerment of frontline workers	Focus on near zero defects and control of gains once achieved

TABLE D-2 Proactive Hazard Analysis Approaches

	Healthcare Failure Mode and Effect Analysis (adapted from FMEA)	Hazard Analysis and Critical Control Points
Origin	U.S. military, 1949, and NASA, 1960s	Pillsbury for NASA, 1959, to ensure safe food for astronauts
Purpose	To evaluate potential failures and their causes, pointing to actions to eliminate or reduce them	A systematic approach to the identification, assessment, and control of hazards
Core methodology	1. Define HFMEA™ topic. 2. Assemble HFMEA™ team. 3. Describe the process. 4. Conduct failure analysis. 5. Evaluate actions and outcome measures.	1. Conduct a hazard analysis. 2. Identify critical control points. 3. Establish critical limits for each CCP. 4. Establish monitoring requirements. 5. Establish correction actions when a CCP deviation occurs. 6. Establish ongoing verification procedures. 7. Establish record-keeping procedures.
Key example	U.S. auto manufacturing (FMEA)	Food manufacturing and services
Health care example	VHA	Medical device manufacturing
Strength	Adapted specifically for health care; model for JCAHO proactive risk assessment requirement	International standard in food sector; close interface with public-sector regulation; empirical evidence of effectiveness

Hazard and Operability Studies	Probabilistic Risk Assessment
United Kingdom—chemical industry, 1960s	Aviation industry
A team-based, systematic, and qualitative method to identify hazards (or deviations in design) in process industries	A tool to assess the contribution of multiple failures and combinations that may lead to catastrophic occurrences
1. Will someone be harmed? Who? In which way? How severely? 2. Will processes performance be reduced? In which way? How severely? What will impact be? 3. Will costs increase? If so, by how much? 4. Will there be cascading effects where deviation leads to other deviations? If so, what are they?	1. Development of a fault tree to visualize risk. Three elements: basic events, "AND" gates, "OR" gates. 2. Probability predictions are added to fault trees.
Chemical industry	Aviation, nuclear power
Telemedicine in European Union	Environmental health risk assessment
Compels parties to assess potential difficulties and devise mutually agreeable solutions	Models all combinations of failures that may lead to adverse events

advocates of each approach have examples where each has been used to achieve safety improvements. TQM is the earliest of the three approaches; the other two, Toyota Production System and Six Sigma, acknowledge their debts to TQM/CQI principles and techniques.

Total Quality Management/Continuous Quality Improvement

TQM/CQI is the earliest application of the scientific method to process improvement. TQM techniques have been applied widely in U.S. and Japanese manufacturing and in other organizations facing competitive challenges in a disciplined approach to enhance customer satisfaction. CQI is TQM applied within health care.

The method requires organizational leaders to establish improvement goals and to choose projects that can achieve specific improvements. Cross-functional teams devise a flow chart of a process under study and use data to understand variations from quality. The methodology regards errors as products of poorly designed systems, not as the fault of individual workers or "bad apples." Once teams have developed a sophisticated understanding of a process, they start a four-step practice:

1. *Plan* an intervention/experiment to improve the process.
2. *Do* the hypothesized intervention.
3. *Study* the results from the intervention.
4. *Act* on the results—if favorable, by institutionalizing the intervention; if unfavorable, by testing another intervention.[3]

Organizations with robust CQI programs have many improvement teams working at all times. TQM was introduced to Japanese manufacturers in the 1950s by Deming, Juran, and others and to U.S. manufacturers in the late 1970s and 1980s. Berwick and others proposed TQM as an alternative to traditional quality *assurance* under the term "Continuous Quality Improvement." CQI may be used to improve many organizational features beyond clinical quality, including patient satisfaction, error rates, waste, unit production costs, productivity, market share, and more. In the early 1990s, the Joint Commission on Accreditation of Healthcare Organizations (JCAHO) embraced this new paradigm and included CQI activities in its requirements for accredited institutions.

Fifteen years after its introduction, however, CQI has not lived up to its promise to "cure health care." Reviewing CQI's history in 1998, Blumenthal and Kilo found accomplishments and disappointments.[4] Among the former is a changed mind-set from assurance to continuous improvement, abandoning blame by focusing on system defects, creating a customer focus, motivating improvement projects across the nation, and educating thousands of health care workers in improvement techniques. Among its shortcomings has been an inability to identify a dramatically changed health care institution despite manufacturing examples such as Toyota; other problems include the failure to make deep inroads into clinical quality and a scant literature documenting sustained improvement.

CQI has been eclipsed by other methodologies, including the Toyota Production System, Six Sigma, and reengineering. Still, CQI remains the predominant quality improvement philosophy and methodology in the health care industry today.

Toyota Production System

Lean production focuses on elimination of waste—of materials, time, idle equipment, and inventory—to improve productivity and profits by improving material handling, inventory, quality, scheduling, personnel, and customer satisfaction. The core methodology as applied at Toyota is captured in four rules:

Rule 1: All work is highly specific as to content, sequence, timing, and outcome.

Rule 2: Every customer-supplier connection must be direct, and there must be an unambiguous yes-or-no way to send requests and receive responses.

Rule 3: The pathway for every product and service must be simple and direct.

Rule 4: Any improvement must be made in accordance with the scientific method, under the guidance of a teacher, at the lowest possible level of responsibility.

A key feature is the empowerment of line workers to implement design changes and to halt a process to avoid errors—turning workers into problem solvers. Although some initially thought Toyota's success was tied to cultural differences between Japan and the United States, the company's success in implementing the strategy in its North American plants neutralized that criticism.

Alcoa used the process to achieve one of the safest manufacturing sites for workers in the nation. Its head, former U.S. Treasury Secretary Paul O'Neill, helped establish the Pittsburgh Regional Healthcare Initiative in 1998, bringing stakeholders together to pursue perfecting the region's health care system—using the Toyota Production System (see case studies section later in this appendix). The initiative focuses on three goals:

1. *Patient safety:* Reducing hospital-acquired infections and medication errors to zero.

2. *Clinical initiatives:* Achieving breakthrough performance in cardiac surgery, depression, diabetes, orthopedics, and obstetrics.

3. *Perfecting patient care:* Redesigning organizations to allow everyone to learn from errors and problems.[5]

Six Sigma

Six Sigma is a quality program that seeks to improve processes so that no more than 3.4 mistakes occur per million opportunities. One commentator describes its approach as "much like that of Total Quality Management, perhaps with a more aggressive goal." Proponents suggest that the relentless focus on error reduction provides a structure and focus missing from other QI techniques. Six Sigma has a five-step improvement cycle corresponding to the acronym DMAIC with the aim to continuously reduce defects:

1. *Define* by identifying problems, clarifying scope, defining goals.

2. *Measure* performance against requirements, gather data, refine problems/goals.

3. *Analyze* by developing hypotheses, identifying root causes, analyzing best practices.

4. *Improve* by conducting experiments to remove root cause, testing solutions, measuring results, standardizing solutions, implementing new processes.

5. *Control* by establishing standard measures to maintain performance and correcting problems as needed.

In 1984, Motorola engineers invented Six Sigma, named for a statistical measure of variation (1 Sigma reflects 690,000 defects per million opportunities; 2 equals 308,000; 3 reflects 66,800; 4 reflects 6,210; 5 reflects 230, and 6 reflects 3.4). The strategy achieved prominence in the 1980s at IBM and became widely known in the 1990s at General Electric, which claims dramatic error reduction and savings from its Six Sigma program. GE has applied Six Sigma to its medical device manufacturing division and to its employee health benefits program. GE also initiated its own Six Sigma health care consulting organization.[6] The University of Virginia Health System and Virtua Health in New Jersey are two examples of health care adapters.

Chassin provides examples where medical care performs below one sigma, as in the documented 79 percent—or 790,000 out of 1 million—of eligible heart attack survivors not receiving beta-blockers. He also notes how the anesthesia community reduced deaths from rates of 50 per million in the 1980s to as few as 5 today. A proposed advantage of Six Sigma over TQM is the former's focus on defects from perfect versus the latter's focus on improvement from variation in a mean.[7]

2. Proactive Hazard Analysis Tools: FMEA/HFMEA™, HACCP, HAZOPS, PRA, RCA

PHA tools tend to be more prescriptive and to have more record-keeping and other requirements than QI tools. These requirements, justifiable when the objective is safety, are more onerous than needed for nonsafety improvement projects. Root Cause Analysis, though not explicitly proactive, is described here for comparative purposes.

Failure Mode and Effect Analysis/Healthcare Failure Mode and Effect Analysis

FMEA is a tool used in manufacturing to evaluate potential failures and their causes and to prioritize potential failures according to risk, pointing to actions to eliminate or reduce the likelihood of occurrence. The Veterans Health Administration (VHA) pioneered the adaptation of FMEA and other industrial process control tools to patient safety, developing the HFMEA™ for use in health care settings. This section describes HFMEA™ more than FMEA. Five steps are involved in an HFMEA™ analysis:

1. *Define the HFMEA™ topic*, including a clear definition of the process to be studied.
2. *Assemble the HFMEA™ team*, which should be multidisciplinary and include subject matter experts and an adviser.
3. *Graphically describe the process* with a flow diagram, numbering each step, identifying the area on which to focus, and identifying all subprocesses.
4. *Conduct a failure analysis* listing all possible failure modes, determining the severity and probability of each, using a decision tree to determine if the failure mode warrants further action, and listing all failure modes where the decision is made to proceed.
5. *Evaluate actions and outcome measures* determining which failure modes to eliminate, control, or accept; identifying an action for each failure

mode to be controlled or eliminated; identifying outcome measures to test the redesigned process; and identifying an individual to complete the action.

FMEA was developed in the U.S. military in 1949 to determine the effect of system and equipment failures[8] and was used by the National Aeronautics and Space Administration (NASA) in the 1960s to predict failures, plan preventive measures, estimate the cost of failures, and plan redundant systems in the Apollo space program. In the 1970s, U.S. manufacturers began using the tool in automotive and other plants, and automakers established industrywide FMEA standards in 1993. In 1998, the VHA established the National Center for Patient Safety to create a culture of safety in its hospital system. In collaboration with Tenet HealthSystem, VHA leaders developed the HFMEA™ as "a systematic approach to identify and prevent product and process problems before they occur."

In July 2001, JCAHO implemented a new standard requiring all accredited hospitals to complete at least one "proactive risk assessment" of a high-risk process per year. The standard (LD.5.2) requires eight actions by hospitals:

1. Select at least one high-risk process.
2. Identify steps where failure modes may occur.
3. Identify possible effects on patients.
4. Conduct a Root Cause Analysis to determine why failures may occur.
5. Redesign the process to minimize the risk to patients.
6. Test and implement the redesigned process.
7. Monitor the effectiveness of the new process.
8. Implement a strategy to maintain the process.

VHA hospitals have proceeded the furthest in using HFMEA™ although many hospitals across the nation are now using this tool in meeting the new JCAHO standards.

Hazard Analysis and Critical Control Points

HACCP is a systematic approach to the identification, assessment, and control of hazards. While some definitions directly refer to food—reflecting the near exclusive use to date of HACCP in food production and service—the process is usable in the manufacturing, distribution, and use of any product or service that may experience safety problems. A "critical control point" is a point, step, or procedure at which control can be exercised to prevent, eliminate, or minimize a hazard. Seven steps form the core of the HACCP approach:

1. *Conduct a hazard analysis* preparing a list of steps in a process where significant hazards occur and identifying preventive measures.

2. *Identify critical control points*—steps at which controls can be applied to prevent, eliminate, or reduce a safety hazard to acceptable levels.

3. *Establish critical limits* for preventive measures associated with each identified critical control point.

4. *Establish monitoring requirements* for each critical control point and procedures to monitor results to adjust the process and maintain control.

5. *Establish corrective actions* to be taken when a critical limit deviation occurs.

6. *Establish procedures to verify* on an ongoing basis that the HACCP system is working correctly.

7. *Establish record-keeping procedures* to document the HACCP system.

HACCP was developed in 1959 by the Pillsbury Company to ensure the safety of food in the new U.S. space program. In 1973, the U.S. Food and Drug Administration (FDA) mandated the first use of HACCP by regulation for all low-acid canned foods after a public outcry over a botulism outbreak in canned soups. Following other foodborne illness outbreaks in the early 1990s, FDA expanded HACCP requirements for seafood and for fruit and vegetable beverages and is now considering HACCP for all foods under its jurisdiction. In 1997, the U.S. Department of Agriculture began implementation of HACCP in all meat and poultry operations under its jurisdiction. HACCP has also become the international food production and service safety standard.

Empirical research has demonstrated the effectiveness of HACCP in reducing levels of foodborne pathogens in food production and service in a wide array of settings. HACCP differs from the other QI/PHA approaches because of its significant and longstanding interface with public-sector regulation. The broad use of the tool results from government mandates more than voluntary compliance. Studies also have revealed weaknesses and gaps in HACCP implementation in the United States, demonstrating that effective implementation requires sufficient resources for regulatory authorities.

Hazard and Operability Study

HAZOP is a team-based, systematic, qualitative method to identify hazards (or deviations in design intent) in process industries. The study begins with the team considering all ways a process might deviate from desired performance using guide words such as *more, less, none, part of,* and *other than* to ensure consistency and reliability. A team—typically one whose members designed and operate a facility—considers the consequences of each deviation from operating conditions by asking key questions:

- Will someone be harmed? Who? In which way? How severely?
- Will the performance of the processes be reduced? In which way? How severely? What will the impact be?
- Will costs increase? If so, by how much?
- Will there be any cascading effects where this deviation leads to other deviations? If so, what are they?

After this process, the team develops an action plan to eliminate or minimize deviations and their consequences. The technique seems to work because key parties to the process are present—designers and operators, as well as builders and maintainers. The HAZOP approach has been helpful in avoiding breakdowns in contractual relationships arising from lack of understanding of what elements are truly important and susceptible to unrecognized threats; it compels both parties to assess potential difficulties and devise mutually agreeable solutions. Another advantage is that it encourages the team to consider less obvious ways in which a deviation may occur. The HAZOP process was developed by ICI Ltd. in the United Kingdom in the 1960s to assess potential hazards of chemical plants to their operators and the public. Its use has been adapted for a range of other industries, including water.

Probabilistic Risk Assessment

The PHA tools already described are designed to eliminate or mitigate potential hazards or failures emanating from a single cause. Reliability and safety analysts in the aviation and other high-risk industries realized a need for a tool to understand multiple failures or combinations of failures that could lead to catastrophic occurrences. PRA was identified as an analysis tool that allows risks to be visualized in ways not possible with FMEA, HACCP, or HAZOP by adding two additional benefits: hierarchical modeling through fault trees and the assignment of probabilities. The fault tree framework graphically illustrates risk and reliability, and the assignment of probabilities allows regulators to establish threshold limits of risk and to specify safety and reliability standards.[9] Unlike the other tools presented herein, PRA does not include process steps to operationalize its use for managers and workers. This tool, instead, may be used in combination with other approaches as a powerful addition to identify elements of a process most critical for safety improvement.

PRA has been used most frequently to assess risks in catastrophic, low-probability events such as nuclear power plant meltdowns, space shuttle accidents, and earthquakes. In recent years, analysts have begun to explore its applicability to estimating environmental health risks.[10] More recently, analysts have begun using PRA to model high-impact, low-frequency iatrogenic injury events in medical care. Marx and Slonim suggest FMEA and Root Cause Analysis (to be described) "are limited in their focus to a single failure or single event" and "are not designed to assess the combinations of risk that, for example, may occur in the medication delivery process between the physician, the pharmacist, the pharmacy technician, the unit clerk and the dispensing nurse. . . . PRA, by comparison, would identify all combinations of failures including the initial profiling error and the failure of safety nets that might otherwise prevent the adverse event."[11]

Few specific examples are available of PRA used for patient safety. The most extensive is an application to anesthesia patient risk described later in this appendix.

Root Cause Analysis

RCA is a qualitative, retrospective approach to error analysis that is widely applied to major industrial accidents. Root Cause Analyses search out latent or system failures that underlie adverse events or near misses. In 1997, JCAHO mandated use of RCA in investigation of sentinel events in its accredited hospitals. Key steps in an RCA include formation of interdisciplinary team, data collection, data analysis—establishing how and why the event happened through identification of latent and active failures, and identification of administrative and systems problems for redesign. Although regarded as retrospective, effective RCAs point toward correction of systems problems to prevent future errors or near misses. Because RCAs are uncontrolled case studies, they may be tainted by hindsight bias.

III. KEY COMMON PRINCIPLES AND ATTRIBUTES OF QI/PHA METHODOLOGIES

Literature review and interviews with quality experts lead to the conclusion that the QI and PHA approaches described here have more similarities to than differences from each other. The essential feature of each is the application of the scientific method to process analysis, management, and improvement. This approach is rooted in the statistical analytic tools developed by Shewhart in the 1930s, applied in war production in the 1940s, introduced to Japanese manufacturing by Deming and Juran in the 1950s, and adopted by U.S. manufacturers beginning in the 1970s and 1980s.

Each tool has attributes distinguishing it from the others. These features merit study and consideration by potential users. No empirical literature has proven any single approach to be "the best," though HACCP has undergone more rigorous scrutiny than any other methodology.[12] Each can be— and most have been—used in health care settings to perform hazard analysis. QI and PHA tools also may be used in combination; for example, at Virtua Health in New Jersey, FMEA is used for planning purposes to identify a high-risk, hazardous procedure on which to use Six Sigma to implement and sustain a process improvement.[13] Tools developed outside of medical care must be adapted to fit the requirements of this sector. Any QI/PHA tool will undergo some adaptation to fit into an organization's culture, structure, and individual requirements.

Key features found in all or at least one of the methodologies are identified as follows:

Features Common to All QI/PHA Approaches

- Scientific approach to process analysis/system improvement
- Decision making driven by data
- Process focus: Use of flow diagrams
- Improvement focus rather than reliance on external standards
- Preventive orientation: Fixing quality problems or hazards before errors are committed
- Interdisciplinary team focus

Features Common to All QI Tools

- Customer focus (internal and/or external) as determinant of quality

Features Unique to Specific QI Tools

- Waste reduction focus: lean production
- Empowerment of frontline workers: lean production
- Reducing errors to near zero: Six Sigma
- Focus on control phase to maintain improvement: Six Sigma
- Companion methodology to overcome organizational resistance (change acceleration process): Six Sigma

Features Common to PHI Tools

- Proactive identification of potential safety hazards and control mechanisms

Features Unique to Specific PHA Tools

- Development of hazard score matrix: HFMEA
- Significant interface with public-sector regulation: HACCP
- Identification of Critical Control Points for ongoing hazard measurement and prevention: HACCP
- Tool develops status as international standard: HACCP
- Asking leading/open-ended questions to identify hard-to-identify hazards: HAZOP
- Ability to analyze multiple or combinations of failures: PRA
- Hierarchical modeling through fault trees: PRA
- Assignment of probabilities: PRA

In researching this report, the authors were struck by the extent of experimentation in the medical community—in the United States and beyond—in adapting and applying these QI and PHA approaches to patient safety problems. We were unable to identify any central "clearinghouse" to enable health professionals to become familiar with these different approaches and to learn lessons from their adaptation through case studies or other methods. *We suggest that the health care community—especially professionals and institutions interested in patient safety and harm reduction—would benefit from the existence of a central resource or clearinghouse on experimentation using various structured improvement tools and methodologies.*

Key Principles to Identify Critical Control Points: Conceptual and Methodological Considerations in Design and Evaluation of Risk/Hazard Identification, Assessment, and Management Strategies in Health Care

Central to all QI/PHA approaches is the use of the scientific method in the analysis, management, and improvement of work processes. Research by Ackoff suggests that in any system a small set of subprocesses accounts for the "identity of the system." He defines a system as a whole that contains two or more parts satisfying five conditions:

1. The whole has one or more defining functions.
2. Each part in the set can affect the behavior or properties of the whole.
3. There is a subset of parts that is sufficient in one or more environments for carrying out the defining function of the whole; each part is separately necessary to carry out the defining function.
4. The way the behavior or properties of each part affects its behavior or properties depends on a behavior or property of at least one other part.
5. The effect of any subset of parts on the system depends on the behavior of at least one other subset.[14]

The third condition posits that each system consists of a small number of *essential* processes without which the system itself cannot function.

Research by Batalden and Mohr applies this insight to medical care, demonstrating that medicine also consists of distinct and identifiable "core processes" that can be mapped, analyzed, and improved.[15] Moreover, in many clinical specialties and subspecialties, the Pareto Principle holds: A small number of core processes account for a high proportion of total work performed within each specialty. James observed that in respiratory therapy five key processes (such as oxygen therapy) account for as much as 90 percent of total work; in physical therapy, four key processes account for the same overall volume of activity.[16]

Examining medical care through the lens of key processes provides a helpful way to consider systemic improvement. One potentially fruitful way to do this is through medical specialties. For example, anesthesiology is acknowledged as the leading medical specialty worldwide in addressing patient safety. A medical malpractice crisis in the 1970s galvanized anesthesiologists at all levels, including grassroots clinicians, to address patient safety by incorporating new technologies, standards, and guidelines and to confront problems relating to human factors and systems issues. As part of this effort, in 1985 the profession established the Anesthesia Patient Safety Foundation, the first such initiative in organized medicine.[17] As a result of their improvements, some have pegged the death rate from errors in anesthesiology at about 5 deaths per 1 million opportunities, which now approaches Six Sigma level. A recent literature review casts doubts on that level of success,[18] though there is broad agreement on dramatic improvements in safety that have led to dramatic decreases in malpractice premiums.[19]

A core requirement in applying any QI/PHA tool effectively to improve patient safety is to build data, measurement, and control systems around key processes. HACCP demonstrates that every process contains multiple Critical Control Points that will vary, process to process. Two preconditions are necessary to identify Critical Control Points in medical care: first, the identification of core processes, and second, the availability and accessibility of data. Then it becomes more feasible to identify Critical Control Points and to eliminate or minimize hazards.

Since the publication of *To Err Is Human*, most interventions to enhance patient safety have focused at the institutional level—hospitals, nursing homes, and clinics. As institutions seek to incorporate patient safety initiatives, a key challenge is to win the attention and support of physicians. The identification and control of Critical Control Points in medical care, along with the striking example of anesthesiology, suggest that a parallel—and potentially more successful—approach to rigorous PHA may be through medical specialties and subspecialties in addition to institutional strategies. One clear advantage, demonstrated by the anesthesiology experience, is the potential application of systems improvements on a global basis.

Recent developments in organized medicine support this direction. Brennan reports that the European Federation of Internal Medicine, the American Board of Internal Medicine, and the American College of Physicians/American Society of Internal Medicine have recently outlined a draft physician charter with new major principles and professional responsibilities. The third draft responsibility suggests a new commitment to improve the quality of care not just for individuals but for all patients collectively, a notion Brennan refers to as a new "civic responsibility." He writes: "The failure of the quality measurement/improvement movement to reach its full potential may reflect the relative failure of the profession to undertake, as a civic activity, the effort to ensure the quality of care defined broadly. . . . Civic professionalism suggests that the professional should be leading the way, not being brought along by regulations. . . . For this step, we must likely turn to the various specialty societies. . . . If we are to be serious about educating practicing physicians about professionalism and quality, we must rely on a strong confederation of specialty societies and groups."[20]

IV. APPLICABILITY OF HAZARD ANALYSIS AND SYSTEMS APPROACH TO ADVERSE EVENT PREVENTION

Croteau and Schyve[21] identify essential steps in Proactive Hazard Analysis to prevent adverse events:

1. Identify a high-risk process.
   a. History of adverse outcomes;
   b. Identified in the literature as high risk;
   c. Has several characteristics of a high-risk process;
   d. New process;
   e. Proposed redesign (such as in response to a sentinel event).
2. Create a flowchart of the process as designed.
3. Assess the actual implementation of the process (e.g., different locations, shifts).
4. Identify where there is, or may be, variation in the implementation of the process; that is, what are the failure modes?
5. For each identified failure mode, what are the possible effects?
6. Assess the seriousness (i.e., the "criticality") of the possible effects (e.g., delay in treatment, temporary loss of function, patient death).
7. For the most critical effects, conduct an RCA to determine why the variation (the failure mode) leading to that effect occurs.
8. Redesign the process and/or underlying systems to minimize risk of that failure mode or to protect the patient from the effects of that failure mode.
9. Conduct a PHA on the redesigned process with special attention to how the redesigned steps will affect other steps in the process and whether they will continue to achieve the beneficial things that the previous design could do.
10. Consider simulation testing of the redesigned process.
11. Consider a pilot test of the redesigned process.
12. Identify and implement measures of the effectiveness of the redesigned process.
13. Implement a strategy for maintaining the effectiveness of the redesigned process over time.

The identification of failure modes and quality management deficiencies must lead to the development and institution of reasonable interventions to prevent adverse events. Multidisciplinary teams composed of an equitable mix of frontline health care workers (e.g., clinicians, safety/facility personnel, environment services) and mid- and upper-level management must promote a pervasive, patient-centered safety culture of adverse event prevention, not individual blame. In keeping with James Reason's "swiss cheese model of error," PHA and quality management programs must identify "latent" errors as well as the more apparent "active" errors. Systems redesign to prevent all such errors should then be based on a balanced utilization of evidence-based technology, training, ongoing education, and consensus standard operating procedures (SOPs) and "best practices," keeping in mind each human's inherent cognitive (e.g., memory recall) and physical (e.g., fatigue) limitations.

Lastly, health care must recognize that adverse event prevention is an ongoing process. Each new system intervention brings with it a whole new set of potential failure modes and contributing factors that should be similarly proactively analyzed and prioritized for intervention. This, combined with the ever-widening scope of system complexities due to an aging patient population, increased numbers of the immune compromised, and the need to "fast track" new and more effective technological advances in medicine, raises the need to handle health care's current "patient safety paradox" with an organized, proactive collective consciousness.

V. DATA REQUIREMENTS AND MEASUREMENT TOOLS TO SUPPORT EACH METHODOLOGY

How can data be employed to do prospective identification of risk points without waiting for a near miss? Pareto charts (histograms), run charts, control charts, and scatter grams are among the more widely used tools to exemplify performance data. Despite the inherent strong points and weaknesses of a respective tool, the reliability, defensibility, and reproducibility of the underlying performance data must be paramount. To maximize the accuracy and precision of such data and to facilitate standardized use throughout all health care, performance measures must be the result of a well-thought-out process to maximize efforts to exceed customer expectation and consistent error and failure definition.[22]

To facilitate and standardize measurement, Chang proffers an error taxonomy consisting of four subclassifications of error: impact, type, domain, and cause. The "impact" classification deals with the outcome or effect of the error; the "type" concerns the visible process that was in error; the "domain" is where the error occurred and who was involved; and the "cause" is the factors and agents that bring about error. Establishing subclasses for respective errors can not only help in defining and standardizing performance measures, but more importantly, it significantly facilitates the identification of corresponding failure modes and consequently the use of PHA and QI methods. Consistently (i.e., globally) defined errors across an entire health care setting enable a collective patient safety consciousness to address potential errors proactively, rather than retrospectively. Retrospective analysis, although necessary and insightful at times, is still retrospective—relying on performance measures of accidents/incidents or near misses, which themselves are the products of, or promote, hindsight bias and a host of other potential unwanted consequences.

VI. CASE STUDIES

Continuous Quality Improvement

Two studies illustrate the promises and shortcoming of CQI.

Concerns about the quality of health care in France led to the creation, in 1991, of a national agency for health care quality, Agence National pour le Développement de l'Evaluation Médicale (ANDEM). In 1997, ANDEM became Agence Nationale pour l'Accréditation et l'Evaluation en Santé (ANAES). Between 1995 and 1998, ANAES sought to increase hospital management's awareness of CQI and to study its implementation in public hospitals. In 1995, a call was issued for projects on patient safety concerns such as nosocomial infections and incidents after anesthesia and blood transfusions. A second call for projects issued in 1996 was open for all project types. Selected projects received a financial incentive of between $10,000 and $80,000. Juries were composed of 12 to 14 individuals with experience in quality selected projects.

From 260 first-round project applications, 29 were selected and 26 were evaluated. Nine projects addressed prevention of nosocomial infections, five addressed medical records management, five addressed anesthesia safety, four addressed blood transfusion safety, four addressed drug dispensing safety, and two addressed controlling violence in psychiatric units. At evaluation, 38 months after initiation, 61 percent of the patient safety projects had met their objectives, and more than 50 percent of participating hospitals had established new CQI projects following the initial one. Half of the project team leaders considered that, at the time of the final evaluation, their main performance indicator (e.g., number of falls, number of nosocomial infections) had begun to evolve satisfactorily. Overall evaluation of this project is limited by the noncomparative nature of the study, which was managed by highly motivated individuals in institutions that voluntarily applied to participate.[23]

By contrast, a randomized controlled trial called Improving Prevention through Organization, Vision and Empowerment (IMPROVE) was conducted by two competing health maintenance organizations (HMOs) in the Minneapolis–St. Paul area to test the hypothesis that an HMO can use CQI to stimulate private primary care clinics to develop better delivery systems for eight clinical preventive services: blood pressure monitoring, Pap smear, cholesterol monitoring, tobacco use cessation, breast examination, mammography, influenza vaccine, and pneumococcal vaccine. Forty-four clinics were randomized with follow up involving 3,136 patients from the control clinics and 3,295 from the intervention clinics. The intervention was conducted between September 1994 and June 1996.

All 22 intervention clinics established improvement teams, and all training sessions received excellent evaluations. At the end, 94 percent of the 114 clinic team members reported being very satisfied or satisfied with their experience. Results showed no significant difference between intervention and control clinics on any of the clinical measures except for blood pressure. Except for two small differences between the intervention and control clinics, CQI failed to produce any significantly greater improvement in the intervention clinics during the trial. "Our study raises questions about whether CQI is the right model for making these changes."[24]

Hazard Analysis and Critical Control Points[25]

Morrison Management Specialists, a member of the Compass Group, is a leading provider of food service expertise to the health care industry. Morrison services approximately 500 health care facilities nationwide, including hospitals, long-term care facilities, and senior dining communities. Mary Ivins, Director, Dining on Call, is responsible for Morrison's program that provides patients with room service–style food delivery and for implementing and overseeing Morrison's food safety policies and procedures.

Morrison's use of HACCP is pivotal to minimizing foodborne illness risks and maximizing quality service. She sees the results from using HACCP as favorable but admits that Morrison's biggest challenges are ongoing education and training of employees in proper food service procedures and simplifying the HACCP process.

Because many food preparation processes and subprocesses are similar, Morrison uses HACCP to identify as many hazards as possible throughout the entire food production process—from receiving food products from vendors, through holding, storage, cooking, and preparation, through service to the patients/residents, visitors, and workers. Ivins points to a number of types of entrees in which HACCP has made a significant impact in reducing the risk of foodborne illness. She believes HACCP has been used to safely prepare ground meat and chicken in a way that prevents diseases, including *E. coli*, salmonella, and campylobacter; to use luncheon meats safely; and to develop methods to ensure the safe cold storage of hot foods.

To keep the program on track, Morrison uses a comprehensive system of internal and third-party auditing with customer service feedback. Critical Control Points and corresponding acceptable physical constraints are established for each part of the process. Temperature, holding/storage time, storage location (e.g., raw food stored below cooked foods), labeling criteria (e.g., name and expiration date), as well as strict guidelines for cleanliness, disinfection, and hygiene of both the facility and food service workers are all important criteria within Morrison's HACCP compliance process. Morrison also audits its vendors by checking and documenting the temperature of a minimum of 10 percent of all potentially hazardous foods at the time of delivery by the vendor.

Morrison's regional directors of operations are responsible for ensuring that each account is monitoring and documenting compliance with HACCP guidelines. Quality assurance management plays a key role, including keeping a policies and procedures manual readily available, posting food safety signage and professional information, and providing a certified food safety manager at each site. All monitoring and documenting are vital to complying with current HACCP guidelines and in determining if the processes and HACCP should be modified to mitigate variations of existing or newly identified hazards.

Ivins sees the long-term gains from Morrison's use of HACCP as the comfort of knowing the company is serving quality, safe food to patients/residents, clients, and employees and a well-educated supervisory and service staff.

Hazard Analysis and Operability Studies

HAZOP has been successful in identifying security threats in certain safety-critical information and communication technology systems.[26] CORAS[27] (risk assessment of security critical systems) has used HAZOP for information security risk analysis involving medical databases and telemedicine. Areas include (1) authentication procedures (e.g., password policies, authentication mechanisms); (2) threats related to unauthorized change of information while produced, transmitted, or stored; (3) threats related to availability of service and information; and (4) threats related to network availability.

Whether used with or without other PHA techniques, HAZOP is an integral part of the CORAS risk management process, specifically the identification of threats involving confidentiality, integrity, and availability for a Web-based telecollaboration service. In at least one proactive risk analysis, CORAS used both fault tree analysis (FTA) and HAZOP. After identifying the threats using HAZOP, the threats were inserted into three fault trees (confidentiality, integrity, and availability) to better visualize the interrelationships among the respective threats.

Prior to conducting a HAZOP, CORAS identified areas of relevance on which the risk assessment and specific security aspects should focus, as well as worst-case threat scenarios. These "targets" and aspects—as well as the experiences of previous assessments—facilitated selection of guidewords for the HAZOP. CORAS's process also uses diagrams (use-case diagrams, sequence diagrams, collaboration diagrams, activity diagrams) of the most important issues. The HAZOP is run as a structured brainstorming session with participants who include developers, providers, and end users (e.g., hospital/medical staff). The diagrams and the HAZOP table are shown on side-by-side screens as the HAZOP is conducted. This enables the team to focus on each threat to be assessed. Although the HAZOP session was used to identify threats, consequences and frequencies also were assessed.

Eva Skipenes, Security Adviser, Norwegian Centre for Telemedicine comments:

> "The HAZOP method is very useful to identify and document threats and unwanted incidents, and to gather as much information as possible from different participants. It is easy for nontechnologists to follow this method, but it requires good planning (choice of guidewords, choice of which aspects to focus on, and which detail level to use). A good result also depends on the availability of important stakeholders, like the users of the system/service, and the providers (both technical and, for example, medical service providers). A HAZOP often identifies threats at very different levels of detail. The use of fault trees afterwards to identify the relationships among the identified threats was very useful."

Skipenes adds that CORAS and NTS will use HAZOP again. NTS is using it for risk assessment of telemedicine services and information security at primary health care centers in North Norway.[28]

Failure Mode and Effect Analysis

The Detroit Medical Center (DMC) in Michigan has successfully used FMEA to identify and mitigate a number of patient safety issues throughout its health system. One such endeavor was initiated as a result of a nationally publicized event concerning "gaps" in the recall process involving Olympus bronchoscopes at a major teaching hospital. The failure of a recall notice to be delivered from a teaching hospital's loading dock area to the clinical areas where the bronchoscopes were used on patients led to contaminated bronchoscope use in patients and subsequent nosocomial infection. Prompted by this report and the potential for use of recalled equipment and drugs in patients if the recall process fails, Tammy S. Lundstrom, M.D., and associated staff at DMC prioritized their current recall process for FMEA. DMC's "recall-FMEA" is based on internal near-miss data and/or events that have been reported in the media from throughout the United States or from other event databases, such as JCAHO Sentinel Event Alerts or Institute for Safe Medication Practices.

DMC's recall-FMEA team is composed of staff from stakeholder departments, including logistics, pharmacy, operating room, invasive procedure areas, materials management, environment of care, epidemiology, purchasing, and respiratory therapy. A core group was chosen to perform the actual FMEA with input from affected areas. Criteria considered for inclusion in the recall-FMEA team included:

- People who have experience with the recall process;
- People who regularly perform steps in the recall process;
- People who have no experience with the process (a reality check);
- A subject matter expert (procurement personnel in charge of recall process);
- Quality department facilitator.

DMC gathered relevant information related to the recall process, including current internal procedures/policies/guidelines related to recalls, a search for any external or professional society guidelines and best practices, development of a professional organization resource list, and interviews of key staff and departments regarding the current process.

Next, DMC developed a process flow chart. Because the recall process itself is such a huge undertaking, the team narrowed the scope of the FMEA to include only that part of the process related to internal departmental responses to recall notices, with the understanding that once this FMEA was completed, the scope would be expanded. Likely failure modes were identified and scored for criticality by assigning a hazard score related to severity of the failure mode and probability of the failure mode (each using a 1 to 4 rating). Subprocesses with a total hazard score of 8 or greater were chosen for redesign. A total of 15 subprocesses were identified, of which 11 had a hazard score of more than 8. Six of these involved the internal departmental response and therefore were chosen for improvement efforts. For example, internal processes involve delivery of DMC recall notices via e-mail notification. The failure mode included involved departments failing to receive the e-mail notification; the likely cause identified was failure to include the appropriate department/individual on the department's procurement e-mail notification list. The effect was that the involved department/individual would not know of the recall, and faulty equipment/drugs would be used on patients. The solution was to identify a point person in purchasing who would be responsible for maintaining the notification list. That procurement staff member was responsible for contacting department heads at all facilities to verify names of point people in each department with the ultimate responsibility of responding to the e-mail recall notice. Redundancy is built in by including department heads, and list maintenance is performed on an ongoing basis to ensure accuracy.

DMC's ability to identify multiple processes and subprocesses as likely fail points in its current recall process, and therefore potential unexpected clinical events involving patients, was decisive in DMC considering the FMEA to be a success. This success was facilitated by DMC's decision to narrow the scope of the FMEA to include only a portion of the recall process, with the goal to expand the scope once the initial subprocess was rectified. The first phase of the recall-FMEA was started on October 9, 2002, and completed on December 10, 2002. Action items were scheduled to be closed out by the end of April 2003, and the next phase of the recall process will be targeted for improvement.

The FMEA has resulted in DMC improving the timeliness and accuracy of its targeted recall notification. The response rates to recalls (e.g., whether a product was not used, returned to logistics, or pulled for pickup) increased by a factor of three over the previous recall notification process. Efforts are ongoing to refine the process further in order to have response rates of 100 percent.

Dr. Lundstrom considers the recall-FMEA a success. She stresses that "although the FMEA process is time consuming, prioritization of improvements through narrowed scope and hazard scoring focuses improvement efforts on the critical elements." Dr. Lundstrom and her staff would use the FMEA process again.

Healthcare Failure Mode and Effect Analysis

Failure mode and effects analysis helps to anticipate what can go wrong with a high-risk health care process and to apply measures to prevent the error. Industries such as aviation, aerospace, and automotive manufacturing have long used failure mode and effects analysis to prevent accidents from occurring, but there is only one model specific to health care. That model, called Healthcare Failure Mode and Effects Analysis, was developed by the Department of Veterans Affairs (VA) National Center for Patient Safety and first put into practice in 2001.

The VA's HFMEA™ model is a five-step process that involves selecting a topic for analysis, selecting a team to do the analysis, mapping a flow chart of the high-risk process, identifying failure modes within the process, and, if necessary, redesigning the process.

In its first application of HFMEA™ the VA asked its 163 medical centers to use HFMEA™ to analyze their contingency plans for their computerized, bar-code medication administration systems in the event of a power failure or other interruption to the system. The process was a valuable exercise, VA officials say, and revealed vulnerabilities to facilities' contingency plans and prompted facilities to make changes to prevent problems from occurring.

For example, some facilities learned that they wrongly assumed that data backups of their computerized bar-code systems were performed more frequently than every 24 hours. In the event of a power failure, newly entered data such as a change in a patient's medication may not have been included in the data backup, and the patient could be at risk of receiving an incorrect medication order. HFMEA™ teams recommended redesigning the process by requiring more frequent data backups of their facilities' electronic medication records and providing a mechanism to let staff know when the backup is completed.

The HFMEA™ process helped the teams identify other gaps in the contingency plans by asking the following questions:

• Do caregivers know how to access and use their contingency plans for the medication administration system?
• Is a process in place to stop new referrals to a unit, if necessary, when the electronic medication administration system is unavailable?
• Is there a procedure to request additional staff if necessary to help implement the contingency measures?
• What process is in place to ensure that once the electronic system is restored, any information about a patient's medications that is recorded manually during a power failure is available to caregivers?

- How are new medication orders recorded while the electronic system is unavailable, and how are they entered into the system when it is restored?
- How much data from the patient's medication history should be provided when paper backup records are needed?
- Without some parameters on the amount of information needed from paper backup records, several facilities realized they could end up with complete paper records of 100 or more pages for some patients.

Although the HFMEA™ teams addressed the same topic, each designed its own solutions to the questions raised by the analysis. VA facilities are now on their own to select topics for a proactive risk assessment in 2003. Topics selected include reporting of laboratory or radiology results, patient identification procedures, and patient backlogs for procedures. The VA's first experience with HFMEA™ also provided the agency with additional lessons to improve the process for proactive risk analysis. Some of the lessons learned from the VA's first application of HFMEA™ include the following:

- Assign an HFMEA™ team member the task of mapping the flow diagram before the team's first meeting. This ensures that the team moves in the right direction from the start.
- Ensure that the steps to a process are numbered and the subprocesses are lettered. These simple measures help to keep the HFMEA™ team organized and prevent the team from overlooking potential failure modes.
- Limit the flow diagram of the process to no more than 10 to 12 steps; otherwise the diagram gets too large.
- Make testing of proposed changes a formal part of the HFMEA™ process. Testing can evaluate whether any of the proposed changes introduce unintended consequences.

Additional information and tools for HFMEA™ are available from the VA National Center for Patient Safety Web site (http://www.patientsafety.gov).

Probabilistic Risk Assessment

In the only published study of Probabilistic Risk Assessment and patient safety that we could identify, Dr. Elisabeth Paté-Cornell extended PRA—called "engineering risk analysis"—to the study of anesthesia patient risk to show how this tool can incorporate human and organizational factors to support patient safety decisions before complete datasets can be gathered and in cases where key factors are not directly observable.[29]

In assessing the risk of severe anesthesia accidents, technical failures such as machine malfunctions can be easily identified and corrected. Indeed, most of the progress in improving anesthesia safety over the past 25 years has been attributed to identifying and correcting technical risks. Risks attributable to human errors are more difficult to detect, characterize, and anticipate because statistical samples are seldom available, such as the risk of injury due to substance abuse by the anesthesiologist. Gathering these data is difficult.

Accidents are divided into scenarios formed of "basic events," and a Bayesian approach is used to assess probabilities and consequences of each type. Probabilities are developed from three sources: existing datasets, analysis of basic engineering properties of the systems, and expert opinions. Expert opinions, when well defined and encoded, provide essential information that could not be obtained in time to support urgent decisions.

Seven initiating events were identified: breathing circuit disconnect, esophageal intubation, nonventilation, malignant hyperthermia, inhaled anesthetic overdose, anaphylactic reaction, and severe hemorrhage. Probabilities per operation were assessed. Experts identified types of problems that could affect the performance of anesthesiologists and the rates of occurrence. Analysts then recomputed the probability of each patient accident for each problem type:

- Problem-free: 0.53
- Fatigue: 0.10
- Cognitive problems: 0.04
- Personality problems: 0.04
- Severe distraction: 0.03
- Drug abuse: 0.03
- Alcohol abuse: 0.04
- Aging/neurological problems: 0.03
- Lack of training: 0.12
- Lack of supervision: 0.04

Figures show estimated probability of the state of the anesthesiologist per operation.

Experts identified policies to decrease the probability of each problem. The distribution of practitioner problems was then used to compute the anticipated benefits from each measure. Whereas alcohol and drug problems had been at the forefront of concerns at the outset of the study, the more immediate and less visible problems were supervision of residents and problems of incompetence. The results were "interesting" because they did not correspond to the initial motivation of the sponsors (the Anesthesia Patient Safety Foundation), who were concerned about drug abuse and behavioral problems. "The major contributors to the problems are much closer to home and the most beneficial measures are mundane, such as better supervision of residents and periodic retraining of all practitioners so that they get familiar again with situations that they may have forgotten because they only rarely occur."

Root Cause Analysis

A recent article in the Quality Grand Rounds series as presented in the September 3, 2002, issue of the *Annals of Internal Medicine,* deals with a patient who suffered multiple adverse events consistent with cascade iatrogenesis. This case raises two important quality issues: Can health care improve the reliability and accuracy of interpretations of diagnostic tests, and should health care regulate the introduction and use of new technologies? It also brings to light limitations to routine use of RCA to identify remediable errors or to better prevent those system errors when the causal pathway to an apparent adverse medical outcome has not been definitively established. In this case there is a question as to whether RCA would yield improved systems for patient care. Despite multiple opportunities to identify errors in the patient's care, the decisions or circumstances associated with these adverse events contributed to the outcomes in *uncertain ways* and are not easily classified as clear-cut errors. If the recommendations of such an ill-conceived RCA are based on unreliable assessment of causality, a Root Cause Analysis can do more harm than good.

In the case, a 40-year-old woman with a history of type B aortic dissection, renal insufficiency, poorly controlled hypertension, erratic adherence to prescribed treatment regimen, and cocaine use was to be evaluated for dyspnea and swelling of her left breast and arm. At initial presentation, the findings seemed consistent with deep vein thrombosis of the upper left extremity and pulmonary embolism associated with a hypercoagulable state due to possible left-sided breast cancer. In contrast to the initial read (by a radiology resident) of a spiral computed tomography (CT) scan as negative for pulmonary emboli, the attending radiologist identified segmental emboli in the lungs, chronic type B aortic dissection, and a huge pericardial effusion when reading the scan the next morning. Based on this read, the patient was treated with intravenous heparin and oral warfarin. Mammography revealed no evidence of breast cancer and ultrasonography of the left arm found no deep venous thrombosis. After one week of hospitalization, another attending radiologist, one with expertise in imaging pulmonary emboli, reevaluated the original CT scan and found it to be negative for pulmonary emboli—a read consistent with the initial read by the radiology resident. The authors point to this portion of the case as highlighting the need for a general strategy to improve the reliability of radiographic interpretation and introduce new medical technologies (i.e., spiral CT scan) instead of using more well-studied, albeit more resource-intensive, diagnostics such as ventilation perfusion scanning or pulmonary arteriography. The authors see the diagnostic uncertainty regarding the use of the spiral CT scan as pointing to an apprehension, namely the appropriateness of integrating new health care technologies prior to sufficient supporting evidence.

With pulmonary embolism having been ruled out, physicians debated whether pericardiocentesis under cardiographic guidance should be performed in an effort to explain the patient's dyspnea and arm and breast swelling. Unfortunately, the patient's anticoagulant therapy had not been discontinued in time to permit the procedure to be performed on the more desired day, Thursday. Instead the pericardiocentesis was performed on a Friday evening by another competent cardiologist with a full complement of catheterization laboratory personnel. Because of some of the patient's pre-existing complications and the formation of a hemopneumothorax during the process, the patient went into cardiac arrest with pulseless electrical activity. The patient was successfully resuscitated after 10 minutes and a pericardial window and pleural and pericardial drains were surgically inserted.

Using RCA, one is inclined to look at the decision to perform pericardiocentesis. Was it wrong to perform the procedure? Was it wrong to perform the procedure on a Friday evening? The authors suggest the decision to go ahead with the pericardiocentesis, even if problematic in retrospect, does not suggest a clear preventive solution to the breakdown in decision making. In contrast, the failure to discontinue the anticoagulation therapy in a timely manner is an error of omission. In retrospect and knowing the outcome already, an observer could be tempted to label the pericardiocentesis an error of commission, arguing that watchful waiting would have been a more reasonable alternative because the patient's symptoms were stable. But watchful waiting could still lead to cardiac arrest due to tamponade over the weekend, implicating an error of omission. This is a good example of an RCA influenced by hindsight bias and a case where the overall outcome of the patient may not have been improved by any intervention that would prevent the decision to conduct pericardiocentesis.

Several evenings after the patient seemingly recovered from the cardiac arrest and pericardial window insertion, she developed right-sided pleuritic chest pain and relative hypotension. Two days earlier, based on the unlikelihood of recurrent pericardial effusion (with the pericardial window in place), the patient's mediastinal drain was removed. Again considering the possibility of pulmonary embolism and in an effort to diagnose the patient, the residents initiated intravenous heparin and a repeat spiral CT scan. Later that same morning, the patient's attending physician discontinued the anticoagulant medication. An emergency echocardiography revealed a large thrombus in the pericardium compressing the left atrium of the heart. The patient subsequently suffered a second cardiac arrest with pulseless activity while undergoing the echocardiography. An emergency sternotomy was performed; then the pericardial clot was evacuated and a laceration of the left ventricle was repaired. On the second day in the intensive care unit, the patient developed R-on-T phenomenon, followed by torsade de pointes tachycardia and subsequent pulseless ventricular tachycardia, requiring intubation, defibrillation, and amiodarone therapy. Laboratory results revealed the patient's renal function and metabolic acidosis had worsened, requiring dialysis.

Although the authors indicate that the decision to discount tamponade and restart anticoagulation therapy may have been the worst decision of the case, it may be difficult even here to get a consensus opinion on whether the decision was an "error" and whether such a system error could be prevented under the circumstances. The authors suggest that the resident's error is more likely from not knowing his own skill limitations and not seeking a competent supervisor to help in making the decision, which represents an important policy issue throughout health care. The patient eventually recovered and was discharged after a 27-day hospital stay, with more than $200,000 in hospital charges and the need for long-term dialysis.

Six Sigma

Virtua Health, a not-for-profit community hospital system in southern New Jersey, adopted Six Sigma in 2000 to achieve operational goals. One of its first six projects, conducted between January and June 2001, sought improvements and error reduction in anticoagulation therapy. Specifically, the hospital sought to reduce errors related to incorrect pump settings, incorrect use of pumps, delays in obtaining and reacting to activated partial thromboplastin time (aPPT), dosing errors, and mixing errors. Other QI activities, including RCA, failed to address the overall performance of the anticoagulation process in quantitative terms.

The improvement team used the Six Sigma DMAIC process: *define* the process to address, *measure* how the current process is performing, *analyze* key factors driving the process, *improve* the process, and *control* the process to sustain progress. The team defined safe and effective anticoagulation capability as the project goal:

1. First aPTT after bolus above therapeutic threshold;
2. aPTT in therapeutic range at 24 hours;
3. Interval between aPTTs until two consecutive are in range;
4. Low platelet counts noted and addressed;
5. Low hemoglobins noted and addressed.

The team's analysis revealed 92 steps required to reach completion of the first dose adjustment—and that system complexity hampered staff performance, with few elements in place to prevent errors by staff. The team determined that simplifying and error proofing the process were the greatest opportunities to increase safety. The following chart shows the steps taken in the improvement phase:

Six Sigma Anticoagulation Improvements: Virtua Health

Process Step	Deficiency	Intervention	Anticipated Benefit
Weighing patients	Done on admission only 48% of time	Bed scales purchased	Easier to weigh patients
Lab–pharmacy data link	No prior system to monitor efficiency	All patients on heparin included in automated review, with manual review of charts identified	Detection of otherwise silent process failures; ongoing comparison to target performance
Heparin hold for aPTT >240 seconds	Unclear definition of start time for 6-hour interval	Clarification with physicians	Decreased process variation
Physician called for aPTT >240 x 3	Unclear which physician group to call	ID of physician group responsible for heparin order on initial order sheet	Decreased miscommunication

Six Sigma Anticoagulation Improvements: Virtua Health

Process Step	Deficiency	Intervention	Anticipated Benefit
Preheparin lab studies	Inconsistency among nurses and physicians on holding heparin until results received	Clarification with physicians; default is do not wait for labs with hold option for physician	Decreased variation in nursing practice
Infusion pumps	Occasional incorrect setting leading to dosage error	Programmable pumps with drug personalities and maximum drip rate settings	Avoidance of extreme overdosage due to pump-setting errors
Use of unfractioned heparin	Complex process with complexity-related failures	Substitute low-molecular heparin	Fewer complexity-related errors

The control phase includes creation of visible metrics used by process owners to ensure gains are sustained. Study authors note their work "is not a research methodology, and the findings of this project should not be interpreted in the same light as a rigorous clinical research paper. The focus of this paper is to describe an approach for identifying opportunities for improvement and taking action that leads to results that matter to patients in a framework that is achievable in the typical community hospital setting."[30]

Toyota Production System

The Pittsburgh Regional Healthcare Initiative (PRHI) is a collaborative effort by institutions and individuals that provide, purchase, insure, and support health care services in Southwestern Pennsylvania. The initiative aims to achieve "perfect patient care" in six counties in the Pittsburgh Metropolitan Statistical Area with the following goals:

- Zero medication errors
- Zero health care–acquired (nosocomial) infections
- Perfect clinical outcomes, measured by complications, readmissions, and other patient outcomes in the following areas:

- Invasive cardiac procedures (cardiac bypass surgery, angioplasty, and diagnostic catheterization)
- Hip and knee replacement surgery
- Repeat cesarean sections for women with no clinical indications for them
- Depression
- Diabetes

The initiative calls these goals "the most aggressive and ambitious performance goals in American health care." It seeks to redefine the patient as the "client" in health care, as opposed to the physician, the insurer, or the payer in the current environment, by reallocating resources based on each patient's needs. "In effect, the patient 'pulls' the resources he or she needs. This system—derived from the Toyota Production System—is capable of adjusting to and meeting varying patient needs quickly and flawlessly."[31]

A Learning Line is a small hospital unit organized around the principles of TPS. At the point of patient care, the people doing the work are the experts and focus on the shared goal of meeting patient needs, one patient at a time. When a problem hinders work, the full-time team leader takes the lead, researching the problem by first determining what happened and asking the question "why" five times to determine the root cause. As the origins become known, the workers closest to the problem design solutions immediately, testing them with scientific methods. The team leader is free to pull assistance as needed to the point of patient care from the manager, the director, the chief executive officer, even trustees. Proponents suggest this approach enables health care professionals to spend more time providing frontline caregiving by wringing inefficiency out of the system; inefficiency is estimated to consume 33 to 50 cents of every health care dollar.

At the Veterans Administration Pittsburgh Healthcare System, one Learning Line team addressed the issue of antibiotic-resistant infection by attempting to increase compliance with procedures to halt the spread of infection and act on PHRI's goal of zero nosocomial infections. In seeking to understand the root cause for infections—asking "why" five times and observing workers at close range—the team leader discovered one reason workers had trouble complying with infection control procedures: Some rooms had gowns and some did not, and stock outs occurred daily. Workers on the Learning Line established who would be responsible for restocking gloves, how often supplies would be checked (daily), and how the cupboards would be labeled so any deficiency would immediately become obvious. Within days, gloves and gowns that workers had stashed away became available as the system supported the workers; glove consumption and costs dropped 15 percent as "stashes" disappeared. The unit believes it has already gained ground on the Centers for Disease Control and Prevention's goal of improved compliance as hand hygiene compliance has risen.[32]

Special thanks to the following individuals for their advice and comments on this project: Judene Bartley, Paul Batalden, Donald Berwick, David Blumenthal, Mark Brulin, Mark Chassin, Richard Croteau, Edward Dunn, Karen Feinstein, Robert Galvin, Doris Hanna, Brent James, Molly Joel Coye, Lucian Leape, Tammy Lundstrom, Thomas Massero, Julie Mohr, Thomas Nolan, Elisabeth Paté-Cornell, Paul Schyve, Ethel Seljevold, Kimberly Thompson, Mark Van Kooy, Cindy Wallace, and Jonathan Wilwerding.

REFERENCES

1. Committee on Quality of Health Care in America. 2001. *Crossing the Quality Chasm: A New Health System for the 21st Century.* Washington, DC: National Academy Press. Pp. 41–42.
2. For a discussion of HFMEA/FMEA and HACCP, see McDonough J. 2002. *Proactive Hazard Analysis and Health Care Policy.* New York: Milbank Fund and ECRI.
3. Nolan T. 1996. *The Improvement Guide.* New York: Jossey Bass.
4. Blumenthal D, Kilo C. 1998. A report card on Continuous Quality Improvement. *Milbank Quarterly* 76(4): 625–648.
5. See http://www.prhi.org/ [accessed March 27, 2003].
6. Welch J. 2001. *Jack: Straight from the Gut.* New York: Warner Business Books.
7. Chassin M. 1998. Is health care ready for Six Sigma quality? *Milbank Quarterly* 76(4):565–591.
8. Military Procedure MIL-P-1629. 1949 (November 9). *Procedures for Performing a Failure Mode, Effects and Criticality Analysis.*
9. Marx, D, Slonim A. 2003. Assessing Patient Safety Risk Before the Injury Occurs: An Introduction to Socio-Technical Probabilistic Risk Modeling in Healthcare. *Qual Saf Health Care* 12(Suppl2):ii33–ii38.
10. Green L, Crouch E. 1997. Probabilistic risk assessment: Lessons from four case studies. *Annals of the New York Academy of Sciences* 837:387–396.
11. *Op. cit.,* p. 10.
12. See McDonough, *op. cit.,* for detailed references.
13. Personal communication, Dr. Mark Van Kooy, M.D., Virtua Health Master Black Belt, March 26, 2003.
14. Ackoff R. 1994. *The Democratic Corporation.* New York: Oxford University Press. Pp. 18–21.
15. Batalden PB, Mohr JJ. 1997. Building knowledge of health care as a system. *Quality Management in Health Care* 5(3):1–12.
16. Personal Communication, Dr. Brent James, March 3, 2003.

17. Gaba D. 2000. Anesthesiology as a model for patient safety in health care. *British Medical Journal* 320:785–788.
18. Lagasse R. 2002. Anesthesia safety: Model or myth? A review of the published literature and analysis of current original data. *Anesthesiology* 97(6):1609–1617.
19. Cooper J, Gaba D. 2002. No myth: Anesthesia is a model for addressing patient safety. *Anesthesia* 97(6):1335–1337.
20. Brennan T. 2002. Physicians' professional responsibility to improve the quality of care. *Academic Medicine* 77:973–980.
21. Croteau R, Schyve P. 2000. Proactively error proofing health care processes. In: Spath P. editor. *Error Reduction in Health Care.* New York: Jossey Bass. P. 184.
22. Chang A. 2003. *Joint Commission Benchmark* 5(2).
23. Marguerez G, Erbault E, Terra JL, Maisonneuve H, Matillon Y. 2001. Evaluation of 60 continuous quality improvement projects in French hospitals. *International Journal for Quality in Health Care* 13(2):89–97.
24. Solberg L, et al. 2000. Failure of a continuous quality improvement intervention to increase the delivery of preventive services: A randomized trial. *Effective Clinical Practice* May/June:105–115.
25. Contributed by Mary Ivins, Morrison Management Specialists.
26. Gran, B.A., Winther, R. and Johnsen, O.A. Security Assessment of Safety Critical Systems Using HAZOPs, in Proc. of Safecomp 2001, Budapest, Hungary, September 26-28, 2001. Stolen K. A Framework for Risk Analysis of Security Critical Systems. In supplement of the 2001 International Conference on Dependable Systems and Networks. Gothenburg, Sweden, July 2-4, 2001, P. D4-D11.
27. CORAS is a European Research and Development project funded by the 5th Framework Program on Information Society Technologies by the European Commission. The project began in 2001 and will last through 2003. Eleven partners are involved: five from Norway, three from Greece, two from England, and one from Germany. One Norwegian participant is the National Centre for Telemedicine (NST), whose mission is to contribute to making effective health services available to all. Formerly the Norwegian Centre for Telemedicine, NST was designated the first World Health Organization Collaborating Center for Telemedicine in July 2002.
28. Personal communication, e-mail from Eva Skipenes, Security Adviser, Norwegian Centre for Telemedicine, to Luke Petosa, Director, ECRI's Center for Healthcare Environmental Management. Sent March 17, 2003.
29. Paté-Cornell E. 1999. Medical application of engineering risk analysis and anesthesia patient risk illustration. *American Journal of Therapeutics* 6(5):245–255.
30. Van Kooy M, Edell L, Scheckner HM. 2002. Use of Six Sigma to Improve the Safety and Efficacy of Acute Anticoagulation with Heparin. *Journal of Clinical Outcomes Management* 9(8): 445–453.
31. Pittsburgh Regional Healthcare Initiative. 2001. *PHRA Scorecard 2001–2003.* [Online]. Available: http://www.prhi.org/publications/member_pubs.htm [accessed April 25, 2003].
32. Pittsburgh Regional Healthcare Initiative. 2002. *On the Learning Line: Case Studies from the Perfecting Patient Care Learning Lines in Pittsburgh-Area Hospitals.* [Online]. Available: http://www.prhi.org/pdfs/Learning_Line_Booklet.pdf [accessed April 25, 2003].

G

Australian Incident Monitoring System Taxonomy

Health Incident Type	Component Factors

Therapeutic agents
  • Medication
  • Intravenous fluids
  • Oxygen and gases
  • Blood and blood products
  • Nutrition
 	
Therapeutic devices and equipment services and infrastructure
  • Equipment or therapeutic device
  • Infrastructure and services
  • Buildings, fittings, fixtures, and surroundings
 	
Injuries and pressure ulcers
  • Falls
  • Injuries unrelated to falls
  • Pressure ulcers
 	
Clinical processes or procedures
 	
Nosocomial infections
	• Factors: Environmental
	• Factors: Organizational
	• Factors: Human
	• Factors: Subject of incident
	• Factors: Agents
	• Agent
	• Incident type
	• Incident problem class
	• Person involved
	• Timing of incident
	• Timing of detection
	• Method of detection
	• Preventability
	• Factors that minimized or aggravated severity of incident
	• Outcome for subject of incident
	• Severity of outcome for subject of incident
	• Consequences for organization
	• Short-term response or action taken
	• Subsequent response or action taken
	• Resource impact
	• Risk level

Continued

Health Incident Type	Component Factors

Behavior, human performance, violence, aggression, security, and safety
- Behavior and human performance
- Violence and aggression
- Safety and security

Logistics, organization, documentation, and infrastructure technology
- Logistics and organization
- Documentation
- Information technology

Specialist domains (completed)
- Anesthesia
- Intensive care
- Obstetrics
- Hyperbaric medicine, etc.
- Hospital pharmacy
- Retrieval medicine
- Retail pharmacy

Other sources of data
- Complaint cases
- Coronial cases
- Medico-legal cases
- Literature and media reports
- Consumer reports
- Occupational health and safety reports

- Narrative(s)
- Time, date, location
- Persons reporting incident

Specialist domains to be developed
- Hemovigilance
- Ambulance services
- Surgical specialties
- Internal medicine specialties
- Neonatal intensive care unit
- Ophthalmology
- Orthopedic surgery
- Gynecology
- Radiotherapy
- Domiciliary care
- Other areas as required

Index